Attachment and Sexual Offending

Understanding and Applying Attachment Theory to the Treatment of Juvenile Sexual Offenders

T0236642

Attachment and Sexual Offending

Understanding and Applying Attachment Theory to the Treatment of Juvenile Sexual Offenders

by

Phil Rich, EdD, MSW
Clinical Director,
Stetson School, USA

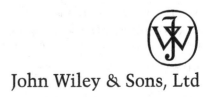

John Wiley & Sons, Ltd

Copyright © 2006   John Wiley & Sons Ltd, The Atrium, Southern Gate, Chichester,
West Sussex PO19 8SQ, England

Telephone (+44) 1243 779777

Email (for orders and customer service enquiries): cs-books@wiley.co.uk
Visit our Home Page on www.wiley.com

All Rights Reserved. No part of this publication may be reproduced, stored in a retrieval system or
transmitted in any form or by any means, electronic, mechanical, photocopying, recording, scanning or
otherwise, except under the terms of the Copyright, Designs and Patents Act 1988 or under the terms of a
licence issued by the Copyright Licensing Agency Ltd, 90 Tottenham Court Road, London W1T 4LP, UK,
without the permission in writing of the Publisher. Requests to the Publisher should be addressed to the
Permissions Department, John Wiley & Sons Ltd, The Atrium, Southern Gate, Chichester, West Sussex PO19
8SQ, England, or emailed to permreq@wiley.co.uk, or faxed to (+44) 1243 770620.

Designations used by companies to distinguish their products are often claimed as trademarks. All brand
names and product names used in this book are trade names, service marks, trademarks or registered
trademarks of their respective owners. The Publisher is not associated with any product or vendor mentioned
in this book.

This publication is designed to provide accurate and authoritative information in regard to the subject matter
covered. It is sold on the understanding that the Publisher is not engaged in rendering professional services. If
professional advice or other expert assistance is required, the services of a competent professional should be
sought.

Other Wiley Editorial Offices

John Wiley & Sons Inc., 111 River Street, Hoboken, NJ 07030, USA

Jossey-Bass, 989 Market Street, San Francisco, CA 94103-1741, USA

Wiley-VCH Verlag GmbH, Boschstr. 12, D-69469 Weinheim, Germany

John Wiley & Sons Australia Ltd, 42 McDougall Street, Milton, Queensland 4064, Australia

John Wiley & Sons (Asia) Pte Ltd, 2 Clementi Loop #02-01, Jin Xing Distripark, Singapore 129809

John Wiley & Sons Canada Ltd, 22 Worcester Road, Etobicoke, Ontario, Canada M9W 1L1

Wiley also publishes its books in a variety of electronic formats. Some content that appears in print may not
be available in electronic books.

Library of Congress Cataloging-in-Publication Data

Rich, Phil.
    Attachment and sexual offending : understanding and applying attachment theory to the treatment of
juvenile sexual offenders / Phil Rich.
        p.   cm.
    Includes bibliographical references and index.
    ISBN-13: 978-0-470-09106-7 (cloth : alk. paper)   ISBN-10: 0-470-09106-1 (cloth : alk. paper)
    ISBN-13: 978-0-470-09107-4 (pbk : alk. paper)   ISBN-10: 0-470-09107-X (pbk : alk. paper)
    1. Teenage sex offenders.   2. Attachment behavior.   3. Psychotherapy.   I. Title.
    RJ506.S48R527   2006
    616.89′00835—dc22   2005009733

British Library Cataloguing in Publication Data

A catalogue record for this book is available from the British Library

ISBN-13 978-0-470-09106-7 (hbk)   978-0-470-09107-4 (pbk)
ISBN-10 0-470-09106-1 (hbk)   0-470-09107-X (pbk)

Typeset in 10/12 pt Times by SNP Best-set Typesetter Ltd., Hong Kong

Dedication

I repeat here a dedication from a previous book, but it is no less meaningful now than it was when I first wrote it.

This book, then, is first and foremost dedicated to the victims of sexual abuse. Their victimization is a personal and social tragedy. I add to this a dedication to those children who grow up disconnected in their own families and, in many cases, disconnected from their society. Their loss is our loss as well.

The book is also dedicated to the leadership and staff of the Stetson School in Barre, Massachusetts, a residential treatment program committed to the best possible treatment of children and adolescents who engage in sexually abusive behavior. Stetson remains a remarkable working environment, and a combination of remarkable people in a remarkable field.

Contents

About the Author

Phil Rich, EdD, MSW, LICSW is the Clinical Director of Stetson School, a residential treatment program for juvenile sexual offenders and sexually reactive children in Barre, Massachusetts. He received his MSW in 1979 and his doctorate in applied behavioral and group studies in 1992, and has practiced as a clinical social worker for over 25 years. He has served as the program director of five residential and day treatment programs, and has worked extensively with troubled adolescents and adults in residential, inpatient, day treatment, and outpatient settings. He has 12 published books, including *Understanding Juvenile Sexual Offenders: Assessment, Treatment, and Rehabilitation*, published by John Wiley & Sons.

Acknowledgments

I have many people to thank, including John Wiley & Sons for the many opportunities they have given me over the past few years to write down my ideas and perspectives and get them out of my head. I must also acknowledge my appreciation for the opportunities for professional growth provided to me by the Stetson School, a program committed to the well-being and improvement of its clients, as well as the quality of its staff. There are too many people at Stetson to personally acknowledge, but I do wish to acknowledge our clinicians, who are certainly the hardest working, most committed, and most skilled group of clinicians I have worked with. I have learned much from our clinicians, and appreciate the ideas that have flowed during clinical supervision and in clinical staff meetings.

In particular, I want to thank Charlie Tousignant, a Stetson clinician, and Joanna Smith, our Assistant Clinical Director, who both showed great interest in my work, as well as helping me to frame early chapters of this book. I also want to thank Joanna for many stimulating and probing conversations about attachment and its meaning, many of which are reflected in ideas fleshed out in various chapters.

It is especially important to me to acknowledge my great thanks to Kathleen Lovenbury, the Executive Director of Stetson School, and Kerry-Ann Cornwell, our Program Director, not only for their leadership and absolute commitment to their work, but for who they are as people. Both Kathleen and Kerry-Ann have offered me their unflagging support and encouragement, have given me the time both to write and attend and present at numerous conferences, and, above all, have shared with me their insights, their great humor, and their friendship.

Many thanks also to Claire Ruston, Assistant Editor for Psychology at John Wiley & Sons, who has graciously facilitated the process of this book and been very supportive, as well as Gillian Leslie, the Publishing Editor, and Ruth Graham, Project Editor. Thank you each, very much. Thank you also to Mary McMurran of Cardiff University, who is also a Series Editor for Wiley and provided very useful comments on the manuscript, as well as support.

Thank you to colleagues who were willing to review this book, pre-publication, not only for their time and effort, but also for their support, not to mention their many contributions to our field.

As always, I thank Bev Sevier, my wife and long, long time friend, for her good humor and constant support, and for her own very important work as a special education teacher. I'm not sure what my life would be like without Bev being there with me. I also want to thank my daughter, Kaye Sevier, whom I have acknowledged many times in previous books and who is now on the edge of adulthood, for the many hours she spent typing up my notes, and say thanks once more for being a wonderful and interesting person, active and interested in the world about her. Kaye, an amazing person herself, faces amazing adventures ahead.

Introduction

In work with sexual offenders—juvenile and adult—it has become increasingly common to link disturbed or underdeveloped early attachment relationships to the later development of pathology. There is an increasing assumption that such deficits of course exist, with an almost implicit supposition that the onset and maintenance of sexually abusive behavior is fueled by what we might call "attachment deficits."

However, the idea that a poor attachment is, or may be, a link between childhood experience and the later onset of sexually aggressive behavior is not new. It has been developing over the course of the past decade, most notably in the work of Marshall, Hudson, Ward, Smallbone, and colleagues. Nevertheless, the idea has taken increased hold in the last few years, with increasing discussions and research studies that hypothesize direct links between attachment difficulties and the onset of sexually abusive behavior. As it became clear to me how much time and effort was going into discussing the role of attachment in conference workshops, journal articles, and book chapters, I realized that I needed to learn more about attachment theory and its application to the treatment of juvenile sexual offenders. Hence this book is as much about attachment theory as it is about juvenile sexual offending.

In fact, as any discussion of attachment and juvenile sexual offenders has to be nested within a larger understanding and discussion of attachment theory itself, the first half of the book is significantly about attachment theory. The second half is focused on the relationship between attachment and *juvenile* sexual offending, but it's difficult to do that without also focusing on adult sexual offenders. In part, this is because most of the limited research on attachment and sexual offending has been conducted with adult rather than juvenile offenders, but it is also impossible to separate the two populations, particularly because attachment is both a phenomenon of early childhood and a facet of human psychology that operates throughout the life span. Further, because adult offenders were, of course, children before becoming adults, we can assume that if disturbances in attachment are a factor in adult sexual offending then they must also be a factor in the onset of juvenile sexual offending, at least in those juveniles who continue to perpetrate sexually abusive behavior as adults. Even in those adults who first engage in sexually abusive behaviors as adults, and not as juveniles, it is clear that disturbances in attachment must have also been present during their adolescence.

This is because the patterning of attachment styles is considered to be a phenomenon that first appears in infancy and early childhood, following a developmental progression throughout childhood and into adolescence and adulthood. Indeed, the idea of *disturbed* attachment falls within the specific realm of developmental psychopathology, implying a distortion or disturbance in normative and expected infant, childhood, or early adolescent development that is a direct or indirect antecedent to the later appearance of psychopathology.[1]

THE GOALS OF THE BOOK

The overarching goal of this book is to describe and discuss the nature and impact of attached relationships and social connectedness on the development of juvenile sexual offending. In order to accomplish this broad goal, several steps are required, each of which serves as an independent, but linked, goal.

The first goal is to explain and critically explore the ideas of attachment theory, including its strengths and limitations. One of those limitations lies in the nature of attachment theory as a *developmental* psychology with a primary focus on infancy and early childhood, and a secondary, but nonetheless significant, focus on the attachment in adults. In fact, the vast majority of attachment theory covers early childhood and picks up again in early adulthood. Between these poles, the transformation of attachment from its childhood origins to its adulthood equivalent is not clearly defined. As such, our understanding of attachment in prepubescent children and adolescents lies in a poorly researched limbo. Although we see the presumed outcomes of attachment relationships by mid-childhood and into adolescence, it is not clear what attachment actually means or how it works in that age group, and even if the concept, as described by attachment theory, is relevant in adolescence and adulthood.

Accordingly, the second goal is to define and describe attachment in such a way as to make it a more comprehensible and durable concept that can help us to better understand what we mean by attachment in pre-teens and adolescents, including the nature, quality, and experience of attachment during adolescence. Closely linked, the third goal is to understand how the attachment model is of use in understanding the impact of early patterns of attachment on the adolescent psyche, including its influence on self-appraisal, social interactions and relationships, and the capacity for emotional and behavioral self-regulation. The goal here is to better understand the nature of early and ongoing attachment experiences as an influence on mental schemata in the adolescent, in attachment theory referred to as the "internal working model."

In principle, the internal working model contains the mental templates for self-image, self-agency (the capacity for self-efficacy), representations of others and the external world, patterned scripts and strategies for interpreting and responding to stimuli and demands, and the capacity to mediate and regulate cognitive, affective, and behavioral responses. As it is postulated that the internal working model develops and changes throughout the life span (hence, *working* model), how does the attachment experience in

---

[1] The reader should remain aware of the distinction between "psychopathology," or the development of mental health disorders, and "psychopathy," or the development of significant antisociality, as both are discussed in the book, and represent different diagnostic sets.

adolescence influence the current mental schema that contains these templates? It is reasonable to presume that feeling secure about self, others, and circumstances is a requisite for the development of effective social skills, including the capacity to face and master complex situations, tolerate difficulty, regulate affect and emotion, and build healthy and satisfying social relationships. Of central importance, then, is understanding in the child, adolescent, and adult the level and quality of internalized security that guides interactions and behaviors. Thus, the third goal is to more clearly understand in pre-teens and adolescents the cognitive and emotional schema, embedded behavioral patterns and internalized scripts for action, and elements of personality that may result from early and ongoing attachment experiences. In effect, the goal is not only to describe the "natural history" of attachment as it evolves from infancy through childhood and into adolescence, but to understand the manner in which it *continues* to shape cognition, affect, behavior, and social relationships during adolescence.

The fourth goal is an obvious one, exploring the relationship that exists between attachment experiences, internalized schema, and the development of sexually abusive behavior in children and adolescent (and subsequently, adults). Central to that question is whether there is any substantial difference in the attachment experiences and patterns of three group of adolescents: (i) a non-clinical population (teenagers who do not get into substantial trouble and are not diagnosed with significant mental health disorders); (ii) troubled but not sexually abusive adolescents, including those who engage in conduct-disordered behaviors or are charged with non-sexual criminal offenses; and (iii) juvenile sexual offenders (recognizing that this population is itself a diverse and non-homogeneous group). Of special concern is whether attachment difficulties are in some way particularly related to the onset of sexually abusive behavior, or more generally a risk factor for antisocial behavior *but not specifically related to sexual offenses*. That is, do attachment difficulties represent a developmental vulnerability that predisposes some individuals towards antisocial behavior but is otherwise unrelated to the onset of sexually abusive behavior, or do they form a significant factor in the development of sexually abusive behavior?

In the first case, assuming that attachment difficulty *is* a risk factor for conduct disorder but not sexually aggressive behavior, other, more pertinent, risk factors are required to fuse and catalyze early experience and eventually lead to sexually abusive behavior. In this case, attachment difficulties are but one risk factor among many, not particularly relevant to later sexual aggression. However, if attachment difficulties themselves represent a risk factor that is *directly* linked to the onset of sexually abusive behavior, with other factors playing a catalyzing but nonetheless secondary role, then such deficits represent a direct pathway to sexual offending behavior. This would represent an important step in our understanding of and ability to predict sexually abusive behavior, at least in the case of sexual re-offense.

The fifth and final goal of the book is to consider implications for the evaluation and treatment of attachment-related difficulties and pathologies, and particularly, of course, in the treatment of sexually reactive children and juvenile sexual offenders. If attachment is directly or indirectly implicated in the development of antisocial and/or sexually abusive behavior, and we can more fully understand what we mean by attachment in pre-teens and adolescents and how it affects their ongoing behaviors, we can develop and apply an attachment-informed framework for evaluation and treatment. Such a framework can help us to recognize and address both non-pathological and pathological concerns resulting from early difficulties and disruptions in the attachment process, as well as ongoing attachment experiences that impact current cognition, affect, and behavior, including continuing moral development and sense of social connection and relatedness.

Above all, however, my general goal is to better understand the population of sexually troubled children with whom we work, and help to educate and train professionals in our field, myself included, in how better to work with these youths. As is always my orientation in writing, my intention is to present information, perspective, and theory in a way that synthesizes and challenges, as well as enlarges and illuminates, current ideas. I hope I am able to do this in a way that promotes critical thinking. This means analyzing and carefully evaluating what we are reading and hearing, seeking confirmatory and contradictory ideas, weighing them one against the other, and linking different ideas and perspectives. Not least of all, critical thinking requires imagination and creativity as we form and re-form our own thoughts and beliefs, applying these to the reality of our work. I invite readers, then, to think critically about the ideas I present in this book, and, indeed, about the book itself.

RELEVANCE OF ATTACHMENT THEORY

I began my research for this book with the suspicion that attachment theory would prove to be important and useful in our work, but not the answer we seemed to be looking for. In a previous book, I described our search for the "Factor X" that will explain to us *why* juvenile sexual offenders become juvenile sexual offenders. It was then, and remains, my sense that there are a myriad of reasons, too complex in their effects and in their interactions with one another, for us to ever fully comprehend why one troubled child engages in sexually abusive behavior and another does not, or why some juvenile sexual offenders desist before they become adults and others become sexual offenders in adulthood. The idea behind Factor X, however, is that if only we knew more, and if only our theory was richer, we could decipher the mysteries behind human behavior. This belies and undercuts our stated notion that sexual offenders, be they juvenile or adult, are a heterogeneous group. Nevertheless, we seem to believe "secretly" that they are, actually, a homogeneous group, and if we can just put our finger on Factor X we can nail the homogeneity factor that can explain everything. I find no Factor X in this book.

The conclusion of this book I'll give away from the start. I conclude that attachment theory is an important and very useful, although flawed, theory that has great applicability to understanding and working more effectively with our population, but attachment status does not distinguish juvenile sexual offenders from other troubled adolescents, any more than it discriminates between adult sexual offenders and other adult criminal groups. It is other factors, other elements, other forces, and other experiences in the lives of youths that, together with attachment, act to shape, rather than determine, developmental pathways and behaviors. Attachment, as an early experience in child development, sets the pace for and is tied to many later developmental events, but on its own is just another player, albeit an important one.

Finally, I conclude that we are not likely to bring about change in the youths we treat through cognitive-behavioral or psychodynamic treatment, individual or group therapy, family therapy, or even the underlying common factors that account for effective therapy.

We will most likely bring about change through the connections, the attachments, and the driving force of relationships and social relatedness. Attachment theory describes for us *how* those connections are made. Applying an assessment and treatment framework informed by attachment theory helps us to see how attachments have formed in any particular individual, how damaged attachment may have contributed to the pathway taken by that individual—including a pathway leading to sexually abusive behavior—and how attachment re-formed may help to create a more socially connected and less antisocial person capable of engaging in self-regulation, moral behavior, and a life style that does not include the victimization of others.

CHAPTER 1

The Relationship of Attachment to Juvenile Sexual Offending

In attachment theory, the term "attachment" is actually a multidimensional construct rather than a word with a single fixed meaning, separating into attachment *experiences*, attachment *patterns*, and attachment *strategies*. There is a link between these dimensions of course, and attachment patterns and strategies develop out of earlier attachment experiences and later come to affect current attachment experiences. However, although they operate interactively and simultaneously to define attachment as a whole, each dimension represents a different aspect of attachment, each with its own meaning. Indeed, this is one of the difficulties in describing "attachment," per se.

The word itself has come to be synonymous with being attached, or having a sense of social connection and the ability to *become* socially connected. Yet "attachment" describes only an abstract concept, actually realized through the *experience* of attachment, the manner or *pattern* in which the experience of attachment is manifested, and scripts or *strategies* by which the seeking and maintenance of experienced attachment is implemented. In its grammar, "attachment" is a verb (to attach oneself to), an adjective (to have an attached relationship with), and a noun (an attachment exists between them). To this end, attachment is a process, an organized set of procedures, *and* a state of being. The attachment concept, then, is operationalized as a subjective experience, a style or pattern, and an approach or strategy. We seek evidence of attachment through self-report, the assessment of classifiable styles (patterns) of attachment, and/or manifestations of attachment-seeking (or maintaining) behavior.[1]

Each of these elements not only begins to define what we mean by attachment, but also makes clear that use of the attachment label in exploring, classifying, and understanding human behavior requires different observational and measurement procedures for different dimensions of attachment, and at different stages in human development. The simple and often off-handed manner in which we describe "attachment," and describe individuals as attached or not attached (or securely or insecurely attached), is both inadequate and ill-informed. Attachment is no less complex and abstract than any other psychological con-

---

[1] Or, according to attachment theory, the activation of the attachment behavioral system.

struct or phenomenon of human behavior, and should be considered, explored, and understood in this light.

ATTACHMENT IN THE ADOLESCENT

It is not even clear if "attachment" in adolescence is the same phenomenon as "attachment" in infancy and early childhood. Certainly, by adulthood "attachment" has taken on a different meaning and relates more to romantic relationships, the parenting role, and, more loosely, other adult affiliative–social relationships. Adolescence, then, beginning in late, pre-pubescent childhood and extending to early adulthood, serves as a transitional period, bridging the developmental gap between the infant and childhood form of attachment and the adult variant, or outcome, of attachment. Adolescence, along with its many other related roles in cognitive, affective, moral, and social development, is presumably the period during which attachment is redefined and transformed, and in which the attachment experience takes on an entirely different meaning, fuels significantly different behavior, and serves substantially different purposes than childhood attachment.

Through cognitive and affective development and the unfolding of the biological and neurological sequence, during adolescence the experiences of childhood metamorphosize into something quite different, becoming crystallized in the still developing ego as aspects of personality. No longer the biological, evolutionarily driven survival tool hypothesized by attachment theory to be driving the behavior and psychology of the young child, as with human development in general attachment in adolescence is also transformed. Although attachment theory does not provide a clear description of attachment in adolescence, it presumably becomes the proving grounds in which the sense of security and self-confidence derived from early attachment experiences turns into the self-directed behavior, self-image, perceptions of others, social relationships, and behaviors that will increasingly define the adolescent and shape his or her adulthood experiences of self and others.

By adolescence, early attachment experiences and the sense of being attached are folded into mental representations and displayed in behaviors that do not resemble the internalized attachment experience and external behaviors of infants and pre-school children. The mental schema described by so many psychologists, built in part upon early attachment experience, is the key to what attachment becomes and how it contributes to and perhaps drives perceptions of self and others, emotional life, social interactions, behaviors, and self-regulation. Conceptualized by attachment theory as the mental schema by which early attachment experiences are hard wired into the central nervous system, embodied in the "internal working model" are the individual's experience of the world, sense of self and others, and strategies to make sense of, implement, and manage social interactions. In most models of mental schemata, this metaphysical mental map serves not only as the center of all intentional action but also as the location of the ego, or sense of selfhood. It is this internal working model that is probably the best target for understanding the impact of attachment on the development of selfhood and the transformations in "attachment" that occur during the transition from childhood to adolescence, and again from adolescence to adulthood.

THE LINK BETWEEN RESEARCH AND THEORY

Regardless of increasing truisms that imply or assert that the development of pathology in sexual offenders is linked to underdeveloped attachment in children, there is little evidence that the existence of attachment deficits has any *direct* connection to the development of sexually abusive behavior in children or adolescents, and hence adults. Despite the attractiveness of the position and its appearance as having explanatory power, the idea that poor attachment experiences serve as a developmental pathway to juvenile sexual offending remains specious at this time. This is not to say that attachment difficulties do *not* play a role,[2] whether major or minor, but merely that we must put such ideas into a context informed by a broad understanding of attachment, sexually abusive behavior, and evidence that links the two, rather than simply interesting and intuitively attractive theory, let alone our great need to understand and be able to categorize all human behavior.

Evidence of attachment deficits and a link to juvenile sexual offending is drawn largely from investigations into the attachment status of adult sexual offenders, but even in this domain such evidence is both limited and questionable. In many ways, a critical review of the research with adult sexual offenders suggests that, despite the use of empirical research designs, there is a confirmatory bias. That is, research seems to be used to confirm a priori theory almost uncritically, rather than discover, test, or evaluate it. In fact, it is not uncommon to read in much of the present research (which is quite sparse and often conducted by the same group of researchers, or built directly upon the work of these researchers) that although the data do not *yet* support the theory, there is nevertheless good reason to believe that attachment deficits *are* key, and it is simply a matter of time, better research design, and improved measurement processes until evidence supporting theoretical assumptions *is* discovered. For instance, despite acknowledging the many limitations reported in most studies, Mulloy and Marshall (1999) write that they continue to be sure that "despite the problems . . . there appears to be no doubt that attachment styles are an important area of dysfunction in sexual offenders" (p. 106). Similarly, Smallbone and Dadds (2000) write that "notwithstanding these limitations, these results indicate that childhood attachment may play some role in the development of coercive sexual behavior" (p. 13). It is as though we have decided that it *is* there (the attachment deficit link) and we will find it, if not now then soon.

It may be true that difficulties and disruptions in the experience of early attachment and the development of satisfactory and nourishing social relationships contribute significantly to the onset of coercive and abusive sexual behaviors in some men, and this idea has both obvious face validity and intuitive appeal. But, so far, this is just an attractive theory that seeks to answer disturbing and complex questions for which we have few other answers.

In fact, there is limited support that the attachment classifications of adult sexual offenders differ significantly from those of non-sexual criminal offenders or non-offenders (i.e., the general population). Accordingly, research has so far engaged largely in a theoretical assumption that attachment deficits *do* exist and that they *are* significantly linked to the development of sexually abusive behavior (in men, at least), despite failing to find strong

---

[2] Indeed, it is my conjecture that attachment *does* play a part in the development of sexually abusive behavior, but fills just one part, not the whole cast.

or consistent proof for this attractive idea. Even across similar studies, researchers have failed to demonstrate any consistent or predictable outcomes that support attachment deficit or related hypotheses, although tend to focus on almost any data that even minimally support the already assumed presence of attachment deficits. In most cases, other data from the *same* research could just as easily suggest that differences in attachment deficits are no more apparent in sexual offenders than in non-sexual criminal offenders, or even the general public. Even when researchers do provide some evidence for their hypotheses in this area, a more critical look at the data shows flaws and weaknesses. This approach, in which research supports theory rather than seeking to understand the problem, is characterized by Andrew Lang, the late nineteenth-century Scottish writer, who is credited as saying that some use research as an drunken person uses a lamp post—for support, rather than illumination.

Reviewed in Chapters 11 and 12, it is as though research studies grab onto the small details that support the theory, rather than the data that do not. These supporting data, even if slim, are used to move us towards a conclusion that researchers seemingly have already reached. In politics, this is called "spin."

THREE RISKS IN ASSESSING ATTACHMENT IN JUVENILE SEXUAL OFFENDERS

Aside from a critique of adult sexual offender research, as mentioned, attachment research in adolescent sexual offenders is even more rare than the relatively sparse research into attachment, social relatedness, and empathy in adult sexual offenders, and is just getting underway at this point. We face three risks, then, if we draw our conclusions from the current research and theory.

Risk One: Failure to Discriminate between Adult and Juvenile Sexual Offenders

We may assume that the same patterns, experiences, and/or strategies of attachment and social connectedness that have been or may be found in adult male sexual offenders also apply to juvenile sexual offenders, although we already know that juveniles are different from adults, and juvenile sexual offenders are different from adult sexual offenders.

We have already come to recognize essential differences between the two populations (juvenile and adult sexual offenders) in most aspects of their sexually abusive behaviors, including motivations, context, and targets, as well as developmental level. It is important to recognize that similar differences will also be found in their experience and level of attachment, which presumably plays a different role during adolescence, is still developing, and is in transition between the childhood variant of attachment and its adult counterpart. It is not only a mistake at this juncture to assume that we have actually proven something about attachment in adult sexual offenders, when we actually have not, but it would be an even bigger mistake to simply transfer what we believe we know about attachment in adult sexual offenders to the realm of juvenile sexual offending. We have already learned not to transpose or overlay our ideas about adult sexual offenders onto juvenile sexual offenders.

Risk Two: Failure to Discriminate among Juvenile Sexual Offenders

We have also learned that juvenile sexual offenders are not only different from adult sexual offenders, but are different from one another and are a heterogeneous group. Nevertheless, the attachment concept is so attractive and intuitively obvious that we may assume homogeneity in the level of attachment and social connectedness across the population, and thus assume a common source of difficulties and causes of sexual offending in juveniles. Here we may come to assume similar experiences, similar responses to those experiences, and similar cognitive, emotional, and behavioral patterns across the entire population of sexually reactive children and sexual offenders.

Given the already elevated level of discussion about attachment deficits in sexual offenders and its presumed application to juveniles, as well as to adults, it is somehow as if we have unlearned what we have previously learned about the level of heterogeneity among sexual offenders, including juvenile sexual offenders, and the lack of a single-point, homogeneous developmental pathway.

Risk Three: The Uncritical Acceptance of Ideas

We face a third risk if we continue to uncritically accept ideas about attachment and its application to the assessment and treatment of juvenile sexual offending, without waiting to better define the ideas of attachment theory and understand how they may influence the development of sexually abusive behavior. Here, the risk is that we may begin to labor under the misapprehension that we have found a cause of sorts—one of the "Factor X" (Rich, 2003) reasons that we seek to explain why juvenile sexual offenders engage in sexually abusive behavior, and what distinguishes them or, at least, their developmental path, from the path of non-sexually abusive youth. We seem to insist, and perhaps this is endemic to the larger field of psychology, that there are universal answers and causes and that if only we had a stronger and more complete theory we would discover those mysterious factor X's that we want to believe specifically drive cognition, affect, and behavior in one direction or another.

In fact, one of the unfortunate elements that seems common to sex offender work is that we seek out and hold onto ideas, sometimes accepting unproven ideas as empirically proven "fact." If repeated with enough frequency and certainty, ideas, even if poorly informed and sometimes erroneous, may harden into "conventional wisdom," shading into dogma in the words of Chaffin and Bonner (1998). On a similar note, Laws, Hudson, and Ward (2000) describe as "received wisdom" the widely accepted view that the cognitive-behavioral/relapse prevention model is the most efficacious model of treatment despite the fact, as they point out, that we have no substantial evidence to demonstrate the efficacy of such models.

Our willingness to accept and latch onto unproven solutions for difficult problems perhaps stems from our understandable need to turn to researchers and leaders in our field for answers, expecting direction to be forthcoming and thus sometimes easily and uncritically adopting their views. Relevant also to the acceptance of weakly proven ideas is the way that information is passed around in the field, like the game of telephone in which the original message is corrupted and distorted by the time it reaches the final player. Our desire to figure things out and help kids, both the perpetrators and victims of sexually abusive behavior, only serves to further exacerbate this situation in which we yearn for straightforward and obvious answers to complex and highly problematic questions. The risk, then, is that unproven and even poorly researched ideas will be proliferated and adopted before their time.

However, the crux of this problem is that many practitioners fail to read enough source material, are overly dependent upon others for answers, and fail to exercise critical thinking about the quality, content, focus, and outcome of the published research. Out of such a combination—the need for answers, the assumption that others have answers, and the sometimes uncritical willingness to accept the repetition of ideas as evidence that the ideas are correct and/or efficacious—we face the risk of misunderstanding and distorting interesting and promising ideas and techniques, and amplifying them into factual and proven explanations of pathology and treatment. Hence, they become mythologized.

A WORKING DEFINITION OF ATTACHMENT

Although I've described the attachment construct as multidimensioned, it is nevertheless awkward and laborious to keep repeating the complexity of the construct. Although in Chapter 2 we more fully explore attachment theory and its implications, it is now time to provide a working definition of attachment that can be easily used, recognizing this working definition as short-hand for a construct that is not easily defined or described, and has at least several dimensions.

Unless specifically describing a single dimension, such as attachment classification, attachment behavior, or the subjective experience of being attached, I will generally use the word "attachment" to describe the sense of social connection that one individual has to another *and* the sense of social relatedness or belonging that an individual has to a larger reference group. In fact, I've already used the term "social connectedness" to describe at least one manifestation of "attachment," almost as a description of what we generally mean when we say that someone is attached. Indeed, it may be that "attachment" is really just another way of describing social connectedness.

In this sense, attachment includes relationships that involve primary attachments, such as the child–caregiver relationship; important and sometimes unique relationships that involve affection and presumably some form of intimacy and special connection; relationships, such as friendships, that are more generally affiliative; and a more pervasive sense of relationship or belonging to a larger social group (e.g., society itself). Each of these relationship types involves an emotional bond of some kind, even if not permanent, and each of these relationship experiences, although varied, can be thought of as demonstrating a sense of and capacity for social and emotional connection, with the "most" attached relationships reserved in childhood for primary caregivers and later in life for romantic partners and one's own children. With a broad and working definition of attachment that allows us to more easily discuss what we mean by attachment, we vastly expand the meaning beyond the narrow definition assigned in attachment theory.

However, this working definition of attachment, even if only a temporary device to help us to work further into the book, does not match the definition that is bedrock to attachment theory. In attachment theory, the only relationships considered to be "attachment" relationships are those between child and primary caregivers (attachment theory allows for more than one attachment relationship), and the "attachment bond" is reserved for *only* this special form of relationship. Attachment relationships are differentiated from all other close relationships, which are referred to as *affiliative* relationships, although these also contain affectional (emotional) bonds. Thus, the attachment relationship is a special and relatively unique form of affectional relationship, most typically between mother and child and somehow transferred in adult life to romantic partners (although never fully explained how). Attachment, then, is a special form of relationship, as noted, most typically between infant and mother, and any variation on or expansion of that concept may compromise our attempt to apply "classic" attachment theory to the study of juvenile sexual offenders. By altering the meaning, and therefore our understanding, of "attachment" as a construct, we risk substantially changing some of the core ideas of attachment theory (which may not be a bad thing).

THE LIMITATIONS OF ATTACHMENT THEORY

The principles, ideas, and limitations of attachment theory are reviewed and discussed in detail in Chapter 2, but for now it is important to recognize that the attachment relationship in infancy and early childhood is reserved for only a few primary caregivers, and most typically the mother (and, secondarily, the father), as well as other possible close caregivers. Furthermore, the attachment bond is not shared between two people (the child and mother, for instance), but is a bond experienced by the child *towards* its mother (or other primary caregiver), borne of physical, and later psychological, dependency. In the attached relationship with a mother, the *child* experiences the attachment bond which therefore resides within the individual and not the couple, and the mother experiences a complementary *caregiver* bond. In the ideal infant–mother relationship, therefore, the child demonstrates attachment behaviors, whereas the mother demonstrates caregiver behaviors in an attuned and complementary relationship. Attachment theory, then, understands and treats only *certain* relationships as attachments.

It is not that it is difficult to hypothesize and recognize the lasting influences of attachment on children, adolescents, and adults, or to classify individuals by a recognizable attachment style (securely attached or insecurely attached, for instance). In fact, attachment theory clearly describes the development of predictable and stable emotional and behavioral patterns and, in effect, personality, as the outcome of early attachment. However, attachment theory does not make clear how, or into what, "attachment" transforms past early childhood and into adolescence, or even what we mean by "attachment" in adolescents; how, or if, attachment influences other affiliative relationships; and why, and how, some of these affiliative relationships may later be transformed into adult attachment relationships (given the special nature of attachment relationships). It is also not clear exactly what secure or insecure attachment means, and particularly when it is possible for a child to experience a secure attachment to one caregiver, and an insecure attachment to another. Is the child, then, secure or insecure in attachment?

When we expand the meaning of attachment, as I have done, so that what we are talking about is narrower and more closely resembles our general and intuitive understanding of attachment in both daily life and in general, we, at the same time, lose the fine tuning and narrow wavelength allowed by attachment theory. As described, the construct of attachment in attachment theory refers to a very limited and very specific relationship, reserved for relationships only with primary attachment figures. This is a critical point to make, not because it is confusing to use other definitions of attachment, but because if we apply *attachment theory* to the field of sex offender specific evaluation and treatment, then we must either use the definition of the attachment relationship that is bedrock to and provided by concepts of attachment therapy as they now exist, or work towards a redefinition of attachment that both meets our needs and does not violate the principles of attachment theory.

In fact, the literature of attachment theory is vast and extremely well defined (although not without its weaknesses and significant contradictions), and perhaps much more so than many other fields within developmental psychology, such as the study of empathy, intimacy, or morality in which concepts are still wide open to debate and sometimes quite vague. Unlike other models of psychological functioning, such as object relations theory, where there is no cohesive center to the theory thus allowing flexibility and the inclusion and application of other ideas, attachment theory is so well defined and with such a clear center that it allows little in the way of flexibility around the use of terms and ideas.

This is precisely one of the difficulties in applying attachment theory to sex offender work, or any other form of psychopathology for that matter. For the most part, attachment theory is a developmental and not a clinical psychology. Accordingly, most of its applications are based on observation and analysis and geared towards explaining, understanding, and modifying the processes of early childhood development, rather than treating conditions that emerge in later life, least of all pathology.

THE LIMITATIONS OF STUDIES IN ADULT ATTACHMENT

All forms of developmental psychology address the social and mental development of *children*, rather than adolescents or adults. This creates inherent problems in applying the ideas of a such a psychology to any slice of life other than early childhood, and is as true for attachment theory as for any other form of developmental psychology. In attempting to expand the attachment relationship beyond early childhood and into the entire life span, attachment theory begins to confuse what is actually meant by "attachment," as it most certainly is not the same in adulthood as it is in infancy and early childhood.

In fact, it is in early to mid-childhood that the attachment relationship can be most easily seen and understood. Adults obviously have no need for the physical protection offered and learning processes facilitated by the attachment relationship. Attachment theory hence postulates that in adults the need for attachment and the feeling of safety experienced through early attachment relationships is somehow transformed into romantic relationships with other adults, which in some cases are variants of, and may rightfully be considered as, attachment relationships. Herein lies one of the significant limitations of attachment theory because it is unclear on how this transference of infant to adult attachment occurs, what "attachment" actually means in such a relationship, the role that adolescence plays in that transformation, and, consequently, the meaning and quality of attachment during adolescence.

In fact, most of the study of adult attachment addresses patterns of attitudes and relational behavior in adults, inferred either from interviews or questionnaires and self-reports (rather than direct observation, the means by which childhood attachment is assessed, analyzed, and inferred). In fact, although adults are classified into attachment categories based on their answers to measurement instruments (interviews or paper and pencil questionnaires), what is being measured is not always clear. For instance, the Adult Attachment Interview (AAI) is the instrument most commonly used to comprehensively evaluate adult attachment, but it actually analyzes in adults the residues of their childhood experiences with their parents, rather than attachment itself, at least insofar as attachment theory defines attachment. Other instruments, most of which involve paper-and-pencil questionnaires and self-reports, measure attitudes and ideas about social relationships, commitment, intimacy, mutuality, and so on, from which patterns of attachment are inferred and categories assigned. Thus, as attachment theory does not really describe the meaning of attachment in adulthood, and certainly does not have the means to recognize and assess attachment in adults through observation and experiment (as it does in childhood), inferences about attachment are mostly derived from the spoken narratives of adults during the AAI or the attitudes and ideas presented through questionnaires and other paper-and-pencil instruments.

Although adult attitudes and ideas about attachment are undoubtedly very much affected and partially determined by early attachment relationships, we are nevertheless no longer measuring "attachment relationships" as defined by attachment theory itself. In many ways, in adults we are actually exploring and examining the *outcomes* of attachment, rather than attachment itself, whether such outcomes come in the form of self-image or are lived out in romantic, committed, casual, hostile, or distant relationships. Of note—although we have developed processes for conceptualizing and assessing attachment in children and alternative processes for conceptualizing and assessing attachment in adults—there are no widely developed processes for conceptualizing and assessing attachment in adolescents.

RESOLVING THE LIMITATIONS: THE INTERNAL WORKING MODEL

For the reasons stated, the decision to expand the construct of "attachment" to a more general and far reaching set of social relationships and social relatedness is both risky and has great import when we discuss the construct in light of attachment theory. This is partly so, not only because attachment theory is very clear on the nature and meaning of childhood attachment, but also because, despite insisting that attachment relationships are evident throughout life, it fails to provide a clear base for understanding attachment in adolescence and adulthood—the very age ranges in which we are most interested as we study juvenile and adult sexual offenders.

However, if we choose to redefine and expand attachment, knowing that the concept falls outside that offered by attachment theory, it becomes an easier concept to operationalize and understand as it plays out in the longitudinal development of self-image, social connections, and the patterning of behaviors. In fact, it may well be that when we attempt to measure "attachment" in adolescents and adults, we are really talking about two separate but related constructs, both sequelae of early attachment experience: (i) an internalized experience of emotional security, and (ii) a sense of social connectedness.

Actually, the issues and limitations of attachment theory are already addressed and resolved in the attachment theory concept of the internal working model (IWM), which itself is conceptualized as a derivative of the attachment process. However, at the inception of the internal working model (that is, the point in time at which internal representations of self and the surrounding world begin to develop), attachment experiences fuel the further development of the internal working model and the IWM, in turn, shapes the experience and outcomes of the attachment process. This reciprocal and mutual process results in attachment experiences and the internal working model being fused into a synthetic whole, in which attachment is reflected in the IWM and, at the same time, the IWM is a reflection of the attachment experience. Hence, the issues and limitations of attachment theory are resolved, although semantic issues remain (e.g., the use and meaning of the term "attachment"), when the focus is on the internal working model as the engine that translates and drives attachment experiences throughout life, rather than "attachment" itself.

The primary limitation, then, is not in the general principles of attachment theory, but in the focus on "attachment" per se, rather than the internal working model. In fact, it may be the focus on attachment over the life span, rather than a focus on the IWM over the life span, that is the most significant weakness of attachment theory in application. This is easily overcome, however, by focusing not on the attachment concept but on the internal working model. As an actively shaping ingredient of the attachment experience and the result and embodiment of that experience, it is the internal working model and not attachment that is most instrumental in the development of a sense of self and others. This makes it far easier to discuss attachment in the broader terms described in this chapter, knowing that we are really interested in the evolving role and operations of the internal working model as the shaper and evaluator of ongoing attachment experiences and attached relationships. This certainly eliminates semantic difficulties around the use of the word attachment and other related conceptual difficulties (described in Chapter 2), providing a focus that can overcome confusion as we follow the development of attachment through the life span.

THE CONSTELLATION OF HUMAN EXPERIENCE

In addition to ideas, presumptions, and hypotheses about attachment found in the sex offender specific literature, other aspects of human interactions, emotional connections, and relationships are also discussed, sometimes frequently. As we explore the constellation of subjective experiences that both underpin and are influenced by human interactions, in addition to the experience of attachment it is equally important to explore the concepts of empathy, intimacy, morality, and remorse, and the experience of self-efficacy and social competence. Indeed, more than simply "other" elements that are perhaps closely related to attachment, these other intrapsychic structures may even be components of or stem directly from the attachment experience.

Moreover, it seems likely that each one of these elements, attachment included, is probably incorporated into the internal working model or ego, once again strengthening the perspective presented here that it is the internal working model, or mental schema of self and others, that is really the focus on interest in understanding and treating juvenile and adult sexual offenders.

THE INTERNAL WORKING MODEL: THE SUBJECT OF EVALUATION AND TREATMENT

The internal working model, once again, is seen as the container, assimilator, and synthesizer of experience and the source of thought, reflection, and action. As a result, the internal working model is also the subject of evaluation and treatment. As we cannot go back in time to actually observe past attachment experiences, the only other courses of action are either to observe current behaviors and interpret these as the reflections of prior attachment experience, or to gain access to perceptions of past attachment experiences through narratives that reflect internalized experiences (and, thus, the internal working model where such experiences are stored). This is actually what the Adult Attachment Interview aims to do in using the carefully designed, structured interview process to unlock the IWM and its interpretation of past attachment experiences with parents. Similarly, as we cannot return to the past to change early attachment interactions and transactions, we can only try to work with the IWM in order to change internalized ideas and perceptions of past experience, and embed and internalize new experiences.

In this way, as the internal working model is believed to be not just a psychological concept but the result of hard-wired synaptic connections, we can hope to establish in the individual new ways of experiencing self and others in both the metaphysical mind and in the neurobiological hardware of the brain, through the formation and retention of new synaptic connections. In Damasio's terms (1994), the way in which we understand and respond to the world is captured and reflected through the patterned firing of familiar synaptic circuits. Our experiences are reflected in "dispositional representations" that exist on a neurological level, acquired through, and therefore modified by, experience.

ATTACHMENT AND THE PATHWAY TO SEXUALLY ABUSIVE BEHAVIOR

It is hypothesized in the sexual offender literature that attachment deficits in some way function to create sexually coercive and abusive behavior. The presumption is that difficulties or disruptions that damage the attachment process also lead or contribute to later emotional disturbances and dysfunctional behaviors that, in these cases, set in motion a pathway to sexually abusive behavior.

However, it's clear that the sources of attachment deficits affect the lives and developing psyches of many more children than just those who later engage in sexually reactive or abusive behavior. It is thus recognized that disrupted or damaged attachment alone is not *the* cause that lies behind sexually abusive behavior. In such a model, attachment difficulties serve as an early developmental vulnerability that is exacerbated, amplified, and triggered into later sexualized behaviors by other risk factors, including other subjective experiences, personal abilities and skills, the social environment, life events, and personal behaviors that for some individuals coalesce to form the crucible from which sexually abusive behaviors emerge.

However, in any model proposing that sexual aggression results from or is in some way prompted by early attachment experiences, two requirements must be met. (1) It is important that the model should hypothesize not only the relationship between attachment problems and later sexually abusive behavior, but also explain the pathway from early attachment experiences to sexual aggression and the special conditions that turn some individuals with attachment deficits to sexually abusive behavior but not others. In other words, the model must explain why, for many who share virtually identical experiences, sexually abusive behavior is not *always* the outcome. (2) The model must demonstrate that attachment difficulties directly contribute to the development of sexually abusive behavior in particular, rather than to criminality or antisocial behavior in general.

In the present state of our research, with reference to each requirement, taken separately and together, we do not have such a model.

CONCLUSION: THE LIMITATIONS AND UTILITY OF THE THEORY

Despite much discussion about attachment in the sexual offender literature and at sexual offender conferences, we have not yet been able to make any definitive statements about the role of attachment in the development and treatment of sexually abusive behavior. Nevertheless, the attachment construct already shows signs of being greeted as the next "white horse"on the treatment horizon, carrying an artificial and premature promise of answers to a field in which there seems to be an insistence on discovering universal answers and producing simplistic tools to address complex and convoluted problems.

I hope, through this book, to make a contribution in moving forward our understanding of the attachment construct and its implications for evaluation and treatment, and at the same time help to rein in our sometimes exuberant adoption of ideas whose time has not yet come. I previously described my goals as providing a clear overview of attachment theory and disordered attachment, the application of attachment theory to the etiology of juvenile sexual offending, and the implications of attachment theory for the evaluation and treatment of juvenile sexual offenders. Beyond these goals, however, a primary goal is to urge practitioners to think critically and carefully before assuming a position as their own, and to always rethink earlier ideas.

The good news is that, even as we continue to explore the nature of attachment in sexual offenders, it is reasonable to apply what we *already* know about attachment and can safely generalize about its implications for social relatedness. In asking, quite simply, "Is attachment really just another way of describing social connectedness?", we can visualize aspects of evaluation that probe that very question and conceptualize treatment interventions that will move juveniles and adults in treatment closer to a position of social connection and relatedness. By viewing troubled behaviors through the lens of attachment theory and building our understanding, evaluation, and treatment on a framework informed by attachment theory, we can begin to build and add to our existing treatment a model of therapy that is attachment-informed. I hope to show the reader that, despite what we do not know about attachment and limitations in our sex offender specific research, we can nevertheless see attachment theory as a useful tool for the purposes of both evaluation and treatment.

CHAPTER 2

The Foundations of Attachment: Attunement and Human Connection

Schore (1999), describing the development of learning and self-regulation through the synchronous relationship that exists between mother and young child, considers attachment theory as fundamentally a regulatory theory. However, developed by John Bowlby (1969), attachment theory is unlike other theories of psychological development, psychoanalysis, and object relations, essentially defining attachment as a *biological* and not a psychological process. We begin the chapter with the idea that attachment theory is unique among theories of developmental psychology in that the establishment of cognitive and psychological processes are secondary to the unfolding and enactment of natural and innate biological tendencies and behaviors, and built upon those processes. From this perspective, attachment is first an evolutionary process, driven by instinct alone and enacted without subjectivity or intention, and is only later a psychological experience.

Central to attachment theory, the phenomenon of attachment is no different from the experience of any animal born vulnerable into a potentially hostile world, initially requiring protection and later guidance for continued survival. The development of a recognizable human psychology[1] is nevertheless secondary to unconscious and instinctive behavior and is itself the product of evolutionary determinism. One might argue simply that being an animal comes first, and, in human beings, psychology follows, including the *subjective* experiences of attachment and selfhood. This can be compared to Maslow's (1968, 1970) well-known and simple hierarchy, shown in Figure 2.1, in which psychologically higher order needs and behavior are not experienced or activated until more basic physical needs and goals are first met and achieved.

However, the "unconsciousness" of attachment theory does not resemble the unconscious described by classic psychoanalysis. Indeed, Holmes (2001) writes that "attachment behaviors are no more or less unconscious that are, say, our digestive processes" (p. 24).

---

[1] An organized and discernible set of cognitive processes, and eventually self-consciousness, that is the essence of what it means to be human.

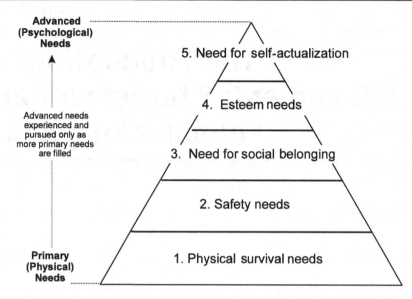

Figure 2.1   Maslow's (1970) Hierarchy of needs

THE DEVELOPMENT AND ORIGINS OF ATTACHMENT THEORY

Bowlby's interest in ethology and the work of Conrad Lorenz and other animal scientists led him along a path by which he fashioned a theory that coupled human behavior, and the psychology behind human behavior, with a model of animal science. Added to this, Bowlby injected cybernetics, or a model of environmental communication and responsiveness in which, through some form of interactive feedback, a set of controls in the environment activate and deactivate systems, or in this case, human behaviors.

Comparing attachment theory to both psychoanalysis and object relations theory also places the theory in its own philosophically evolutionary chain. That is, like other theories of its time, attachment theory was born of psychoanalysis, and was closely connected to object relations theory, another offshoot of classic psychoanalysis. Indeed, Bowlby, a psychoanalyst, described the development of attachment theory as a variant of object relations theory (Bowlby, 1988, p. 29). Accordingly, as he developed and described his theory, Bowlby paid great attention to the ideas of Sigmund Freud, and although straying far away clearly showed great deference to Freud and maintained some connection with Freudian theory, perhaps not wanting to stray too far or alienate himself from psychoanalysis, the center of psychotherapy at that time. A reading of Bowlby's important trilogy on attachment (1969, 1973, 1980) shows the care he took to recognize and describe Freudian ground and carefully and respectfully describe differences, even as he disassembled and refuted classic psychoanalysis.

Bowlby rejected the ideas of classic psychoanalysis, and many of the primary psychological drives and constructs it postulated. He accepted and built upon a number of basic premises, but developed them in entirely different directions. Holmes (2001) writes that Bowlby "developed attachment theory both as an extension of and in opposition to psychoanalysis" (p. 66). For instance, Bowlby rejected entirely the idea that infant behaviors are driven by a primary feeding urge and a subsequent psychological attraction towards the breast, and that the infant soon after, in the earliest years of development, begins to engage in eroticized ideas and sexualized fantasies (or, for Melanie Klein, aggressive and destructive urges centered about the breast). The accompanying psychoanalytic belief is that all other human ideas, needs, attractions, and relationships are secondarily derived from this primary drive. Similarly, Bowlby did not believe that the infant engages in outward manifestations of internalized and primitive sexual or aggressive fantasies, or is even capable of constructing such fantasies. Neither did he believe that phobia and trauma drive development, parental relationships, and self-identity. Instead, Bowlby argued that "food plays only a marginal role in a child's attachment to his mother" (Bowlby, 1979, p. 116), and that attachment behavior is a primary drive that develops independently from feeding and is primary (and not secondary) to feeding. Rather than an offshoot or derivative of the feeding process or erotic or destructive fantasies, Bowlby plainly saw the "function of attachment behavior (as) protection" (1969, 1979), changing in intensity and direction over the course of development, but developing most clearly between 5 and 12 months and most strongly during the second and third years of life.

Unlike Freud and Klein, who believed that fears and phobias were unrealistic infantile fantasies developed and projected out of primitive sexual or destructive ideation, Bowlby considered fear to be natural, normative, and necessary. He considered the presence of fear to be neither infantile nor psychologically abnormal. On the contrary, Bowlby considered the absence or hyperactive presence of fear to be the concern: "it is not the presence of this tendency in childhood or later life that is pathological; pathology is indicated either when the tendency is apparently absent or when fear is aroused with unusual readiness and intensity" (1973, p. 84). Rather than viewing the attachment behaviors of children as evidence of fantasy and neuroticism, Bowlby believed "the propensity to show attachment behavior is a healthy characteristic and in no sense infantile" (1979, p. 116).

ATTACHMENT THEORY AND OBJECT RELATIONS

Although it is clear that Bowlby's attachment theory is an object relations theory, it is based on a different set of premises from those postulated by Klein and Fairbairn—virtually originators of and certainly leaders in object relations theory in their era. Bowlby saw attachment as a biological process and *the* primary drive, with all else following, including his ideas about how the external world is absorbed into and mentally mapped by the mind. This is the essence of any object relations theory—that is, how the developing child comes to understand objects in the external world, be they people or things, and in the internal world of the mind build mental representations of those objects, the self, and the relationship between self and objects. In the psychoanalytic world, objects are those people, parts of people, or things that psychologically influence cognitions, behaviors, and representations of the world, and through which instinctual drives are achieved and needs satisfied. However, whereas classic psychoanalytic theory sees objects as merely the medium through which primary feeding, sexual, or aggressive drives are discharged, in object relations theory it is the object *itself* that is central, and "object relations are . . . the determining factors in development" (Buckley, 1986, p. xii), thereby making object relations theory a true theory of relationships. Where psychoanalysis was a theory of internal processes, conflicts, and fantasies, in object relations theory "psychology . . . resolve(s) itself into a study of the relationships of the individual to his objects" (Fairbairn, 1952, p. 60).

Another important, and central, point of departure from classic psychoanalysis lies in the hypothesized development of internal representations of the world, a central feature of all object relations theory. In attachment theory the mental schema is the result of social construction, or the interaction of individuals with their environment and the product of experience. This is distinctly different from the special role assigned by traditional psychoanalytic theory to feeding as the means by which objects are introjected and translated into mental representations. Bowlby (1979) described "the replacement of the orally derived theory of internal objects by a theory of working models of world and self that are conceived as being constructed by each individual as a result of his experience, that determine his expectations, and on the basis of which he plans" (p. 115). Following and further defining these lines of difference, Bowlby eliminates "dependency" and "independence" as merely secondary drives (contingent upon the primary drives of feeding and sex), and replaces them with the concepts of attachment, trust, reliance, and self-reliance.

Peter Fonagy (2001a, pp. 8–9) further distinguishes between attachment theory and object relations theory. In object relations theory, he writes, the goal *is* the object, around which all behaviors are organized. In attachment theory, however, the goal is really not the object at all, but the experienced state of security ("felt security") that results from a physical (and later, psychological) relationship with that object. This leads to, and is satisfied by, the establishment of an internalized representation of mother and the emotional experience of physical proximity, and hence security. However, despite Fonagy's assertion that this separates attachment theory from object relations theory, it is precisely this internalization of an object (mother) and a relationship to that object, that defines attachment theory *as* an object relations theory. Indeed, Holmes (2001) writes that "attachment theory has always accepted that it is essentially a variant of object relations theory" (p. 21).

In fact, the idea that the external world is internalized, or absorbed into the mind, is basic to any theory that accepts consciousness and cognition as the basis for human behavior. In such models, the mental map is made up of internal schematic representations that pattern or help to make predictable external reality and mental scripts that guide both relationships and action. In attachment theory, and lying at its heart, this mental map is known as the *internal working model*, containing the templates required to make sense of, respond to, engage in, and manipulate the environment. It is the construction and contents of the internal model that is central to any understanding of selfhood and how the attachment experience is played out through social behavior.

The Root Elements of Attachment

Through combining ethology, cognitive development, cybernetics, and human psychology, Bowlby defined the formation of attachment as an evolutionarily designed, biological system that protects life in its earliest stages and later promotes mastery, thus paving the way for continued survival and reproduction. In practice, illustrated in Figure 2.2, attachment theory can be conceptualized by five key components that combine to produce a working system of attachment in children, adolescents, and adults.

1. *Primary and multiple biological processes.* A set of evolutionarily established physiological or behavioral systems whose processes are hard wired and located in the central nervous system, designed to first keep the infant safe from harm and later to promote physical and mental growth, and;
2. *Interactive behavioral systems.* Discrete behavioral systems, of which attachment is only one, each with different purposes and processes, that influence and combine with one another to produce a higher order of functioning than mere survival, and;
3. *Cybernetic control mechanisms.* Behavioral systems responsive to specific stimuli found in both the environment and within the central nervous and endocrine systems that are engaged in a feedback loop to determine when behavioral processes are activated and later deactivated, thus maintaining homeostasis (an even/balanced state of being), and;
4. *Goal-oriented and corrected cognitive processes.* The emergence of higher cognitive (that is, not strictly physiological) processes that are not unique to humans, which create the capacity for understanding and manipulating the environment, recognizing and establishing goals, and designing and organizing a set of behavioral strategies for both achieving those goals and adjusting behaviors accordingly, and;
5. *Higher cognitive human development.* The capacity for language, and the conscious self-awareness it allows, that organizes and transforms the attachment system in humans into consciously experienced emotional events and accompanying behavior, and orients the drive for attachment towards lifetime affectional relationships. This advanced human development of attachment nonetheless remains a biological primary drive, and serves to enhance both reproduction and the survival of the next generation through the development of the sexual and the caregiver behavioral systems.

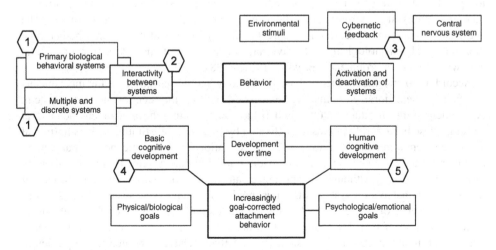

Figure 2.2   The interaction of five key components of attachment

Attachment as Instinct: Biological Behavioral Systems

As described, attachment theory recognizes attachment as an essentially instinctive, or hard-wired and inevitable, process designed for survival. In humans, the idea and experience of attachment is transformed into something beyond survival through the human experience of consciousness and self-awareness. Of this, Ainsworth, Blehar, Everett, and Wall (1978) write that "the predictable outcome of a child's attachment behavior is to bring him into closer proximity with other people, and particularly with the specific individual who is primarily responsible for his care" (p. 6). Critical to understanding attachment theory, they note also that "it is under very unusual circumstances that an infant or young child encounters conditions such that his attachment behavior does not result in the formation of an attachment" (p. 9). That is, attachment almost always forms, whether adaptively or maladaptively, securely or insecurely, or with strategies for maintaining proximity that are organized or disorganized. "Detachment," for instance, is a particular reflection of the attachment experience and does *not* reflect a lack of attachment. The idea that attachment is instinctive, and is virtually certain under any condition, becomes the basis for questions about the *form* that attachment takes and deficits or disorders of attachment, rather than a *lack* of attachment.

Bowlby (1969) describes behavior typically considered to be instinctive as: (1) following a recognizable pattern and course in most members of the same species; (2) involving a predictable *sequence* of behaviors rather than a *single* response; (3) contributing to the preservation of the individual or species; and (4) naturally present so that examples of the behavior occur even when learning opportunities are rare or not present. Bowlby is asserting that "instinct" is more correctly understood as an in-built (hard-wired) behavioral *system* rather than a specific behavior. Rather than being predetermined and specific, individual behaviors that derive from the behavioral system are driven by an inherited *potential*, hence the actual form of the behavior is shaped by the specific environment into which the instinctive behavioral system is introduced. Here, Bowlby builds the ground for the mutual and reciprocal relationship between nature and nurture in which we see behavior, psychology and, eventually, personality emerging as a synthesis of both inborn tendencies (nature) and environmental influence (nurture), rather than one or the other: "The antithesis 'innate versus acquired' is unreal . . . every biological character, whether it be morphological, physiological, or behavioral, is a product of the interaction of genetic endowment with environment" (Bowlby, 1969, p. 38).

According to attachment theory, based in biology and not psychology, the mechanisms for natural behavioral systems are embedded within the central nervous system. Attachment is the product of one such behavioral system—the attachment behavioral system. These behavioral systems are activated by both internal stimuli, such as hormonal levels, and environmental stimuli, and the activation of a specific behavioral *system* results in the appearance of specific *behaviors* related to that system. This is an important distinction to make. Although, for instance, attachment behaviors are the product of the attachment behavioral system, they must not be mistaken for the system itself. Accordingly, the absence of the related behaviors does not signify the absence of the behavioral system. Absence of fear, for example, does not mean that the fear behavioral system is not present, it simply means the system is not active. Behaviors related to the particular behavioral system are terminated when stimuli have desisted or other conditions are met that deactivate the system. The behaviors disappear, but the behavioral system remains. Such behavioral systems, including attachment, are present from the cradle to the grave (Bowlby, 1979, p. 129). This explains why the appearance of detachment does not signify a *lack* of an attachment behavioral system, but simply a variant of a deactivated system.

Bowlby defined behavioral systems and resulting behaviors as "environmentally stable" if the system is activated in similar ways throughout the species, even if environmental conditions vary or change. Because the human child is born in a completely vulnerable manner, dependent upon others for protection in its earliest months, attachment theory proposes that infants are evolutionarily equipped with an environmentally stable behavioral system that will maintain proximity to a primary caregiver, resulting in predictable and consistent behaviors (attachment behaviors). In the earliest activations of the attachment behavioral system, these comprise sets of basic and purely physical behaviors (sucking, clinging, following, crying, and smiling). Between 9 and 18 months of age these evolve into a more sophisticated, but still rudimentary, set of attachment behaviors driven by self-agency and cognitively derived goals, and infant behaviors are modified and corrected by the child in order to meet these goals.

In short, a *behavioral system* represents an innate (instinctual or unlearned) propensity for the individual to behave in certain ways when triggered by a specific stimulus. In the case of the attachment behavioral system, the propensity, or the goal, of the behavioral system is to maintain proximity to the caregiver (the attachment figure). The behavioral system, then, is a biologically loaded spring waiting to be released. As obvious as it may seem to state this, the actual *behaviors* of the behavioral system are those that are exhibited once the behavioral system is activated. Once the behavioral system is deactivated (conditions have been met), the behaviors disappear, although the behavioral system remains in the biological background, inactive but present.

INTERACTING BEHAVIORAL SYSTEMS

On the other side of the relationship equation lies the behavior of the primary caregiver—usually, of course, the mother. That is, the caregiver behavioral system is the evolutionary adult complement to the child's attachment behavioral system, or maternal behavior in this case that allows the child and mother to adapt to one another. However, from a neurobiological perspective, attachment is not merely an emotional or cognitive experience. Chemical transmitters are, in part, responsible for the maternal bond and the neuropeptide oxytocin, released during both female labor and lactation, is often associated with the maternal and generally affectional bonding process (Carter, Lederhendler, & Kirkpatrick, 1997; Giovenardi, Padoin, Cadore, & Lucion, 1997; Insel, 2000; Panksepp, Nelson, & Bekkedal, 1997; Turner, Altemus, Enos, Cooper, & McGuinness, 1999; Uvnäs-Moberg, 1997), an essential component in any complementary infant–mother attached relationship. To this end, Holmes (2001) describes the attachment bond as a complex psychophysiological state.

However, attachment theory is concerned less with the *act* of attachment per se, and more with the contribution of attachment to human growth in general. In effect, attachment theory presumes that the ultimate psychology of individuals derives from three related systems that interact with one another during early childhood. The *attachment*, *exploration*, and *fear* systems together serve to modulate and regulate the child's behavior, out of which develops the internally developed and neurologically "hard-wired" internal working model through which the child, and eventually the adolescent and the adult, finds representations of self and others, serving as the template for all experiences of the world, its interactions, and its relationships.

As such, attachment is not the result of a psychological drive or a by-product resulting from the satiation of other needs, such as food or sex, but is in itself a primary physical drive in which security and safety are actively sought. Hence, if attachment needs are not met, then exploration behaviors will not ensue, except in unusual circumstances. In fact, it is the *absence* of attachment behaviors, coupled with other behaviors in an otherwise well-adjusted infant, that suggests secure attachment, rather than a display of attachment behaviors. Just the opposite, if attachment behaviors are exhibited, at that moment at least, the attachment behavioral system is active because the child is feeling insecure, uncertain, and/or fearful and in need of physical or psychological protection.

DEVELOPMENTAL PATHWAYS IN THE REARING ENVIRONMENT

The principle of "the environment of evolutionary adaptedness" asserts that the instinctual (innate and hard-wired) qualities of each behavioral system evolve in concert with the environment in which the species evolutionarily developed. These biological behavioral systems are thus suited for survival and reproduction in *those* environments, attachment included. Bowlby (1973) notes, hinting at the roots of developing pathology, "the further the *rearing environment* departs from that of evolutionary adaptedness the more likely are that individual's behavioral systems to develop atypically" (p. 82). Here, we can start to form at least some preliminary ideas about any relationship that may exist between attachment and maladaptive and/or antisocial behaviors as a possible result of rearing a child in an environment that is not protective or nurturing or, worse, is neglectful or abusive. This is not, presumably, the environment best suited for the development of secure and socially capable individuals. This may also help us to make sense of the development of sexually coercive behaviors as we consider the influence of the social environment, as well as the convergence of other behavioral systems that are activated within that environment, such as the sexual, affiliative, and caregiver systems.

There can be no argument about the prevalence of sexual messages in our society that promote sexual behavior for its own sake and for pleasure, rather than for reproduction or the raising of families, and often have little to do with responsible or even contained sexual behaviors. In addition, we are well aware of the neglect and abuse that many individuals who later develop sexually abusive behavior themselves experience in their early years. These attributes of the "rearing environment" may represent a fundamental and important shift in the environment of evolutionary adaptedness described by Bowlby, and may reflect a level of social anomie (social normlessness) in the environment in which our children grow up. This, combined with attachments of an insecure nature, may well have some value in understanding how, for some individuals, an innate drive but failure to achieve attachment may also drive engagement in sexually precocious and later sexually abusive behavior.

Nevertheless, as Bowlby's model asserts, although the potential for particular behavior is innate, the actual behavior is the result of the interaction between instinct, individual propensities, and events in the environment. This strongly suggests that potentials and instinctual behavioral drives aside, despite similar starting points and obvious influences, there is no set pathway for any particular behavior and the behavioral outcomes for each individual are the result of many influences. Bowlby (1973), mirroring the biologist C.H. Waddington, refers to this as homeorhesis (stable flow), or the creation of established, albeit individualized, pathways. Homeorhesis describes the process by which forces form and support the trajectory of the developmental channel along which an individual is already moving. Factors found within the individual and the environment combine to "canalize" the present pathway, or maintain the trajectory along that pathway, and there is a self-regulating quality (or inertia) that increases the likelihood that one will stay on that pathway over time. Earlier events, forming and emanating from the pathway, establish the path for later events that then have an increasingly high potential to occur, and these in turn further define an increasingly set future pathway.

> Thus the developmental process is conceived as able to vary its course, more or less adaptively, during the early years, according to the environment in which development is occurring; and subsequently, with the reduction of environmental sensitivity, as becoming increasingly constrained to the particular pathway already chosen. (Bowlby, 1973, p. 367)

Kagan (1984) describes the same process as a developmental journey containing many points from which one can move in a number of different directions. However, each choice modifies, even in a small way, the probability of a particular outcome. Once a choice is made, a form of inertia resists any detour from that path and eventually a form is assumed that Kagan describes as "difficult or impossible to change."

However, there are no predetermined pathways that inevitably set into motion any particular behavior, including sexual aggression. Individual pathways are so complex and influenced by so many factors, both subtle and obvious, that we may not be able to define a single pathway, or set of factors or events, that leads to the same behavioral outcome for every individual first stepping along a similar path. Almost like smoke drifting into the air, we cannot predict the eventual pattern of the smoke because it is influenced by a host of subtle factors, of many of which we are unaware. Although many similar journeys with common starting points eventually take significantly different directions, we recognize that once started there is an increasingly and ever more narrowly defined process of self-selection by which the trajectory of the current pathway is strengthened, behaviors become ingrained, and developmental pathways move closer towards inevitable outcomes.

Bowlby (1988) writes "the model of developmental pathways regards an infant at birth as having an array of pathways potentially open to him, the one along which he will in fact proceed being determined at every moment by the interaction of the individual as he now is with the environment" (p. 136). Atkinson and Goldberg (2004) similarly describe as a basic principle of attachment theory a recognition that behaviors and relationships occur within a broad context, in which attachment "is just one of a network of influences, including genetic, physiological, psychological and environmental, that are involved in child development" (p. 15).

The Attachment Bond

Of special note, the attachment system in the child operates in synchrony with what is, more or less, the adult equivalent found in the behaviors that constitute a caregiver behavioral system. Bowlby (1988) describes caregiving as the major role of parents, not only as complementary to attachment behavior but also "regarded in the same light as careseeking, namely as a basic component of human nature" (p. 121). Ainsworth et al. (1978) distinguish between *attachment* as a bond, or in the case of the mother–child relationship an enduring relationship between a young child and his mother, and *attachment behaviors* which serve to form and engage in the bond. However, whereas both the mother and infant hopefully experience an attached relationship, attachment *behaviors* are a feature of and reside within the child and not the adult.

In this regard, the attachment bond technically does not reflect a dyadic relationship between two people (the child and the caregiver), but exists only within the child. It represents the dependency that one individual (the child) has upon another individual (the mother) who is perceived as the caregiver. A child can thus be attached to a person who is not, in turn, attached to the child. The "attachment bond" is a specific type of a larger class of bonds referred to as "affectional" or affiliative bonds, many of which may form during an individual's life, but which are not attachments in the language or intent of attachment theory. This underscores the biological underpinning of attachment, serving the cause of survival rather than social connectivity, per se.

The attachment bond, then, is a special relationship, not to be confused with more general affectional bonds that are part of the larger sociable, or affiliative, behavioral system. Attachment is thus not symmetrical and not simply interchangeable from one individual to another, although the child may form more than one attachment relationship. Bowlby (1969) considers attachment to be limited to the behavior of the child as directed towards the caregiver, and hence limits the attachment bond to the relationship experienced by the child. Recognizing that a bond is a property of two parties, however, he considers that the mutual bond should rightly be called the "attachment-caregiving bond" (p. 366), and Ainsworth (1989) refers to the mother–infant bond, rather than a mutual attachment bond. Nevertheless, this is unwieldy language and in common usage the attachment bond, as used by Schore (2001a, 2001b), reflects the complementary relationship between both parties, rather than the exclusive experience of the child.

Attachment and the Secure Base

Attachment behaviors are embedded within an attachment behavioral system, which, as described, is one of several systems that operate within the infant and throughout life. In particular, Bowlby postulated that *attachment* behaviors operate in a mutual and inverse relationship with behaviors in the organized *exploratory* system of the child in which, when one behavioral system is activated, the other is, in effect, switched off.

Over time, attachment behavior changes. It eventually reflects the partnership between the attachment figures in which attachment and caregiving behaviors meld, and also reflects the increasing capacity of the child to build and act upon attachment strategies that trigger goals for exploration based upon an internalized experience of safety and security.

In this regard, the attachment relationship ideally becomes the "secure base" from which the child explores and emotionally grows, and eventually moves into the larger world outside of the attachment relationship. From the balance between (a) the linked, inverse activation and deactivation of the attachment system and (b) the exploratory system the child derives the secure base that contributes to, and is the embodiment of, the secure (or insecure) internal working model, or the child's internalized representation of the world.

Bowlby and Ainsworth's conceptualization of secure base behavior, beginning sometime around the eighth month, is similar to the "home base" described by Margaret Mahler (Mahler, Pine, & Bergman, 1975). Mahler describes three major phases in the developmental process from birth to about age 3, by which young children engage in the process of separation from parents and individuation of self—a process she believes to be "the first crucial prerequisite" for the development and maintenance of a "sense of identity" (p. 11). Mahler breaks the third phase of separation–individuation (following "normal autism" and "symbiosis") into four subphases that begin at about 4 months. During the second subphase of "practicing," lasting from approximately 10 to 18 months, Mahler's description of the "refueling" process by which children stray away from and return to their mothers during play and early ambulation, using their mothers as a "home base," is similar to the exploration behaviors described by Bowlby and Ainsworth in their conceptualization of the secure base.

However, although similar in concept and content and both addressing similar phenomena observed in young children, exploration in attachment theory does not constitute a developmental *stage* but a behavioral *system* that is in play throughout life, even though taking different forms as the individual ages. The similarity is clear, however: whether a developmental phase or enduring behavioral system, the need for the parent to serve as a safe haven is instrumental in the child's internalization of the world as a safe, predictable, and responsive environment, and that experience is central in the development and emergence of secure identity and selfhood. In both models, also noteworthy is the appearance of these secure/home base behaviors at a predictable age in normative development (instinctually, without requiring learning opportunities to become active), and the inverse connection between attachment and exploration.

The outcome of these developmental behaviors, in which the child requires the parent to serve as a safe and secure platform, also coincides with the first stage of Erikson's (1959/1980) developmental model. Covering essentially the same developmental period of up to 18 months, the first emotional–cognitive goal for the developing personality is the establishment of trust, or confidence in the responsiveness of the environment, including of course, and most of all, caregivers. Erikson writes that "the *amount of trust* derived from earliest infantile experience does not seem to depend on absolute *quantities of food or demonstrations of love* but rather on the *quality* of the maternal relationship" (p. 65).

PRECURSORS TO ATTACHMENT: INFANT–CAREGIVER COMMUNICATION

Although the infant has no cognitive capacity to speak of during the first few weeks of life, it is born with a developed set of perceptual senses. These innate senses are not only the sole means by which the infant can experience the world, but also represent the basis for early attachment—that is, attachment for pure survival, leading gradually, and later in quantum leaps, to the establishment of the secure base and the construction of the internal working model. Schore (2001a) notes that from birth the infant is using its expanding physical and cognitive capacities to interact with the social environment, but in its earliest "proto-attachment" experiences, uses what it has—emerging and maturing motor and perceptive sensory capacities, especially smell, taste, and touch—to interact with the social environment.

Salkind (1994) writes that babies seem almost programmed to respond to human language, and with the exception of eyesight, all perceptual senses appear to be functioning and developed early in life. Of visual perception, Mehler and Dupoux (1994) conclude that the infant is virtually blind at birth, seeing everything as a blur, and they write that it is not until one year of age that infants have the visual acuity of an adult, although Salkind describes visual acuity by 6 months. However, it is clear that unlike eyesight, the auditory acuity of infants is well developed at birth, and it is likely that infants can recognize their own mother's voices by 4 weeks of age. In some studies, discrimination of mother's voice has been hypothesized within 1–2 days of birth (Smith, Cowie, & Blades, 1998). Taste, too, appears well developed at birth and present as early as 3 days, and infants appear to be able to recognize the smell of their own body odor and discriminate by smell their mother's milk (Salkind, 1994). Bowlby (1988) reports that within days of birth an infant is able to distinguish its mother by her smell, voice, and the way the infant is held.

Although visual discrimination is not reliable until after 5 to 6 months of age (Cohen, DeLoache, & Strauss, 1979) or even after the first 6 months (Bowlby, 1988), it seems certain that by 2 months and perhaps earlier, infants are able to distinguish faces from non-faces, and between 3 and 6 months to recognize increasingly more complex facial patterns (Smith et al., 1998). However, the infant is not only recognizing and receiving information *from* the external world, it is also communicating and transmitting information *to* that world.

By 6 months, Yale, Messinger, Cobo-Lewis, and Delgado (2003) report strong evidence that infants express their own emotional states through intentional and coordinated positive or negative facial expressions, the direction of their gaze, and their vocalizations, and that this capacity for coordinated self-expression is central to the development of emerging communication skills. Between 3 and 6 months the infant's developing instinctive capacity for self-expression contributes to an emerging awareness that it can communicate directly with its caregiver; on some rudimentary level, the infant recognizes the utility of facial expressions and vocalization, understanding that it will be recognized and responded to by the caregiver. Biological growth and interactive learning come together, and through the mutual interactions of the two primary players—the infant and the mother—the roots of the attachment and maternal bond begin to develop.

Jahromi, Putnam, and Stifter (2004) found evidence that maternal behaviors intended to regulate their infant's emotional condition also develop and significantly change within the first 6 months, from the primary use of soothing and affection displayed largely through touch to increased use of maternal vocalizing and distraction behaviors. Pure touching behaviors were shown to decrease by infant age, whereas maternal vocalizing and distracting behaviors increased, suggesting that caregivers move from reliance on tactile strategies to more expressive vocalizations as the child ages, because they recognize the increasing and changing capacities of the child for communication. Clyman, Emde, Kempe, and Harmon (1986) write that it is important for parents to ensure early *face-to-face* affective interaction, and that there is reason to believe that looking at the face of another is central to the infant's developing sense of other and self, taking on increasing importance after 6 months of age. They regard as "social referencing" the infant's ability to gather information, and especially to resolve uncertainty, through looking at the face of a primary caregiver.

Face to Face: Attunement and Attachment

Facial engagement, then, becomes a central means for establishing the attachment link, and developing the communicative, learning, and self-regulatory abilities identified by Schore at the start of this chapter. Schore (1994, 2001a) describes sustained mutual gaze transactions between the infant and mother, as well as the mother's facial expressions, stimulating and amplifying emotion in the infant. As noted, Yale et al. (2003) report that the child develops the capacity to use facial and other expressions of emotion by 6 months, and Schore (1994) postulates that the child's internal state is hence communicated back to the mother, and "in this interactive system of reciprocal stimulation both members of the dyad enter into a symbiotic state of heightened . . . affect" (p. 71). He writes that sustained mutual facial gazing represents an intense form of interpersonal communication, providing clues to both parties to the readiness or capacity of the other to receive and produce social information. Tronick, Cohn, and Shea (1986) envision a similar process in their Mutual Regulation Model. The infant's experience of self-efficacy, or "effectance," is promoted through the non-verbal, dyadic mother–child experience in which the relationship itself helps to regulate emotion in the infant.

Although attachment theory holds that attachment will occur in almost any circumstance, it is precisely this interplay between caregiver-behaviors-directed-at-infant and infant-behaviors-directed-at-caregiver that is the essence of the early attachment process. It is the capacity to express ideas and emotions through the communication, the content of the communication, the intensity level of the communication, and the accuracy of response to communication that defines not only the quality of that communication, but the quality of the attachment bond that forms through repeated and sustained communication over time. The capacity to engage in this person–person communication, as well as the capacity to accurately and sensitively communicate and respond, is of course quite different for the parent and the infant. The mother is expected to be capable, contained, and attuned, whereas the baby is expected to be simply expressive at first and, over time, to demonstrate greater precision, accuracy, clarity, and appropriate timing in reciprocal communication, as well as control over emotional expression.

This is why the attachment relationship is one way, and not mutual—that is, the infant is dependent upon the caregiver for safety and instruction, and not vice versa. Nevertheless, it is through this synchronous communication that the baby learns about communication and self-control, for better or for worse, and experiences the external world as sensitive, satisfying, and responsive, or insensitive, incapable, and unreliable. The attuned caregiver provides the empathic recognition, accurate responses, and sensitive guidance required for optimal attachment, whereas the emotional and behavioral interactions of the misattuned, insensitive, or abusive caregiver lead to the development of "nonoptimal" attachment, in Goldberg's (1997) terms.

Through the earliest of communicative experiences, initially dependent on sensory perceptions and manipulations, the infant engages in a direct relationship with its primary caregiver, not only to express and get needs met but also to receive guidance in how to deal with the external world and regulate internal states. In just a few weeks, with the emergence of basic cognitive abilities, the development of attachment takes on another slant, essentially involving "mind reading." More precisely, beginning in early infancy, attachment requires of the caregiver a sensitive and almost intuitive understanding of the child and the ability to recognize and understand its needs. Correspondingly, for the infant, this means experiencing the mother as responsive and accurate in both her perceptions of and responses to physical and emotional needs.

Stern (1985/2000) describes the need of the developing infant for "an other" who can regulate the infant's own self-experience, or a *self-regulating other* (p. 102). He writes that all of the events that regulate the feelings of attachment and security are experiences initially created through mutual interaction with a self-regulating other, even if the other is eventually an internalized representation of a caregiver, or an "evoked companion" as Stern describes it. In describing attunement, or affect attunement, Stern (p. 139) writes that three conditions must be present: (i) *interpretation*, in which the parent is able to read the infant's emotional state from its overt behavior, (ii) *reflection*, in which the parent demonstrates behavior that mirrors the infant's behavior without simply imitating it, and therefore accurately corresponds to the infant's own behavior, and (iii) *recognition*, in which the infant experiences the parental response as corresponding to and congruent with the infant's emotional experience. It is through the interaction of these three processes that Stern contends attunement is achieved, or the transmission of affect states from one person to another without the use of language, and the recognition in both parties that the transaction has occurred. He notes that attunement is not about behavior per se, but those aspects of behavior that reflect internal (affect) states, and he uses the terms "mirroring" and "echoing" to represent those concepts that come closest to affect attunement, or "one person reflecting another's inner state" (p. 144).

Mind to Mind: Mind Reading and Connected Minds

In the optimal attached relationship, then, there is a synchrony of communication in which the mother and child form accurate impressions of one another, what is wanted or needed, and how to respond, and the child in turn is able to experience and recognize the external and internal state of the mother. This is accomplished both through mutual gazing at one other and other forms of overt interaction and communication, and experiencing the momentary and often unobserved sensory signals and motor events that Hofer (2000) has referred to as hidden regulators. Schore (1994) describes "hidden within the dyadic relations between mother and child" (p. 4) split second, but nonetheless crucial, transactions that serve to inform and regulate the experiences, emotions, and behavior of the infant. Of course, it is the caregiver who is "in charge" of this relationship and this communication and the child who is dependent, and thus Polan and Hofer (1999) refer to this attunement as the caregiver's "spontaneous, nonverbal responses to . . . children's expressed emotions" (p. 176). Schore (1999) writes that these visual, prosodic, auditory, and tactile events are transmitted back and forth between and through the faces of the infant and mother, "in a context of affect synchrony" (p. xvii), and thus neurobiologically stored in the internal working model of the child.

As Polan and Hofer (1999) also note, the internal working model of the child is gradually built from the child's interactions, including, and most especially, those with the primary caregivers, creating a mental representation of self and mother "upon which the child's approach to future social interactions is based" (p. 173). From Bowlby's (1973, p. 204) perspective, built into the IWM is the child's experience of whether an attachment figure is accessible and responsive (image of other), and also whether the self is someone to whom anyone, and particularly the attachment figure, is likely to respond (image of self).

The implication in all this, returning to the mind-reading analogy, is that two brains can be tuned to one another. As Schore (2001a) writes, there is a metacognitive brain–brain encounter between mother and child that sustains a relationship and organizes complex states within both brains. He believes that when two brains are engaged in an "affective synchrony," they create a resonance that plays an important and basic role in reorganizing the brain of the adult and creating an enduring organization in the brain of the child. Siegel (1999) addresses this identical idea as he writes that three fundamental principles explain the development and emergence of the mind: (i) through the interaction of neurobiological processes and interpersonal experience, (ii) by the impact of actual experience upon and shaping of the maturing neuronal brain, and, echoing Schore, (iii) through interactional "patterns in the flow of energy and information within the brain and between brains" (p. 2). He writes that "the developing mind uses the states of an attachment figure in order to help organize the functioning of its own states" (p. 70), describing "mental state resonance" as the internal states of two individuals are brought "into alignment."

However, rather than simply assigning this phenomenon to the realm of mysterious psychic occurrence, Schore and Siegel as neurobiologists both consider that the experience of mental attunement at the emotional level corresponds to a physical occurrence at the neural level. This interactive process between mother and child causes brain synapses to fire, forming a specific synaptic connection within each brain. If these pre- and post-synapses fire together often enough they create "long-term potentiation" in the synaptic connection, strengthening that particular synaptic nerve response and thus making it more likely that the same synaptic response will occur more and more easily. This contributes to the development of networks of synaptic connections and the shaping of neural circuits in the brain, a process commonly described by the expression "cells that fire together, wire together."[2] This succinctly describes the translation of external experience into the shaping of the mind, with neural plasticity occurring in the formation and strengthening of new synaptic connections. Damasio (1994) describes mental representations of external events contained in dispositional neural patterns, in which "dispositional representations exist as potential neuron activity in small ensembles of neurons" that consist of patterns of neural firing, acquired and strengthened through learning. "What dispositional representations

---

[2] Often incorrectly attributed to Donald Hebb, the expression "inputs that fire together, wire together" was coined by Bear, Connors, and Paradiso (1996).

hold in store in their little commune of synapses is not a picture per se, but a means to reconstitute 'a picture'" (p. 102). The "self" is thus formed, according to LeDoux (2002), at the synaptic level as the result of the interaction between external events, such as the mother–child experience, and the neural response to and organization of that event.

Required in this process, of course, is the caregiver's capacity to intuit the internal state of the infant, or accurately recognize and be able to metaphorically "read" its mind. The converse is also true, however, in that the developing child must have the capacity to form what is often called a theory of mind. That is, the natural ability to both recognize one's own mind and also recognize that others have minds, and that these minds operate independently from the child's own mind and contain different thoughts and feelings, and generally understand how the "other" mind works.

This means that the child must eventually recognize both similarities and differences between mind-of-self and mind-of-other, and accurately understand motivations, attitudes, preferences, experiences, emotions, and ideas of the other. More plainly, the child must have an awareness and understanding of mental processes and underlying mental states in both self and others. Involving the capacity for metacognition, theory of mind requires the capacity to think about thinking, and more to the point to think about the way *others* think. This capacity is linked to that of self-reflection, and eventually reflection and insight into the minds of others. Siegel (1999, 2001, 2003) describes this capacity of the child to "perceive the subjective experiences of others, and of themselves" (2003, p. 38), or to understand and "read" the mind of the other, as "mindsight," suggesting that this ability may be the cornerstone of empathy and compassion. Indeed, the ability to accurately infer subjective states in other people is a significant element in our understanding of what it means to be empathic, another quality often asserted to be deficient in sexual offenders. "Mind blindness" represents the limitation or incapacity of the individual to recognize or understand the mind of others. At the extreme end, although there are other explanations for the condition, autistic children are considered to lack a theory of mind, and hence are unable to fully recognize or understand their own minds, or the minds of others.

CONCLUSION: ATTACHMENT, ATTUNEMENT, AND CONNECTION

It is precisely this model of attunement and connected brains (or minds) that is central to essential ideas of attachment theory, in which minute, fleeting, and almost imperceptible signals serve as hidden regulators that trigger and influence a synchronous relationship between mother and child, affecting both parties. The same external event—the fleeting look, the gesture, the spoken word, the interaction—is a potentiator, and accordingly creates an event in the brain. In a neurobiological model, this event is a synaptic firing, forming the basis for "hard-wired" neural circuits that embed into the brain memories and representations of events and interactions that occur repeatedly.

Beyond the neurobiology of attachment (the incorporation of attachment at the neural level), we recognize that through the developmental process of attachment and bonding during infancy and early childhood comes the establishment of felt security, the development of theory of mind, and the emergence of a sense of self and others.

The Commission on Children at Risk (2003) has written that "the self-organization of the developing brain occurs in the context of a relationship with another self, another brain" (p. 16). In a relationship that provides security in attachment for the child, brains are tuned into the same things, creating a shared experience and linked reality in the brains of both parties. Here perhaps, in this conceptualization of finely attuned relationships, lie the roots of empathy, even in the precognitive infant. The mother is attuned to and reaches out to the child. The child in turn learns not only about its ability to get its desires and needs met on a basic level, but also about the other (its mother). And, through the eyes of the mother and in her communication, the child discovers in her mind a representation of itself; thus, through discovering the other, the child discovers self.

CHAPTER 3

The Formation of Attachment and the Emergence of Self

In attachment theory, like object relations theory in general, it is clear that early experiences with the caregiving "object," most typically the mother, are central to the development of the individual, and that individual's experience and understanding of self and others. Attachment thus provides the basis for continued development and functioning, including future social transaction, interactions, and relationships. A sense of self-agency and self-efficacy are presumed to be linked to social and interpersonal competence, and hence are central to personal satisfaction and social connectedness. Security in relationships and internalized representations of people, experiences, and expectations are at the same time both the outcome of the attachment experience and the ongoing force that shapes attached relationships.

Before discussing the meaning of security or the development of the internal working model, it is important to first understand the internalization of the attachment experience and, tied to that process, the development of selfhood.

THE MATERNAL ROLE IN ATTACHMENT

Bowlby's great partner was Mary Ainsworth, who operationalized and further developed his ideas and allowed them to be tested in a laboratory setting. She created and developed the "strange situation" as the experimental model by which 12-month-old children could be observed under rigid and controlled conditions (using a stranger to the child as an experimental variable, hence the name). Form this, she derived a model of attachment style, or a set of three defined categories into which the attachment behavior of young children could be classified, later expanded to four categories by Main and Solomon (1986). This classification is still widely used to describe attachment patterns in both children and adults, or at least variations of Ainsworth's original model.

Attachment theorists, then, believe that by one year of age attachment patterns have been formed and are evident, and are generally believed to largely serve as a template for the experience and demonstration of security throughout life. MacDonald (1985) describes the first two years of life as critical to the development of attachment, "providing a foundation for later development" (p. 103), and noting the possibility that children who have not formed secure attachment by age 2 will have difficulties later in life. Basic to the idea of attachment theory is that the role and behavior, and, of course, level of attunement of the mother (or alternative primary caregiver) is absolutely central to the development of these patterned attachment styles. Winnicott (1964) described the role of "good-enough mothering" as that of creating the facilitative/holding environment in which the child develops, and wrote "the ordinary good mother knows without being told that during this time nothing must interfere with the continuity of the relationship between the child and herself" (p. 109). Winnicott (2002) believed that:

> These processes of growth cannot take place without a facilitating environment . . . (which) must have a human quality, not a mechanical perfection, so the phrase "good-enough mother" seems to me to meet the need for a description of what the child needs if the inherited growth processes are to become actual in the development of the individual child. . . . A good-enough mother starts off with a high degree of adaptation to the baby's needs . . . . That is what "good-enough" means, this tremendous capacity that mothers ordinarily have to give themselves over to identification with the baby. (pp. 233–234)

Clearly, Winnicott placed a great deal of emphasis on the role of the mother, placing a huge burden on her for the well-being of the developing child. Similarly, Schore (2001a) considers the co-creation of a secure attachment bond between infant and mother to be the basis of the infant's increasing capacity to cope with stress, both environmental and internal. Schore (1994) describes the mother as the major source of the environmental stimulation that facilitates the maturation of the child's developing neurobiological structures, writing that "affective interactions between the caregiver and the infant (are) imprinted into the child's developing nervous system" (p. 62). Indeed, in addition to serving as a basic principle of attachment theory, almost all of the object relations and ego theorists consider the maternal–child bond to be critical in the development of positive and healthy adaptation and growth in the developing child. From their studies of children in the strange situation, Ainsworth, Blehar, Everett, and Wall (1978) describe six attributes of maternal behaviors related to attunement and the development of secure attachment in their children.

1. Sensitivity–insensitivity to the baby's signals and communications.
2. Acceptance–rejection, or the balance between the mother's positive and negative feelings about her baby and her capacity to resolve her conflicts.
3. Cooperation–interference, measuring the mother's fostering of her child's independence and separateness and the level of direct control she exerts.
4. Accessibility–ignoring, addressing the mother's emotional accessibility to the infant, even she is physically accessible.
5. Emotional expression, or the degree to which the mother shows or lacks emotional expression in her face, voice, or movements.
6. Maternal rigidity, or the extent to which the mother is rigid, compulsive, and/or perfectionistic.

Correlating maternal behaviors with the attachment behaviors of 1-year-old children, Ainsworth concluded that maternal behavior during the first year of life is significantly associated with the development of securely attached children, resulting from maternal responsiveness to infant signals and communications.

> The finding of the studies . . . plainly show that 1-year-olds who are identified as securely attached . . . have experienced and concurrently experience more harmonious interaction with their mothers than those who are identified as anxiously attached, whether avoidant or resistant. Their mothers are more sensitively responsive to their signals and communications and are more keyed to reciprocity.
>
> (Ainsworth et al., 1978, p. 196)

Ainsworth and her colleagues found that the mothers of securely attached children (in group B, today referred to as securely attached) were found to be more sensitively responsive to infant signals and communications than mothers of other children. On the other hand, the mothers of children who were avoidantly attached (group A children, today largely referred to as insecure avoidant) were clearly "more rejecting" than other mothers, frequently felt negative emotions or showed little emotion towards their children, were rigid and insensitive to their children's needs, and avoided close physical contact. These children, upon reunion with their mothers after the brief separation built into the strange situation design, seemed to avoid contact with their mothers, maintaining an emotional and physical distance, and tended to treat their mothers much as they did strangers.

Mothers of group C children were also relatively insensitive to infant signals, but were less rejecting than group A mothers and showed no aversion to physical contact. However, these mothers were inept in holding their babies and showed little affectionate behavior in holding them, focusing more on routine than emotional attachment. Group C children, who were also considered to be insecurely attached, demonstrated ambivalent and resistant behavior at the same time they sought reunion with their mothers, and thus are today typically classified as insecure and anxious, ambivalent, or resistant.

THE DEVELOPMENTAL PROGRESSION OF ATTACHMENT

Bowlby describes the development of attachment, and hence the attachment bond and the contributions of attachment to human development, in sequential phases. Whereas Mahler, Erikson, and others have identified *stages* of infant and child development, in Bowlby's attachment theory it is behavioral *systems* that trigger behavior rather than developmental stages. Nevertheless, Bowlby describes the process of attachment developing through a series of phases, and thus the appearance of certain behaviors in the infant at predictable and specified points in its development. Although attachment theory is not a model of cognitive development per se, a description of the sequential development of attachment makes it possible to recognize the same sort of expected behaviors that are described by other developmental theorists. However, despite its emphasis on lifetime behavioral systems, this certainly implies that attachment may also be understood as a stage theory of development.

In particular, Bowlby (1969) described four phases in the development of parent–child attachment, taking care to note that, as with most stage theories, the phases are approximate only, with no sharp boundaries separating them from one another. Ainsworth later renamed the phases, and her more succinct titles are placed in parentheses and italicized below, next to Bowlby's named phases.

Attachment Phase 1

Orientation and Signals with Limited Discrimination of Figure (*the Initial Preattachment Phase*).

Although Ainsworth describes this phase as lasting only several weeks, Bowlby describes it as lasting between 8 and 12 weeks. Although the infant is attuned to certain environmental stimuli from birth, it is unable to discriminate between people, and initially responds to its mother figure in an undiscriminating manner.

This early stage is similar to Mahler's phase of normal autism, active during approximately the first four weeks of life. During this stage, the infant has no conception of an external world or capacity to distinguish self from others. Physical and emotional needs are gratified outside the infant's awareness, who exists "in a state of primitive hallucinatory disorientation . . . in an *autistic* orbit" (Mahler et al., 1975). In attachment theory, this phase is completed when the baby is able to discriminate between people and begins to recognize its mother figure. Ainsworth et al. (1978) add that is useful to consider this attachment phase continuing until the infant can consistently recognize the mother by means of visual cues, which occurs between 8 and 12 weeks.

Attachment Phase 2

Orientation and Signals Directed Towards One or More Discriminated Figures (*the Phase of Attachment-in-the-Making*).

Between 8 and 12 weeks of age, infants begin to demonstrate recognized discrimination and preference for their mothers (or primary caregivers), following differential responses to auditory stimuli after the first four weeks and to visual stimuli after approximately 10 weeks. The infant begins to clearly differentiate between figures, including both familiar and unfamiliar figures.

This second phase, beginning somewhere around 8 weeks, continues until about 6 months of age. However, Bowlby notes that infants can remain in any of these early phases longer in different circumstances, clearly defining such circumstances as unfavorable for the development of attachment along normative time lines. In her description of the phase as attachment-in-the-making, Ainsworth describes infants as essentially incapable of attachment until reaching the third phase of development, during which they clearly discriminate and actively seek out their attachment figure(s).

Operational from 8 to 12 weeks until about 6 months, attachment Phase 2 is similar to the Normal Symbiotic phase proposed by Mahler. Although the time lines differ, Bowlby and Ainsworth's attachment phases one and two approximate Mahler's autistic and symbiotic phases, and like Mahler's phases cover birth to approximately 5–6 months of age. The primary task of the symbiotic phase (4 weeks to approximately 5 months of age), fitting with attachment theory, is the development of the infant–mother bond and the development of a dyadic system. During this phase, the infant merges with the mother, remaining in an unindividuated state, but begins to demonstrate increased awareness of the external world. The child associates the mother (or other primary caregiver) with the gratification of needs and the elimination of negative stimuli (maintaining, in this conceptualization, Mahler's connection to classic psychoanalysis). Also, more closely aligned with attachment theory, the mother serves to both provide and mediate stimulation, serving as the child's "stimulus barrier," or external filter and model for the development of internal self-regulation.

Hence, Bowlby and Mahler's theories describe infant development occurring during the first 6 months in two phases, during which the infant evolves from an undifferentiated, and, in effect, unconscious, state to a state of dawning differentiation and sense of awareness, serving as the cognitive and emotional backdrop to the formation of attachment. Donald Winnicott, another object relations theorist of that era, describes the first 3–6 months as a period of "absolute dependence," or the holding phase during which develops "the dawn of intelligence and the beginning of the mind as something distinct" (1986, p. 241). During this phase, the infant begins to move from an undifferentiated state of merger with mother to a differentiated and structured state, and hence the experience of objects as external to self. In the effective holding environment, the mother adapts herself and the environment to best fit the needs of the infant which are accurately identified by the "good-enough mother." According to Winnicott, the foundations for the mental health of the child are laid down during the holding process, facilitated by maternal care or "good-enough mothering" (Winnicott, 1986).

Attachment Phase 3

Maintenance of Proximity to a Discriminated Figure by Means of Locomotion as Well as Signals (*the Phase of Clear-Cut Attachment*).

It is during this stage that Ainsworth proposes that attachment "proper" develops. During this phase, which is active from 6 months until the third birthday or into the third year, the child develops a full range of discriminatory and attached behaviors, including apprehension of strangers and separation (from caregiver) behaviors and the child's behavior begins to show organization and self-correction around desired goals. During this phase, again consistent with Mahler's third phase, beginning with the child's increasing capacity for ambulation, and hence self-directed physical movement, the child is active in seeking and maintaining proximity with its caregiver (attachment figure), while also physically moving away from the parent and therefore engaging in exploring the newly extended environment. The development of the secure base (or "home base," in Mahler's terms) occurs during this phase, sometime after the eighth month.

Mahler breaks this phase, which she calls separation–individuation, into four subphases and therefore offers more specificity than Bowlby or Ainsworth. Nevertheless, Mahler's Phase 3 also lasts from approximately 5 months to 3 years. She considers the developmental tasks of the child during this time to be largely those of individuation, which she nicely calls "hatching," consisting of: (i) differentiation of self from mother (*differentiation* subphase, 5–10 months); (ii) experiencing and practicing autonomy (*practicing* subphase, 10–16 months), (iii) the child's increasing awareness of and concern about separation from the mother, and need to both maintain individuality *and* decrease the sense of separation (*rapprochement* subphase, 16–24 months); and (iv) the development of a sense of selfhood and a stable, internalized representation of the caregiver, allowing for both a sense of individuality and connection (*consolidation of individuality and object constancy* subphase, 24–36 months). Although not an attachment theorist, Mahler's concepts actually exemplify the essence of Bowlby's secure attachment: security of self and other, and both individuation and social attunement.

Attachment Phase 4

Formation of a Goal-corrected Partnership (*The Phase of a Goal-corrected Partnership*).

Like Mahler, Bowlby postulates that the child has achieved a sense of object constancy by age 3 but is not yet able to understand its mother's motivations, thoughts, and feelings. Where Mahler's model of connection and separation ends at approximately age 3, Bowlby describes a fourth phase in the development of attachment, beginning sometime after the child's third birthday, developing through till about age 4 when attachment formation is more-or-less complete. In this phase, the child begins to demonstrate a more mature attachment and less egocentrism, is better able to infer the mother's internal experiences (thoughts, feelings, and motivations), and is hence able to establish goals that will both respond to mother and influence her behavior. Bowlby refers to this as a goal-corrected partnership, implying a more intentional and organized, but less egocentric, set of goals, built and carried out in collaboration with the caregiver. By this point, Bowlby postulates that the child's mental map, or internal working model which contains the template for experiencing and understanding self and others, is becoming increasingly more complex and capable. As the child comes to observe and understand the mother's behavior and her motivations, "from that point onwards his picture of the world becomes far more sophisticated and his behavior is potentially more flexible" (1969, p. 267).

Although Ainsworth speculates that attachment proper develops only during Phase 3, Bowlby writes "it is of course entirely arbitrary to say by what phase a child can be said to have become attached. Plainly he is not attached in Phase 1, whereas equally plainly he is so in Phase 3. Whether and to what extent a child can be said to be attached during Phase 2 is a matter of how we define attachment" (1969, p. 268). To this degree, then, the development of attachment, and the internalized sense of security it brings, most clearly occurs and is cemented between 5 months of age and the third birthday, although the ground work is laid from birth onwards.

Attachment, the Emergence of Self, and Social Connection

Stern (1985/2000) presents a conceptually different way to understand the development of both attachment and selfhood. He considers that infants are predisposed to engagement with others, as part of an emergent sense of self, and already have an innate sense of self/other at birth. Rather than the creation of *individuation*, each successive developmental stage is designed to further *connect* with, and not separate from, others. In expressing the view that "the infant's major developmental task is the opposite one, the creation of ties with others—that is, increasing relatedness" (2000, p. xiii), Stern asserts that this perspective minimizes or eliminates the need to conceptualize phases such as Mahler's normal autism and symbiosis. Further, rather than describing each successive stage of development as replacing or subsuming the preceding stage, Stern considers that the emergence of new stages has a more holistic quality, and all developmental domains remain interactive with one another in a dynamic model of human development and interaction.

In Stern's view, internalized objects are neither representations of people nor parts or aspects of others. Instead, he describes object representations as constructions of patterned (repeated) experiences of the interaction of self with others: "what is inside (i.e., represented internally) comprises interactive experiences" (2000, p. xv). Although in 1985 describing the sense of an emergent self, the sense of a core self, and the sense of a subjective/intersubjective self as the first three pre-verbal senses of selfhood, in 2000 Stern writes that he now considers each emerging together, as individual subcategories of a subsuming non-verbal sense of self. Stern (1985/2000) describes five essential phases in the *emergence*, and not the *development*, of selfhood, as he considers the aspect of selfhood to be present at birth. In this emergence, he defines two overarching senses of self: the *pre-verbal* self, emerging from birth to approximately 15 months (which by 2000, Stern was calling the non-verbal self), and the *verbal* self emerging in the normative child between 15 and 36 months. He breaks the pre-verbal/non-verbal self into three individual phases of emergence. The *emergent self*, active until about 8 weeks of age, is the natural and predisposed enactment of self-organizing and environment-orienting experiences. This process contributes to and continues through the second phase, or the emergence of the *core self*, from 8 weeks to 6 months—a period during which, outside of conscious awareness, infants experience a rudimentary sense of agency, coherence, continuity, and affectivity (experienced emotionality).

Although Stern's first two phases of selfhood are coincident with Mahler's phases of normal autism and normal symbiosis, he nevertheless disagrees with Mahler's psychoanalytic drive-oriented perspective and her characterization of the infant as first oblivious and then fused with the mother, both of which lead to Mahler's separation phase. Nor does he agree with Mahler's hypothesis that the third phase is primarily about individuation. Stern considers that infants are "predesigned to be selectively responsive to external social events and never experience an autistic-like phase" (1985/2000, p. 10), and that "there is no symbiotic-like phase. In fact, the subjective experiences of union with another can occur only after a sense of core self and a core other exists" (p. 10). In Stern's conceptualization of the core self, he describes an earlier subphase of "self versus others" (2–6/7 months) as a distinct state of separateness and continued self-organization. This is followed by and overlaps with a "subphase of self with others" (6/7–9 months) in which attachment is more clearly formed and internalized, establishing a sense of union with other, leading into and overlapping with his third phase of developing self.

Stern's third phase in the emergence of the pre-verbal/non-verbal self is that of the *subjective self*, from between 7 months and 15 months, again overlapping with, subsuming, and building upon "self with others," during which infants discover "that there are other minds out there as well as their own" (1985/2000, p. 27). Intersubjective experiences lead to the strengthening of attachment and social connection, and while Stern acknowledges that this remains a period for exploration, autonomy and individuation, he asserts that it is equally devoted to the establishment of intersubjective relationships with others, and hence has as a focal point the establishment of attachment or social connection and union (rather than separation and distinctness).

In the fourth phase of development, starting around 15 months, Stern describes the emergence of the *verbal self*, with the developing capacity to use and understand signs and symbols, and of course language, all of which give rise to conscious thought and self-awareness in a way that was not possible in earlier stages of development, and the increasing capacity for objectivity as well as subjectivity. Finally, by 2000 Stern identifies a fifth stage, developing sometime after the third birthday, implying a further development of both language and a resulting deepening sense of self-history, or continuity, that Stern refers to as the *narrative self*. Rather than just a sense of self derived solely from individual experience, Stern regards the narrative self as a co-construction of individual experience and the shared relationship with caregivers and family members, and as such influenced by experiences of attachment and the self-regulatory and self-correcting capacities endowed by the attachment experience.

Self and Proto-self

Stern's concepts are similar to those of Antonio Damasio (1999, 2003) who asserts that "consciousness is not a monolith" (1999, p. 16). He writes that consciousness not only develops from a rudimentary to a more sophisticated form, but that several levels of consciousness continue to coexist at the same time throughout life. That is, although early *core consciousness* develops in the infant and provides the groundwork upon which *extended consciousness*—"of which there are many levels and grades" (p. 16)—later develops, both forms of consciousness continue to operate once established. Core consciousness is the workhorse of daily self-awareness and cognitive operations, focused on the operations of a single moment, or the here and now, with a single level of organization. It serves as the backbone of daily cognitive operations that involve working memory, planning, problem solving and creativity, and its structure and role remains relatively unchanged across the lifetime of the individual. Out of core consciousness emerges a *core self*, or a constantly re-created sense of self that provides a sense of continuity and selfhood from event to event. Extended consciousness, however, operates at several levels of organization, focusing on and evolving across the lifetime of the individual, leading to a more elaborate sense of self. From extended consciousness comes the self-awareness and narrative self described by Stern, or the *autobiographical self* in Damasio's terms.

The emergent self that Stern describes is conceptualized by Damasio as the *proto-self*. Where Damasio proposes that the autobiographical self results from extended consciousness and that the core self is the product of core consciousness, he describes the proto-self as a preconscious biological precursor, "a coherent collection of neural patterns which map, moment by moment, the state of the physical structure of the organism in its many dimensions" (p. 54). He describes the proto-self as existing outside of, and indeed prior to the development of, self-awareness, without power of perception and holding no knowledge. It is from the proto-self that (core) consciousness emerges. Consciousness occurs, he writes, when the brain not only constructs a mental representation, but "internally construct(s) and internally exhibit(s) a specific kind of wordless knowledge," recognizing and understanding that it has been changed by an external event or object and recognizing the event or object itself (pp. 168–169). As well as describing Stern's emergent self, Damasio is describing internal representation as the point of departure for emerging consciousness, and recognizing a relationship between self and object as a distinguishing feature in the development of selfhood, hallmarks of object relations theory.

Emergence and Attachment Theory

Summarizing and embodying his stages in the "developmental progression of the sense of self," Stern (1985/2000, pp. 26–34) describes quantum leaps in the organization of subjective perspectives. These accumulate and continue to operate throughout life (rather than being submerged in or lost to later developing domains), each of which "remains forever as distinct forms of experiencing social life and self" (p. 32).

1. Domain of emergent relatedness. 0–2 months.
2. Domain of core relatedness. 2–6 months.
3. Domain of intersubjective relatedness. 7–8 months.
4. Domain of verbal relatedness. 15–18 months.

Although clearly disagreeing with Mahler's interpretations of the meaning underlying early human development (despite describing similarities in the chronological sequence and content of behaviors in infants and young children), Stern supposes and supports an attachment perspective. His only strong caveat, however, is that "while attachment is of enormous importance as an index of the quality of the parent/child relationship, it is not, however, synonymous with the entire relationship. There are many other self-experiences regulated by others that fall outside the proper boundaries of attachment" (1985/2000, p. 103).

In fact, Stern's model of an increasing and accumulative and holistic experience of both selfhood and social connection fits closely with Bowlby's conceptualization of the ontogeny of attachment (basically, development from egg to adult), largely summed up by three principles (Bowlby, 1969, p. 268):

1. A tendency for the range of effective stimuli to become restricted. Over time, the things that affect the individual will become increasingly more selective and narrower in content, and even self-selective, tending to shape the individual along a particular attachment pathway (homeorhesis). *Once embarked on a course, and the longer we remain on that course, it becomes increasingly difficult to dislodge us.*
2. A tendency for primitive behavioral systems to become elaborated and superseded by more sophisticated ones. Experience shapes innate behavioral systems, defining and refining them, sharpening and increasing their attunement with their environment. *Experience shapes who we become and how we behave.*
3. A tendency for behavioral systems to start by being non-functional and later to become integrated into functional wholes. Behavioral systems are subsumed into larger and more holistic behavioral systems and internal working models that focus and direct cognition, emotion, and behavior (and relationships). *Our behaviors and attitudes, and*

the dispositional representations and mental models that drive them, become more consolidated, consistent, and functional over time.

THE DEVELOPMENT OF ATTACHMENT AND COGNITIVE CAPACITY

In its application to human psychology, attachment theory, like all developmental theories, presumes the development of self-awareness (consciousness), which in turn presumes the development of increasing cognitive complexity and capacity in the child. That is, it is not possible to conceive of higher orders of intentionality in people, organized strategies to achieve proximity and establish security (i.e., patterns and goals of attachment behavior), or internal working models and mental schemata without recognizing the necessity of the accompanying and required level of cognitive sophistication.

In order to represent and manipulate the world psychologically, the child must be capable of decision making and problem solving *without* resorting to action. That is, in order to use abstract and non-physical symbols, internal representations, and mental processes to accomplish goals through behavior, the individual must be able to recall, understand, and recapitulate past experiences, at the same time as imagining and anticipating the future, including desired and possible outcomes, while considering present circumstances and their likely effect upon the future. These abilities are programmed at birth, but unfold and develop only over time, affected, of course, by the capacity of the individual, but also interactions with the environment. As Bowlby (1980) has written, referring to Piaget, the child is not capable of recalling and using in any complex manner an internalized model of the world before about 18 months of age. In fact, it is almost impossible to discuss any principles of or stages of cognitive development without referring to Piaget, and his seminal work.

PIAGET'S STAGE OF COGNITIVE DEVELOPMENT

Piaget described four stages of cognitive development, taking the child from birth through early–mid-adolescence. In normative development, cognitive capacity evolves from a set of reflexes present at birth in which there is no awareness of internal (self) or external (objects) to a capacity, by mid-adolescence, for abstraction, hypothesis, perspective taking, and decisions informed by an awareness and understanding of the world and its relationships. This unfolding of cognitive capacity is not the result of experience per se, but the product of the developing brain and its neural processes. Nevertheless, central to his ideas Piaget recognized that neural processes unfold into and are completely influenced by the environment. He was not only interested in the effects of the learning environment on the naturally occurring neural processes by which cognitive capacity chronologically unfolds, but recognized that it is impossible to understand cognitive development within each individual without also understanding the mutual interactions of the environment and neural processes.

The adaptation process by which individuals seek equilibrium (or homeostasis) is triggered by states of disequilibrium as new events are experienced by the child, and comprises the twin processes of assimilation and accommodation. As new information is experienced and *assimilated* and incorporated into the child's existing schema, or internal working model, that schema is altered in order to *accommodate* the new information or experience. Thus, the child adapts to the external objective world, and thus returns to a state of equilibrium, through a change and growth in internal subjective mental structures. Cognitive development, then, is very much as Ainsworth et al. (1978, p. 4) described attachment theory: both "programmed" and "open ended," reflecting nature and nurture, or the interaction between genetics and the learning environment.

Piaget (1937/1954; Piaget & Inhelder, 1969) describes four stages in cognitive development, much accepted today. The *sensorimotor* stage lasts from birth to approximately 2 years of age, and covers much of the same period described by Bowlby, Mahler, and Stern (and other developmental psychologists). During this stage, the young child passes from a state of complete undifferentiation, reflexivity, and lack of any form of self-awareness or awareness of others/objects to a recognition and sense of object permanence and rudimentary sense of self, basic competence in developing plans and manipulating the environment to get needs and desires met, and capacity to recognize and use symbols and language. Major changes occur during Piaget's second *pre-operational* stage, lasting from approximately 2 to 7 years of age. Language develops fully during this period, and the child builds on the internal schema (comprising mental representations) that allows a more sophisticated and detailed awareness of self, others, interactions, and social rules, thus allowing consciousness and intentional planning. In attachment terms, during the early part of this stage, the child engages in goal-corrected behaviors.

During the *concrete operational* stage, lasting from approximately ages 7 to 11, the child begins to understand rudimentary abstract concepts, and is thus better able to plan behavior, manipulate the world, and reflect on outcome. Piaget defined the final stage as that of *formal operations*, coming on-line at about age 11 or 12, or around the onset of puberty. From that time on, with the possibility of increasing sophistication, the adolescent is capable of increased abstraction, perspective taking, hypothesis formation, consideration of future-oriented events and possibilities, and the development of ideologies. Although the brain, particularly at the synaptic level, continues to undergo change and development and remains relatively "plastic" (new synaptic connections, and thus new neural pathways, continue to form), nevertheless from mid-adolescence onward the neural and operational capacity of the brain resembles that of the adult, with experience making the difference rather than the further unfolding and emergence of new neural processes and capacities.

Cognitive Development in the Early Stages of Attachment

Piaget thus describes the cognitive development required for the transformation of the attachment of infancy and early childhood into the attachment experience of the older child, adolescent, and adult. He also defined substages of the sensorimotor stage, between birth and age 2 years, or the cognitive stage during which many of the elements inherent in the development of attachment and selfhood develop. Piaget subdivided this stage into the six stages of infancy, leading to the capacity for object permanence, internal representation, symbol recognition, and social interaction, and hence the capacity to intentionally act upon and manipulate the social environment (rather than just being influenced by it).

Beginning with the basic reflexes of Stage 1, by stage 4 (8–12 months) the infant displays more complete acts of intentionality and goal-directed behavior and understanding of cause and effect, and object permanence and other complex cognitive ideas begin to form and coalesce. Piaget writes that during the course of Stages 5 and 6 (12–18 months), the appearance of object permanence and object relations marks the "double formation of a self differentiated from other people and other people becoming objects of affectivity" (Piaget & Inhelder, 1969, pp. 25–26)—meaning that the child is becoming "decentered," or less egocentric, and is able to experience and show authentic affection for others in a less narcissistic/egocentric personal world. By 1 year of age, the infant engages in variations of behaviors that have feedback loops that bring about new and unexpected outcomes, and thus contribute further to both learning and a sense of physical and social mastery. The child is no longer restricted to applying only already established schemata, but can both assimilate and accommodate new ideas and thus alter and further develop the internal working model (schema). This is a forerunner to the more advanced exploration behaviors that are possible only when ambulation (crawling and walking) occurs, as exploration is a prime focus in this development stage. Recall in attachment theory that exploration will not occur in the absence of an experienced sense of security, and also that by this age (12 months) attachment patterns are evident.

From Piaget's stages of development much else can be inferred and elaborated, including the ability to assume different perspectives, the development of moral decision making and behavior, the development of the roots of and capacity for empathy, and, by direct extension, the development of social behaviors and interactions. These areas are, of course, of enormous importance to any discussion of intentional and antisocial behavior in children, adolescents, and adults, including the perpetration of sexually abusive behavior.

The Cognitive Framework for Attachment and Selfhood

Piaget's conceptualization recognizes more than just the development and sequencing of cognitive processes, and the increasingly cumulative, amplifying, and holistic manner in which human cognition develops. It also provides a framework for understanding how these processes unfold into and are influenced by and shape the environment, thus providing a means to experience a sense of selfhood and others. This framework allows other developmental theorists to conceptualize processes of identity and belonging, with cognitive processes serving as the driving engine that makes selfhood possible. In this case, "selfhood" is always contingent upon underlying and parallel developing cognitive processes. At its root, attachment theory is *not* contingent upon cognitive processes, as long as it remains at the primitive and rudimentary biological (animal) level, or the level of Damasio's proto-self. But the moment it takes on psychological development, it too requires a cognitive framework. One might say, however, that in humans, cognitive development cannot help *but* give rise to selfhood and attachment.

ATTACHMENT AND SELFHOOD

By the first year, attachment has developed and is evident, readily observed and measurable by social scientists, as in Ainsworth's strange situation. By age 3, and certainly by age 5, attachment has more clearly formed and been established in patterns that are considered by most attachment theorists to be stable and enduring over time, and into adulthood.

Figure 3.1 compares Bowlby (and Ainsworth), Mahler, and Stern's depictions of the stages of early development, individuation, and attachment/social connection, and also includes a broad overview of Piaget's stages of infant development during the sensorimotor stage of cognitive development. In this depiction of Piaget's early stages there is a focus on the development of object permanence, or the capacity to form and manipulate internalized representations of the external world, and thus be said to have formed a differentiated sense of self as separate from other people and things.

Despite different conceptualizations in each model of the internal processes behind developmental stages, even more striking is the similarity in both general content and time frame, as well as developmental sequence.

Clear from each description of early development, the establishment of attachment and the development of a sense of self not only appear to be complementary to one another, but, more to the point, appear facets of the same essential aspect of human development. That is, attachment (or awareness of and social connection to others) and selfhood (or awareness and experience of self as distinct) mirror one another, and each is found in the other. Attachment is not possible without a pre-existing sense of, or potential for, selfhood on which to hang the experience of attachment and social connection, nor is a sense of self possible without the framework of the other. "Me" or "I" cannot exist without a sense of "you" or "them." The development and experience of individuation that leads to a sense of self, also leads to the connection and attachment of self to others.

The likelihood that attachment and selfhood are interwoven, or even aspects of the same thing, makes it clear that, regardless of which came first, attachment has powerful implications for understanding the development of personal identity, the formation of personality, the manner in which others are experienced, the foundations of social connections and relationships, the development of ideas and attitudes, the creation of behavioral strategies, and finally the enactment of actual behavior. However, whether attachment and selfhood do *not* exist prior to their development in sequential stages or whether they can be said to *already* exist at birth and simply emerge over time, both are nevertheless the inevitable result of human development, almost immediately from birth. It is not a matter of *whether* an individual will attach or develop a sense of self but rather, for each individual, *what* the experience and quality of attachment and selfhood will be and *how* those experiences will play out in the child, and into adolescence and adulthood. The essential difference between attachment theory and the theories of other development theorists is its postulate that attachment, as an evolutionarily designed and biological process, precedes all else and is the subject of primary interest, having fundamental influence over the path along which all other human development follows.

Piaget and Inhelder's (1969, pp. 154–159) description of human development through the development of cognitive structures, describes the essential ideas of not only attachment theory, but of contemporary object relations theory and theories of ego and

Bowlby/Ainsworth Attachment	Mahler Symbiosis/Individuation	Stern Emergent/Narrative Self	Piaget Cognitive Development
Phase 1: 0–8 (12) weeks. Pre-attachment.	Phase 1: 0–4 weeks. Autism.	Phase 1: 0–8 weeks. Pre-verbal/Non-verbal Self. Emergent self. Domain: Emergent relatedness.	Sensorimotor stage: 0–24 months. Substage 1: 0–1 month Basic reflexes. Stage of reflexes. Substage 2: 2–4 months. Primary circular reactions. Stage of first habits.
Phase 2: 8 weeks–6 months. Attachment-in-the-making.	Phase 2: 4 weeks–5 months. Symbiosis.	Phase 2: 8 weeks–6 months. Pre-verbal/Non-verbal self. Core self. Domain: Core relatedness.	Sensorimotor stage: 0–24 months. Substage 3: 5–7 months. Secondary circular reaction. Discovering procedures.
Phase 3: 6–36 months. Clear-cut attachment.	Phase 3: 5–36 months. Separation-Individuation. Subphase 1: Differentiation. 5–10 months.	Phase 3: 7–15 months. Pre-verbal/Non-verbal self. Subjective self. Domain: Intersubjective relatedness.	Sensorimotor stage: 0–24 months. Substage 4: 8–11 months. Coordinating secondary circular reactions. Intentional behaviors, recognition of object permanence.
Phase 4: 36–48 months. Goal-corrected partnership.	Subphase 2: Practicing. 10–15 months. Subphase 3: Rapprochement. 16–24 months. Subphase 4: Object Constancy 24–36 months.	Phase 4: 15–36 months. Verbal self. Domain: Verbal relatedness.	Sensorimotor stage: 0–24 months. Substage 5: 12–18 months. Tertiary circular reactions. Novelty and exploration. Further permanency of objects.
		Phase 5: 36 months. Narrative self.	Sensorimotor stage: 0–24 months. Substage 6: 18 months. Invention of new means through mental combinations. Mental representation .

Figure 3.1 A comparison of developmental models: Bowlby, Mahler, Stern, and Piaget

self-psychology in general. They describe four general factors responsible for the process of human mental development, with the fourth serving as the essential ingredient that consolidates the first three.

1. *Physical development.* Biological processes, and especially the maturation of the central nervous system and endocrine systems (responsible for hormone transmission).
2. *Physical and cognitive experience.* The acquisition of experience through the engagement and re-engagement in actions performed upon objects (involving physical behaviors and cognitive appraisals about the consequences of those actions, rather than experiences in social situations and relationships).
3. *Social learning and interaction.* The process of social interaction and transmission which, although essential, is insufficient by itself. They write that socialization is a process of "structuration" in which the individual contributes to, as much as receives from, the socialization process, and is therefore both a product and shaper of the process. In describing structuration, Giddens (1984) writes that social life neither comprises individual acts nor is determined solely by social forces, but that self-agency and social structure are in a mutual relationship, in which structure is produced by, reflects, and shapes individual behavior. Piaget and Inhelder comment, then, on the interdependence and similarity of the words "operation" and "cooperation."
4. *Equilibration and self-regulation.* Piaget and Inhelder write that the first three factors alone cannot explain human development, and that any explanation of child development must combine into a whole ontogenetic dimension (natural physical development) and a social dimension. Thus, the fourth factor is both assimilative and accommodating, a self-regulatory capacity that adapts to and mediates the pressure of and relationship between biological development and social shaping, seeking and constantly responding to disequilibrium (change) and promoting growth and stability (equilibrium).

Recognizing that the child is both the recipient and instrument of change, and hence is neither passive nor in control, Piaget and Inhelder (1969) write that an internal mechanism is required to maintain balance "in the search for a coherence and an organization of values that will prevent internal conflicts" (pp. 158–159), naming this mechanism as self-regulation: "it is impossible to interpret the development of affective life and of motivations without stressing the all-important role of self-regulation." This process of self-regulation, "both retroactive and anticipatory" (p. 157), is a key process much described by attachment theorists and is perhaps ultimately responsible for the balance between interacting and mutually interdependent biological and social forces. This returns us, then, to where we began the previous chapter, with Schore's (1999) observation that attachment is fundamentally a theory of self-regulation—an idea that may have special relevance when we consider antisocial and sexually abusive behaviors.

THE NATURE OF ATTACHMENT: MULTIPLE MODELS

The idea that attachment is just about regulation, and that attachment theory is simply a theory of self-regulation and how that capacity is acquired, represents just one aspect of attachment theory, and limits a more complete understanding of its processes and effects, and the implications of attachment to human behavior. Lyons-Ruth, Melnick, Bronfen, Sherry, and Llanas (2004), for instance, describe attachment as "the psychological version of the immune system . . . the pre-adapted behavioral system for combating and reducing stress" and attachment theory as "a two-person theory of conflict and defense" (p. 67), an analog adopted also by Jeremy Holmes (2001) who describes attachment as the "psychological immune system." Johnson (2003) adopts a similar view, describing attachment theory as "essentially a theory of trauma" (p. 9), or a model in which human development and personal identity are based on a balance of secure versus insecure, or trauma-producing childhood experiences balanced against the capacity of the individual to accommodate and adjust to trauma. To this end, describing hypothetical outcomes of a non-optimal attachment process, Sroufe, Carlson, Levy, and Egeland (1999) define attachment theory as a theory of psychopathology, as well as a theory of normal development. Here, we might suggest that one element of attachment balances *vulnerability* created or fostered by the developmental process against *resiliency* produced by that same process.

Alternatively, Weinfeld, Sroufe, Egeland, and Carlson (1999) write that "attachment theory is concerned with social behavior and emerging expectations of self, others, and relationships" (p. 84). On a similar note, Moretti and Holland (2003) describe attachment theory as an extension of self-discrepancy theory, organized along the two dimensions of *self-representation* and *standards of self* that children and adolescents assume are the standards of the larger society. They argue that self-image, motivation, behavior, and patterns of attachment are derived from discrepancies between the way individuals see themselves and the way they believe significant others see them, or discrepancies between self-image and perceived social standards for selfhood. Moretti and Holland write that self-regulation (developed through the attachment experience) is derived from congruency or discrepancy between who children would *like* to be and who they think they *actually* are (or how others perceive them, thus connecting discrepancy theory to attachment theory). This is a similar model to Bartholomew's two-dimensional model of representations of self and other (Bartholomew & Horowitz, 1991; Griffin & Bartholomew, 1994), in which attachment status results from complex interactions between dimensions (shown in Figure 7.3, Chapter 7). Weinfeld and colleagues, Moretti and Holland, and Bartholomew all describe attachment theory as a social perception theory, with attachment status resulting from internalized representations and experiences of self and others.

Crittenden's dynamic-maturational model (Crittenden, 2000a; Crittenden, 2001; Crittenden & Claussen, 2000) is also a dimensional theory. She describes attachment status resulting from interactions between the two dimensions of *affectively* driven behavior on the one hand, and *cognitively* driven behavior on the other. Whereas both of these dimensions coexist in a dynamic interaction at any given point in time, Crittenden also describes their interaction within a chronological third dimension, as the individual matures and changes over time. Although Fraley and Spieker (2003) describe Crittenden's model as two dimensional, it is really three dimensional, with attachment patterns, behavior, and communication resulting from a balance between affect, cognition, and chronological development. Thus, Crittenden's model is a theory of dynamic interaction between emotion and cognition as they develop over time, and the interaction between developing emotional and cognitive complexity, biological and social development, and experience over time. It is accordingly a theory of human development in the social environment.

Bowlby's work, of course, remains at the heart of attachment theory, and is a true *psychosociobiological* model in which he describes developing attachment as a process of interaction between biology, the quality of the child-rearing environment, and the developing capacity for mental representation. In this model which emphasizes the interaction between and synthesis emerging from biological, social, and psychological forces, attachment theory describes: (a) the primary status and biological function of intimate emotional bonds between individuals, controlled by processes within the central nervous system that build and rely upon internalized representations of self and other, and (b) the critical influence of the behaviors of caregivers on the development of the child (Bowlby, 1988, p. 120). As described by Shonkoff and Phillips (2000), "human development is shaped by a dynamic and continuous interaction between biology and experience" (p. 3).

SYNTHESIZING ATTACHMENT: THE INDIVIDUAL IN THE ENVIRONMENT

These ideas deserve a final look and synthesis, recognizing that attachment theory is a complex means to describe not only the condition of being attached, but the process that stimulates and by which we seek and maintain attachment and develop a sense of selfhood, and which ultimately may help to understand and explain behavior. Here, by attachment, we refer to both the process that activates the search for attachment (including the urge to seek attachment and the attachment behavioral system itself) and the experience of being attached, or the sense of social connection to important others.

1. Attachment is first biological in origin, initiated by primordial triggers that do not require any consciousness, self-efficacy, or intentionality. Attachment behaviors are activated and deactivated by internal and external conditions, actual or perceived.
2. Attachment behaviors are antithetical to exploratory behaviors but are required for the development of experienced security, which then deactivates attachment behaviors. On their own, attachment behaviors inhibit growth and independence. They are required, however, in order to signal security needs to caregivers, as well as to promote physical (and later psychological) well-being.
3. The fulfillment of attachment needs (and, hence, satisfaction of security needs), through the responsiveness and attunement of caregivers, not only deactivates the attachment behavioral system but also provides the base for an internalized and increasingly permanent sense of safety, hard wired into the central nervous system.
4. Attachment behaviors become less physical and instinctive during the course of early childhood development, and more cerebral and intentional, in concert with the developing cognitive structures and capabilities of the brain. Over time, attachment transforms with respect to needs and goals, and with the physical, mental, and emotional maturity of the individual.
5. Attachment experiences are internalized in the form of felt security and eventually in mental representations of self and others with respect to self-efficacy, self-agency, and self-confidence, and the ability to depend upon others. These experiences of self and

others can be assessed in order to infer a felt sense of security within the individual. Attachment, then, plays a central role in the development of, and may be a counterpart to, the sense and quality of selfhood.

6. Attachment transmits and imparts to the child the capacity for self-regulation through the responsiveness, attunement, and behavior of caregivers, and the experiences, results, and perceptions of attachment determine the quality and capabilities of the self-regulatory system. Some individuals fail to develop a sufficient capacity for self-regulation and continue to engage in insecurity-driven (or pathologically damaged) attachment behaviors, although such behaviors are inhibitory to or deactivate other behavioral systems required for emotional growth and the development of self-confidence.

This synthesis is illustrated in Figure 3.2, following attachment processes from the attachment behavioral system through to the development of self-regulation and resulting self-image, social relationships, and behaviors. Note, however, that although the model shows sequential elements, in reality the process, although developmental, is mostly not rigidly sequential but *interactionally* sequential, in that one element affects, leads to, and depends upon another.

Recognizing that attachment theory presents a coherent, cohesive, and comprehensive theory of human development, it is also able to help us to recognize developmental antecedents to, and perhaps even causes of, later pathology. Because attachment theory proposes a normative path of attachment, it also points to deviations from presumed optimal attachment processes, leading to both adaptation that leads to attachment subtypes and maladaptation that may be linked to the development of psychopathology. In describing attachment theory as a dynamic systems theory of psychopathology, Sroufe et al. (1999) describe social behaviors as patterns within and resulting from social relationships, rather than traits within the individual. Emphasizing the critical interplay between the individual, early experiences, and the ongoing social environment, they write that "early experience often plays a critical role in the developmental dynamic that yields pathology, but this role depends on a surrounding context of sustaining environmental supports" (p. 2). They also recognize and make clear that the early experiences of the child, and what the child thus brings to social interactions, may influence the nature of later experience and the surrounding context.

Sroufe et al. describe the prevailing perspective in attachment theory in which suboptimal attachment is neither viewed as, nor considered to be, a *direct* cause of psychopathology. Instead, attachment difficulties are considered to be significant factors in establishing a developmental pathway along which functional difficulties and psychopathology may later appear. As such, non-optimal attachment is considered to be a developmental vulnerability to later difficulty.

Attachment theory is not without significant problems, however, in some cases lacking clarity and presenting conceptual ambiguity. Indeed, Robert Karen (1994) has written that "attachment theory is by no means without flaws, holes, and huge unanswered questions" (p. 437). Despite noting that attachment theory holds great promise in trauma work, Rebecca Bolen (2000) describes only partial and limited empirical support for attachment theory, writing that the theory is equivocal with many problems in construction, consistency, and empirical proof. Nevertheless, despite its flaws, attachment theory is about

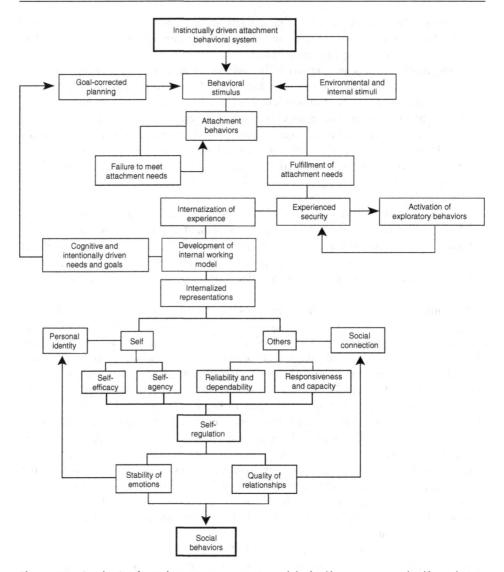

Figure 3.2   Synthesis of attachment processes: A model of self-awareness and self-regulation

nature and nurture, rather than one or the other—the inherited life and the experienced life, and the interactions between them, unified on the neural level, where mind meets matter. Where Chapter 2 began by recognizing and naming the roots of attachment as biologically and evolutionarily deterministic, this chapter ends by recognizing that the human experience of attachment is nevertheless very much determined by social forces at every level, and the constant interaction between environment and genetics.

CHAPTER 4

The Secure Self: Attachment, Self, and the Internalized World

Attachment theory is truly a biopsychosocial theory in that it embraces and integrates these three aspects of human development in understanding the functional psychology of individuals as they move through a world inhabited, driven, and defined by relationships, from the earliest precognitive development of the new born to the socially flooded life of the adolescent and adult.

However, Rutter (1997) notes that the process by which the relationship quality of attachment becomes transformed into an individual characteristic, presumably that of security, remains a "crucial unanswered question," noting that no satisfactory explanation has been found regarding how an early dyadic (attachment) relationship affects or shapes all later relationships. He writes that the "prevailing view at the moment, however, is that the process resides in some form of internalized representation or working model of relationships" (p. 23). Nevertheless, with respect to the view that the attachment process is internalized, Rutter describes the idea of an internal working model as too all encompassing to have much empirical value. Similarly, Dunn (1993) considers the internal working model, at the heart of attachment theory, extremely limited because "it is so vaguely conceived that it can be used to explain almost everything" (p. 105).

In fact, Lamb (1987) concludes that there is little that can be said with confidence about the effect of early attachment status, describing evidence of early attachment and later behavior and performance in the child as "weak and inconsistent" (p. 818). Although written almost two decades ago, Lamb's contention is as true now as it was then. He writes that attachment theorists tend to focus on the enduring, self-perpetuating, and *endogenous* processes that maintain earlier attachment patterns—that is, factors and established patterns within the child that maintain attachment status, rather than *exogenous* (environmental) factors. Nevertheless, in attachment theory this very point *is* considered central to the development of self and social connection, translating into the factor of personal security believed to result from attachment and embodied in the internal working model.

THE INTERNAL WORKING MODEL: REPRESENTATION, SELF, AND OTHER

The development of metacognition is a process also referred to as mentalization. The ability of individuals to reflect upon, understand, and make sense of their own mental experiences and the mental experiences of others is close to Schank's (1999) description of our capacity to "say what we know and know what we think" (p. 254). Metacognition—the ability to mentalize—translates into the capacity for reflective functioning, or self-reflection. In turn, the ability to be *self*-reflective influences the ability to reflect upon and understand the mind of *others*, resulting, in part, in a theory of mind, as described in Chapter 2. However, self-awareness and other-awareness are elemental counterparts in the larger experience of mentalization; although self-awareness contributes to the recognition of mental states in others, the capacity to recognize, reflect upon, and understand the mind of the other is key in developing a sense of self in the first place. In the infant, it is in the mind of the other (the mother) that the roots of self-awareness and selfhood are found, and in this regard awareness of "other" establishes the capacity for, and possibly the origins of, awareness of "self."

Johnson-Laird (1983) writes that human beings understand the world by constructing working models of it in their minds, following Craik (1952) who defined such a model as a small-scale model of external reality within the mind, by which the individual may mentally experiment with various alternatives, react to anticipated future situations, and use knowledge of past events to deal with the present and future. The experience of being with others, including mutual recognition and attunement, quality of interaction, and reciprocal understanding, is formed and stored in the internal working model, which serves as a mental representation upon which ideas about other and self are based. In attachment theory and other object relations theories, the internal working model contains mentalized representations of self and others, and is the basis for personality, self image, and behavior. It also serves as the filter calling up and through which different forms of memory are consciously recalled and reconstructed into a working model of the world,[1] which in turn act as the building blocks for varying levels and systems of schemata and operational scripts that underlie behaviors and interactions in familiar scenarios.

The internal working model is the basis for the grand schemata by which individuals understand themselves and others, as well as relationships between themselves and others. Whether cognizant of their internal working model or not, according to attachment theory (and object relations theory in general), all individuals have an internal working model, and in higher forms of self-awareness (and occasionally through therapy) individuals become aware of and have access to these internal maps. The internal working model begins in the precognitive infant, but is not static. It is a dynamic (hence, psychodynamic) phenomenon that grows and develops, and accumulates and evolves, throughout the life of the individual. The "working" part of the internal working model, suggests constant growth and change over time in internalized representations.

---

[1] As Allen (1995) has written, "no matter how accurately an event may be perceived and stored, when it is remembered, it is not replayed as in a video recorder; rather, it is *reconstructed*" (p. 101). This is similar to Damasio's (1994) perspective, in which dispositional representations are not the holders of pictures, but the means by which picturers are reconstituted.

THE ATTACHMENT RELATIONSHIP AND THE INTERNAL WORKING MODEL

In attachment theory, at the earliest of ages, in precognitive and even pre-emotional stages of development, through the process of being experienced, understood, and accurately responded to by the caregiver, we learn to recognize, understand, and regulate our own internal states. This represents an important prerequisite for further developing an understanding of others (in object relations theory, as objects that exist independently outside of ourselves, but can be incorporated into internalized representations that contribute to the development of selfhood).

Through the robust internalization of security, incorporated into the internal working model, we see the development of resilience, as well as self-modulation. Many writers have described the ability of the secure individual to experience discomfort and failure to get needs or desires met, but nevertheless remain able to deal with the difficulties of life and its demands, and the demands and requirements of relationships within it. The establishment of the secure internal working model also allows the development of mentalization, or theory of mind, and thus the capacity to experience and understand the mind of another, and join with that mind, in a rudimentary and perhaps basic form of empathy. Through this secure union of minds comes both social development and the acquisition of social norms, and hopefully prosocial and moral values. In this model, then, attachment provides the basis for all emotional and cognitive experiences of self and others. In its neurobiological counterpart, attachment is hard wired into the central nervous system, affecting the growth and trajectory of the brain.

The capacity of the attachment figure to accurately recognize and respond to the attachment signals of the child represents more than just the provision of reassurance. Over time it is the primary means by which the internal working model, incorporating sense of self and other, develops and is imprinted in neural circuits, or in the dispositional representations described by Damasio (1994).[2] This involves the process of biofeedback and incorporation, and provides the platform upon which all else develops, or can develop. In this conceptualization, it is both the product of and basis for the assimilation and accommodation process central to Piaget's ideas and observations about cognitive development and growth.

DYNAMIC MENTAL MAPS: MEMORY AND AWARENESS

It is impossible to define any model of internalization entirely as the *product* of something or entirely as the *source* of anything, because it is a mental and abstract embodiment of a constant working interaction with the environment. This interaction is neither *chronologically* static in time, nor *cognitively* static in terms of development. In the first instance, the mental map is not chronologically static in that it is not simply a product or reflection, stored in memory, of some past time or place, but is in constant engagement with the

---

[2] Crittenden (in press) prefers the term dispositional representations to internal working model, because it makes clear the "disposing to action" function of representation, in which neural and mental processing dispose us to behave and think in particular ways.

current environment, remaining connected in time through dynamic memory to past experiences and anticipated or possible future experiences. This characteristic is linked to
episodic memory and an awareness of that form of memory, named *autonoetic consciousness* by Tulving (1985). Episodic memory is the storehouse of actual experience that
can be consciously recalled, rather than semantic memory which is based on facts and
intellectualized recall, and is more complex than the lower form of procedural memory,
which simply stores actions and outcomes without conscious awareness.

Procedural memory is associated by Tulving (1985) with *anoetic* or non-knowing consciousness and is present at birth, or very soon after. On the other hand, the more cognitively sophisticated and later developing semantic memory signifies *noetic* awareness, or
consciousness that allows the individual to be aware of an internal and external world and
engage in introspection, but is more-or-less limited to facts and detail. However, *autonoetic* memory is associated with self-awareness, making it possible, according to Tulving
and colleagues (Wheeler, Stuss, & Tulving, 1997), for the individual to engage in mental
"time travel" and experience (and recall) self in past, present, and future, connecting these
three dimensions of time with a consistent and stable sense of self. "Autonoetic (self-
knowing) consciousness is a necessary correlate of episodic memory. It allows an individual to become aware of his or her own identity and existence in subjective time that
extends from the past through the present to the future" (Tulving, 1985, p. 388). One may
argue that it is precisely this facet of self-aware consciousness that makes possible Craik's
internal model of external reality—a model that incorporates the capacity to envision and
tie together past, present, and future.

MEMORY

Procedural memory is often referred to as *implicit* because it represent a preconscious
awareness, unavailable to conscious recall. For this reason, it is also considered *non-
declarative*. Semantic and episodic memory are both forms of *explicit* and *declarative*
memory because they are accessible to consciousness. Memories, then, are declarative,
semantic, and episodic and they're also non-declarative, procedural, and implicit. In
Tulving's terms, they are anoetic, noetic, and autonoetic. Figure 4.1 provides a simple synopsis and summary of these often interchangeable terms for describing levels or systems
of memory.

Memory system	Direct/ indirect expression	Spoken or non-spoken	Conscious experience	Emotional quality	Self-awareness	
					Capacity for	Level of
Procedural	Implicit	Non-declarative	Unconscious	None	Anoetic	Unaware
Semantic	Explicit	Declarative	Conscious	Flat	Noetic	Factual
Episodic	Explicit	Declarative	Conscious	Interwoven	Autonoetic	Autobiographical

Figure 4.1 Synopsis and summary of memory systems

Spoken or declarative memory, at the moment of becoming declarative, also speaks of the affect that is interwoven into the memory. However, whereas semantic memory is "flat" and more-or-less devoid of evoked emotion, episodic memory is more clearly tied to emotion, sometimes evoked by and sometimes evoking affect. Semantic memory is about nouns—people, places, and things that can be put into words. On the other hand, episodic memories are more like adjectives with their emotional coloring and recall of experiences that can be put into words, Together, semantic and episodic memory are the grammar of memory, the nouns and the adjectives together.

Mental Maps, Memory, and Awareness

The mental map, then, continues to grow and remain dynamic and interactive over time, not simply taking in and storing into memory more experience (Piaget's assimilation), but actively responding to that experience by interpreting possible meaning and changing in its own structural representations (accommodation) and acting back upon the environment to maintain an equilibrium between the internal and external worlds. The mental map both filters and interprets incoming experience and changes in the manner in which it can and does filter and interpret experience.

Just as mental maps are not chronologically static, they are also not *cognitively* static. That is, the system of internal representations continues to grow and become more sophisticated in parallel with the development and acquisition of increased cognitive skills. Over time, the internal model increasingly incorporates and uses cognitive tools that were simply not available at an earlier point in its efforts to understand and manipulate the world, and in ways possible only with the acquisition of higher levels of cognitive awareness. For instance, Bowlby's phase four goal-corrected behavior is only possible at the point where cognitive development allows such a capacity, some time after age 3. This is particularly relevant to the acquisition of different types of memory systems (procedural, semantic, and episodic) and their associated level of conscious awareness.

It is unlikely that episodic memory develops, or can develop, prior to age 2, and more likely age 3, and may not be fully operational until age 4 or later, accounting for the lack of conscious memory of experience prior to age 3 (Wheeler et al., 1997). This development is quite relevant in terms of mental maps because it reflects the interrelationship between: (i) the development of the mental map in terms of its capacity for content (depth, breadth), stability (self-regulation), and reflective function (metacognition), and (ii) developing/emerging forms of memory, related levels of consciousness, and eventually self-awareness and hence the arrival of the autonoetic consciousness of Tulving, the autobiographical self of Damasio, or the narrative self of Stern (Chapter 3).

Although the internal working model is developmental in its growth, it is nonetheless important to recognize that such development is, to a great degree, contingent on its biological origins. That is, the development of autonoetic and self-aware consciousness is able to develop when it does, at around age 3, because of the development of the orbitofrontal region of the frontal lobe that takes place at around that age. The orbitofrontal region is often considered to be the associational cortex of the brain, particularly in the right frontal lobe, as it is in contact with multiple significant regions of the brain, seemingly involved with higher executive functioning on every level. Remembering that

Bowlby considers attachment to be encoded in the central nervous system, the entire concept of mental maps is then considered to have a neurobiological base, with the internal working model embedded into the central nervous system, and perhaps the right orbitofrontal cortex. From this perspective, the internal working model is a neurobiological structure out of which further human cognitive sophistication and psychology emerge.

Internal models, then, or mental maps, are dynamic entities, not only considered to be the source of ideas about self and the world but also "working" models that interact with and change as a result of the environment in which they exist, in turn acting back on that environment through physical and mental activity.

THE NEURAL INTERNALIZATION OF THE EXTERNAL WORLD

Virtually every model that recognizes an internal, cognitive world recognizes the necessity and conjectures one version or another of a mental map, or internalized representations about the world, self-representations, cognitive schemata, or mental models. These models propose that the internal world is developed through interactions with the external world, and that the external world is absorbed and re-created in a neural form within the brain. In the biologically based attachment model, this is no different than the mental map of the bumblebee that allows the insect to consistently find its way between its hive and a flower garden, and further to communicate this map to other bumblebees who then absorb this map of the external world into their own internal maps, in effect passing it from bumblebee mind to bumblebee mind. Of course, one difference lies in the complexity and depth of the internal representations of the world built by human beings, the result of not only greater cognitive capacity but also the human capacity for self-awareness and consciousness. In humans, cognition and consciousness go hand-in-hand. In normal circumstances, we cannot help but be aware of ourselves. Schank (1999) describes this as "the explicit knowing of what we know or think. This is what is generally known as consciousness—that we can say what we know and know what we think" (p. 254).

A second difference is that our capacity for self-aware consciousness leads to the continued and more complex development of the internal map, upon which still further human cognition and psychology is built. In animals the mental map serves to ensure their survival, guide them through the world, and coordinate their actions and social behaviors. In humans the internal map serves the same essential functions, but is additionally capable of self-discovery. Thus, the biological map transcends itself to become a psychological process through which we engage in self-directed planning and behavior, self-reflection, self-appraisal of our successes and failures and, in turn, intentional self-correction (Bowlby's goal-corrected behavior). Through these conscious experiences develops a sense of self-agency and self-realization, from which self-image, self-esteem, and personal identity are in turn derived, all pertinent to any discussion of attachment and selfhood. In addition, the ability for self-realization and self-correction is, of course, the basis for both instruction and therapy, and hence an additional layer of intentional transformation.

The development of the biological mental map results from the interaction between the external physical world and the internal mental world, or the translation of external stimuli into neural patterns. This reflects an interactive neurobiology that is tuned and responsive to the external physical world, and in turn acts upon that external world through the physical activities of the individual. Beyond this, as discussed in Chapter 2, the neurobiology of the individual is attuned to the neurobiology of other individuals in that external world. However, in addition to caregiver–child dyadic relationships, it is also attuned to the neurobiology of other family members, the community, and society as a whole (if communities of people can be said to have neurobiologies), thus, in effect, producing social beings. In this respect, as a process that is both experience *expectant* and experience *dependent*, neurobiology is shaped by others and acts back upon others, tied to a larger social reality.

THE INTERNAL WORKING MODEL AS STOREHOUSE

Bruner (1966, p. 5) describes the internalization of events as a "storage system" that corresponds to the environment. This "stored model of the world" makes it possible for the child to extrapolate beyond bits of individual information, allowing predictions about the future and directing behavior. Bowlby (1980) tells us that such storage occurs, absorbed into internal models, as the result of learning experiences that begin during the first year of life and are repeated frequently (daily) throughout childhood.

Through this process of overlearning (the learning of something until it is performed without conscious awareness), cognitive and behavioral components embedded into the internal working model begin to operate automatically and outside of awareness, as do the rules for evaluating behavior, thoughts, and feelings, which also become overlearned during childhood. This represents the way in which early attachment experiences, overlearned as a result of repetition and woven into the mental map, play out in self image, experience and expectations of others, social relationships, and every other aspect of social life. Metacognition addresses this, as the individual is able to exercise self-reflective thought. Nevertheless, Bowlby is largely addressing preconscious thought here, as well as the wellspring from which cognitive distortions emerge, or the thinking errors typically described as characteristic of sexual offenders.

In addition to containing representations of relationships and social interactions, and templates for behaviors and their anticipated consequences, internal working models also contain *scripts*. Often themselves the result of overlearning or habituation,[3] scripts are mental structures encapsulating previously experienced sequences of events, along with expectations and plans for behavior in future similar circumstances (Schank & Abelson, 1977). The script triggers a predetermined sequence of actions on an automatic basis, operating preconsciously or without intentional thought. Script *rules* that activate scripts depend on ideas, or templates, also contained in the internal working model. Rules, in turn, are contained in *plans* that underlie and organize scripts, closely resembling the strategies described by attachment theory that organize attachment behavior, allowing us to recognize the behaviors as coherent. Of particular importance, Schank and Abelson write that scripts, rules, and plans are developed through episodic experience, with children as "active script constructors, beginning at a very young age" (p. 225). Hence, scripts

---

[3] Habituation involves a general accommodation to common environmental conditions, or becoming accustomed to something through experience so that there is a predictable response, eventually leading to an automatic and often decreased response to the stimulus.

are formed on the basis of early life experience, although modifiable and evolving over time.

Thompson (1999) describes internal representations as self-perpetuating and a source of continuity between early attachment and later functioning. He groups these into four interrelated representational systems, within which representations may change and become further elaborated over time. The internal model serves as the storehouse of these four representational systems, through which expectations about the world and its players are reflected and triggered.

1. *Anticipatory representations* about what may be expected of caregivers, beginning during the first year of life.
2. *Event representations* of attachment-related experiences stored in episodic memory beginning during the third year (although Schank & Abelson [1977, p. 225] report that episodic-derived scripts are available from age 2).
3. *Narrative representations* of self through autobiographical memory in which specific events are sequentially connected, continually built over time, and recalled as an uninterrupted personal narrative, beginning at age 4.
4. *Metacognitive representations* of others and their psychological characteristics, by which the behavior of attachment partners and the nature of relationships is inferred, developing between age 3 and 4.

Hofer (2000), too, writes that once the infant becomes capable of associative memory (memory retrieved by reference to its actual content, or its association to other memories of events or facts), they begin to function at a symbolic level, forming mental representations of caregivers and events based on experience. These interactive memories form the basis of Stern's (1985/2000) model in which "Representations of Interactions that have been Generalized" (RIGs) are described as the basic building blocks from which internal working models are constructed. Stern describes RIGs resulting from direct experience and eventually integrated into the core self, or a preconscious sense of selfhood. In effect, Stern is describing these RIGs as the "atoms" from which the mental map is constructed.

Finally, Bowlby (1973) describes *two* internal working models. The *organismic* model represents internal representations of self, including behavioral skills and capacities, whereas the *environmental* model provides a representation of the environment and the people and things in that external world. Schore (1999) writes that Bowlby is tying together psychology and biology, "describing a theoretical landscape that includes both the biological and social aspects of attachment, a terrain that must be defined in terms of its structural organization as well as its functional properties" (p. xix).

The Nature of Security

Embedded within the internal working model is a sense of security. Unlike Mahler's "working base," which represents a stage through which children eventually pass, the secure base of attachment theory is affixed *within* the mental map, serving to potentially reactivate attachment behaviors and needs at any point. It is from this secure base that a sense of *personal security* develops and is established as the enduring remnant of the early attachment experience, or the endogenous factor described by Michael Lamb (1987). In fact, probably the most important and most significant aspect of attachment theory is that, in terms of psychology, a secure attachment results in the development of a secure and confident personality from which the many fruits include the ability to feel confident, to tolerate and suffer emotional difficulties, to be perceived by others as confident, and to pursue and achieve goals.

Blatz (1966) proposed a security theory that influenced and shaped Ainsworth's thinking about security and the secure base, and she acknowledges that it may even have been Blatz who first used the term "secure base" (Ainsworth, 1988). Although her doctoral dissertation, on the assessment of security and insecurity in young adults, was based on Blatz's theory, Ainsworth and Blatz eventually only agreed on two sets of circumstances necessary for the experience of security in the individual: (1) confidence in the personal capacity to deal with any sufficiently familiar situation, or the presence of another factor or person to address the particular circumstances, and (2) confidence that whatever the consequences of personal behavior they can be adequately dealt with through self agency, or, due to another factor or person, there will be no unacceptable consequences as a result of personal behavior.

However, Blatz described security as the capacity to unequivocally accept the consequences of personal behaviors, without recourse to others, equating security with mental health. Interestingly, he separates "security," which he describes as a state of mind and personal identity, from "safety," which he describes as an attempt or need to escape from personal responsibility, writing that "safety is the antithesis of independent security" (p. 63). Congruent with attachment theory, he defines safety as the search for an agent, or someone outside of one's own self, to provide such safety. However, attachment theory asserts that an enduring sense of security *results* from a sense of enduring safety, and the secure attachment that follows, thus implicating relationship interdependence as essential to security. Blatz, instead, suggests that security is an internalized experience that allows individuals to accept complete responsibility for their own safety without recourse to others, thus implicating *in*dependence, and not *inter*dependence, as key.

Ainsworth (1988) writes that for Blatz the secure base is operational only during early childhood, and is not appropriate as the continuing sole basis of security. From his perspective, security is a purely personal responsibility in which the child comes to depend more and more on itself, until security becomes completely independent of any outside agents. Blatz refers to outside individuals who are needed as "deputy agents," considering dependence on them as a regression to an earlier condition of immature dependent security, or "pseudo-maturity." This is a major point of departure from the attachment theory conceptualization of security. The concept of the secure base, and therefore reliance (not necessarily "dependence") on others, is intrinsic to the idea of the internal working model, and therefore active throughout life. In attachment theory, interdependence is essential to important social relationships. Felt security is the *result* of a balance between social interdependence and independence, rather than a sense of security borne out of pure independence (in which, from Blatz's perspective, the use of others as a source of emotional safety is seen as regressive). Indeed, it is the idea that the secure base experience continues throughout the life span that allows attachment theorists to extend the ideas of childhood attachment into adolescence and adulthood.

Security and Secure Attachment

The very idea of felt security, then, is tied to secure attachment. One feels secure because one can depend on caregivers to recognize, understand, protect, and nurture, and "be there" when needed, and this experience of secure attachment, built into the internal working model, is transformed into felt security. One might say that security and secure attachment are the same thing, tying self (sense of security) to others (secure in capacity to rely on others). In this model, one cannot be secure without feeling securely attached, and vice versa.

In terms of social behaviors, Fonagy et al. (1997a) assert that the basis for moral social behavior is the capacity to recognize and understand (and, I suppose, care about) another person's perspective, and that only through secure attachment can the individual develop such skills, referred to by Fonagy as mentalizing. Fonagy (2001a) describes mentalization, also referred to as metacognition, as central to attachment theory, a reflective function that is innate in most individuals but nevertheless developed through the attachment relationship. He asserts that exploring the meaning behind the actions of others is crucially linked to the child's ability to label and find meaning in its own experience. He further asserts that the capacity to adequately mentalize evolves out of the attachment experience and the child's opportunity to observe and explore the mind of the caregiver, and that severe deprivation undermines the acquisition of mentalization. Fonagy et al. (2000) believe that secure attachment creates an environment for the acquisition of the metacognitive capacity "we believe underpins reflective self-function" (p. 269). This idea is mirrored by Bretherton and Munholland (1999) who write that secure attachment fosters self-reflection, which in turn enhances the ability for perspective taking and facilitates interactive feedback with others.

Attachment Security, Criminal Behavior, and Metacognition

Going further, Fonagy and his colleagues (1997a, 1997b) propose that crimes are committed by adolescents with inadequate mentalizing capacities, who engage in pathological attempts to adapt to a social environment in which mentalization is essential. They describe four ways in which a failure of mentalization (or, perhaps the capacity to form empathy or engage in empathic behaviors) can lead to disengagement of prosocial behavior.

1. Mentalization is intrinsically connected to self-awareness and the formation of personal identity. Therefore, those with limited reflective skills and a reduced ability to envision the mental states of others will also have a less well-established sense of their own identity. This reduces the capacity of individuals to recognize and be in touch with their own thoughts, and therefore accept responsibility for their subsequent behaviors. They "may more readily feel that they are not responsible for their actions because they genuinely lack a sense of agency" (p. 257).
2. Reduced capacity for mentalization may lead to a failure to anticipate or appreciate the consequences of personal behavior to the victims of such behaviors.
3. Reduced capacity for mentalization may contribute or lead to devaluing or dehumanizing potential or actual victims.

4. Limited metacognitive skills may lead to the easy deconstruction and reinterpretation of representational systems, including ideals and values, and thus allow antisocial behavior to be experienced in a self-serving manner by the perpetrator as appropriate and acceptable.

In this conceptualization, the failure of mentalizing not only limits the process of secure attachment, felt security, and the development of affiliative bonds (and may even be the result of a failure to achieve secure attachment), it actually offers the individual an alternative means by which to exercise control over the world and experience competency, and thus a sense of self-regulation, self-agency and self-efficacy. Furthermore, without the reflective functioning provided through mentalization, or metacognition, behavior becomes *reactive* rather than *reflective.*

It is of special note that Fonagy and colleagues (1997a) direct their perspective to adolescents, as it suggests, completely in line with our thinking about juvenile versus adult sexual offending, that adolescents are at a different point in their development, motivated by different things, and far less sophisticated, self-directed, aware, or set in their pattern of behaviors. Fonagy offers a clear method by which to understand how attachment deficits might contribute to a lack of metacognitive capacity which, in turn, limits the development of empathy, sets the stage for the construction of cognitive distortions, and provides an alternative means for achieving a sense of efficacy. Each of these, in different ways, may contribute significantly to engagement in any victim-based crime, including sexual abuse. This ties in with the work of sex offender theorists such as Marshall, Ward, Hudson, and Smallbone, discussed in Chapters 11 and 12, all of whom attempt to tie attachment deficits to sexually abusive behavior, although failing to do so fully or recognizing Fonagy's well-theorized link between attachment, metacognition, and criminality.

Although Fonagy presents a good argument, it not clear whether the key to metacognition is actually secure attachment. He asserts that the path to attachment security both leads to and stems from the capacity of the infant to find itself in the mind of its mother, and to gradually recognize and understand the mind of its mother and itself, hence developing a theory of mind. This is a purely theoretical stance, however, and can be neither proved nor disproved. It also does not mean that there are not other, equal or more powerful, means for developing metacognition, or that later life difficulties do not *obstruct* the natural development of theory of mind rather than earlier life experiences, such as attachment bonding, enhancing its development. After all, the very premise of attachment theory is that certain behavioral systems, presumably including the attachment signaling and communication systems, are innate and therefore require few or no learning opportunities in order to be demonstrated. From this perspective, metacognition unfolds as an innate ability, and does not require the learning opportunities provided through the attachment experience.

Nevertheless, Fonagy asserts that it is a *higher* order of metacognition that fails to develop as a result of insecure attachment (to which he refers as the "agentive mind"), although this premise remains questionable and unproven, albeit attractive. Support for his idea that metacognition is developed further through learning, despite being an innate capacity, is found in the work of Jerome Bruner. In describing the learning process and the development of cognitive skills, Bruner (1966) describes mental growth as a staircase with sharp risers, developing in spurts and rests, writing that growth is initiated only when certain capacities begin to develop. The idea of "readiness," Bruner writes, "is a mischievous half-truth" (p. 27) because we teach readiness or provide opportunities for its nurture rather than simply waiting for it to develop: "Knowing is a process, not a product" (p. 72).

ALTERNATIVES TO SECURITY AND MENTALIZATION

The failure to internalize attachment security is assumed by attachment theorists to set in motion pathways that lead to behavioral, relational, and other functional difficulties. However, there are, of course, alternatives to this idea. For instance, Fonagy's idea that adolescent antisocial behavior results from a lack of both security and metacognition, linked through the attachment experience, fails to recognize social theories that explain the same behavior. Hirschi (2002) describes two theories that explain antisocial or criminal behavior that have nothing to do with mental maps, internalized security, or a lack of mentalization, focusing instead on social stresses that contribute to criminal behavior. I choose to include these ideas here, not simply because they offer an example of alternative hypotheses but more specifically because they offer an alternative that remains tied to the concept of attachment, albeit from a different perspective.

Strain theory hypothesizes that behavioral or criminal deviance results from an inability to fulfill legitimate needs through conformity, whereas control theory focuses on the reasons why people do *not* commit crimes. This theory assumes that inhibitory or controlling factors are absent in those who commit crimes, and that delinquent acts result because an individual's bond to society is weak or broken. Both are models of anomic theory that follow from Durkheim's (1893/1997, 1897/1951) work, proposing that attachment to social values and norms provides the basis for prosocial behavior and engagement. Anomie (normlessness) results in a loosening of social attachment and personal meaning, leading to personal dysfunction and societal decay, including crime. Thus, these social control theories link *societal* level attachment (the individual's bond to society) to deviant and destructive behavior.

Hirschi notes that "since these theories (strain and control theory) embrace two highly complex concepts, the *bond* of the individual to *society*, it is not surprising that they have at one time or another formed the basis of explanations of most forms of aberrant or unusual behavior" (2002, p. 16), and "control theory assumes that the bond of affection for conventional persons is a major deterrent to crime" (2002, p. 83). Certainly, it is not too much of a stretch to apply these ideas to an understanding of the roots of sexually abusive behavior—that is, the acquisition of legitimate social goals (or goals that are perceived as legitimate) through deviant means by individuals who otherwise feel unable to achieve these goals, and particularly when social ties are weak.

Secure Attachment, the Agentive Mind, and Self-in-Society

Alternatives notwithstanding, it is Fonagy's (2004) contention that violent individuals experience deficits in theory of mind resulting from the inadequate integration of two "primitive" modes through which young children experience internal reality, described as *psychic equivalence* and *pretend mode*. In these states, the very young child assumes that it experiences the world as it actually is (psychic equivalence), and there is no separation between internal ideas and the actuality of the world. In *pretend mode*, the child is able to live and imaginatively interact in a totally internal (psychic) world, regardless of the real nature of the external world. Fonagy contends that the child is able to come to grips with and eventually integrate internal and external reality due to the experience of safe and secure attachment and the accompanying mediating influence of an attachment figure who, in those early days, serves as the regulator of internal and external experience. In this conceptualization, the attachment figure serves as a bridge between the psychic and external world of the infant. As disconnected internal realities yield to the reality of, and are integrated with, the external world the result is, in part, theory of mind, or the ability to know and reflect upon mind-of-self and mind-of-other. Presumably, without the experience of a secure base, this process of integration fails to develop adequately or is otherwise limited.

Further, Fonagy asserts that children acquire an understanding of five increasingly complex levels of self-agency, or a sense of self-direction and capacity for action.

1. *Physical agency* results as the child recognizes its capacity to physically manipulate the world, and that it is therefore an agent whose actions can affect and bring about change in the external world.
2. *Social agency* develops alongside physical agency as the child recognizes itself as having, not just the ability to physically affect the word, but also the capacity to communicate with others. As briefly described in Chapter 2, between 3 and 6 months the infant is able to intentionally use facial gestures, gaze, and vocalization to communicate with others, and recognize its capacity to do so (Yale et al., 2003). Fonagy describes this as "knowing that one's communicative displays can produce effects at a distance, in the social environment" (p. 17).
3. *Teleological agency* develops between 8 and 9 months, as behavior that is intentionally goal seeking and designed for purpose.
4. *Intentional agency*, as the further development of mentalization, develops after the child's first birthday and during the second year. Built on prior developing levels of agency, the child recognizes that it is able to act intentionally and can affect not just the behavior of other people but also their focus, and hence their minds. This serves as the precursor to the goal-corrected behavior that Bowlby reports comes on-line sometime after age 3.
5. *Representational agency* develops after age 3, at which point the child develops the ability to be aware of knowledge itself (or, knowledge of knowledge, just as we are able to think about thinking), and thus forms a sense of itself as capable of imagination and representation. By age 6, Fonagy asserts that the development of representational agency, the capability to imagine the world, leads to a sense of coherence in time and space, or "in other words, the *autobiographical self* has come into being" (Fonagy, 2004, p. 18). This autobiographical self is described by Damasio (1999) as the outcome of extended consciousness, and by Tulving (1985) as autonoetic consciousness that conceives of a continuous self existing across and through past, present, and future.

Self-agency, or the "agentive mind" (Fonagy, 2004), is central in our ability to evaluate behavior and form an experience of the self behind the behavior (i.e., selfhood). Nevertheless, Fonagy's five increasing levels of self-agency should not be considered the *result* of attachment, because failure to securely bond does not mean failure to develop self-agency. However, attachment difficulties will, according to Fonagy, result in an impoverished theory of mind which, in turn, will result in a diminished sense of self-agency (and particularly representational agency) and a compromised ability to recognize or be concerned about the effects of self-agency on others. Nevertheless, in describing self-agency, Fonagy is describing a psychological phenomenon that will develop in most children (with the possible exception of conditions such as those lying along the autistic spectrum and other relatively rare neurological conditions). The question is not whether a sense of self-agency will develop, but instead, what will be the depth and the quality of that sense of self-agency, and how will it affect social behavior, interactions, and transactions? For the child who develops a limited agentive mind, Fonagy (2004) hypothesizes a "decoupling" of mind and action leading to possible acts of violence and antisocial behavior that are experienced as "agentless" (p. 36).

In addition, as a sense of self-agency is not an element to be considered standing alone from either self-efficacy or other aspects of experienced selfhood, an additional question regards the interaction between self-agency (the sense of self-direction and capacity to act upon the world) and self-efficacy (the sense of self as capable, competent, and able to effect desired goals), as well as other elements embedded in the subsuming internal working model. Hence, Fonagy's view of self-agency must be considered within the larger context in which self-agency develops and intermixes with other aspects of the internal working model, and, indeed, the social environment.

For instance, many delinquent adolescents have a *strong* sense of self-agency—that is, they feel very much self-directed and capable of acting upon the world, and are aware of their ability to control their world and people in it. This is, of course, one of the very issues addressed by this book—the capacity to experience and demonstrate agency over *other* individuals through the exercise of *self*-agency. Here, in the commission of antisocial behavior, we are presumably addressing *distortions* in self-agency, or deviations from the sense of self-agency that we expect in a socially connected and personally safe society. In fact, these deviations from the norm, skewed by uneven, neglectful, or abusive attachment experiences, may *serve* self-agency, and in many delinquents quite possibly develop into an exaggerated and grandiose experience of self-agency.

In the anomic (normless) world described by Durkheim, such deviations from the norm are considered maladaptive responses to a loss of, or failure to develop, attachment to the larger society, and in strain theory as the use of alternative means to acquire socially desirable goods. However, although self-agency may allow the unattached individual to act upon and manipulate the world, it may be entirely divorced from a sense of self-efficacy, or the capacity to act successfully upon the world or feel satisfied. That is, self-agency may be experienced as empty and devoid of meaning because suboptimal attachment fails to install the important sense of mutual social connection required to derive satisfaction, value, and affiliation from social behaviors and relationships. In this context, self-agency—and particularly the form of exaggerated self-agency implicated in criminal behavior and "taking what you want"—may even be a substitute *for* a sense of self-efficacy. To put it another way, a grandiose sense of self-agency may be an antidote against feeling incap-

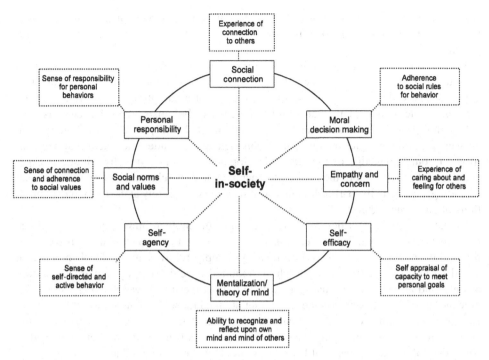

Figure 4.2   Self-in-society: Constellation of elements that contribute to social self

able and powerless. Yet another way of saying this is that optimal attachment experiences instill both self-agency *and* self-efficacy, from which the capacity to act *and* experience a sense of accomplishment is derived.

Self-agency, then, is one element in a well-populated constellation of intertwined internal experiences of self and others. These interacting elements, representing images of self, others, relationships, and social expectations, contribute to the formation of "self-in-society," or the self that is the product of and in constant interaction with internal and external forces, as illustrated in Figure 4.2. The model depicts the self engaged in interactions and transactions with the external world, thus experiencing possibilities for social behaviors, expectations imposed by the external world, and perceptions of meaning derived from contact with the external world. The elements are not static, however, and develop and change incrementally, based on cognitive developments and social expectations, both of which increase over time, creating more stress for the social self, and more solutions.

CRITICISMS OF THE ATTACHMENT PARADIGM

As noted, attachment theory is not without difficulty and has been the subject of criticism for ideas that are sometimes considered weak and ambiguous, failing to recognize multiple routes to selfhood, overemphasizing the importance of the maternal relationship, and seeing the attachment relationship as "one way," thus failing to recognize the infant's unintentional contributions to its own relationships, and particularly the contribution of temperament.

In his essay, "Three Pleasing Ideas," Jerome Kagan (1996) wrote that psychologists want to know how past experience contributes to current psychological processes, and that "the answers to these questions often involve a trio of assumptions of uncertain validity that remain pleasing to a large number of American psychologists" (p. 901). Kagan is critical of this perspective, which he feels is both limited and provides psychology with answers for complex questions that are incomplete and exclude other ideas that can contribute to our knowledge of individual development and diversity. His critique is especially useful as we explore the nature of attachment and its relationship to juvenile sexual offending, and, actually, part of Kagan's critique is aimed squarely at the ideas and assumptions of attachment theory.

In that essay, Kagan criticized the deification of the mother–infant bond as the edifice of human development. This reflects his earlier criticism that object relations theorists of the mid-twentieth century (including Bowlby) simply reformulated "old phenomena in social terms," by asserting that the child "required psychic security and freedom from anxiety, and an affectionate maternal attitude toward the infant was the single most significant factor determining whether the infant attained those precious states" (1979, p. 8). He notes that blame for adult difficulties was "shared with the family of rearing" and "unhappiness, failure, and symptoms in adolescence and adulthood are often explained as being due to absence of parental love during infancy and early childhood" (pp. 8–9).

Nevertheless, rather than simply "using psychoanalytic theory as a scaffold for (its own) theorizing" as Kagan asserted (1979, p. 8), attachment theory has actually spent decades attempting to provide empirical evidence of the maternal connection to a secure sense of social connection and selfhood, as well as the consistency of attachment patterns across the life span. Nevertheless, attachment theory continues to fall short of its goals, and particularly those that: (i) apply experiences in one relationship to all other relationships and (ii) apply early attachment experiences across the life span. In fact, we continue to know far more about attachment and its processes and outcomes in childhood than in adolescence or adulthood. Despite much operationalizing and testing of the theory, then, and descriptions of the "lawfulness"of key attachment principles, attachment theory nevertheless remains theoretical.

Rutter (1997), as described, also asserts that the question of how the early attachment experience becomes transformed into an individual characteristic remains unanswered, following Lamb (1987) who has written that little can be confidently stated about the effect of early attachment experiences and classification with respect to later functioning or attachment status. Critical of the vaguely defined hypotheses and ambiguous construction of studies involving the strange situation, Lamb asserts that outcome data are weak, ambiguous, and speculative and, although interpreted by attachment theorists in a manner that supports theorized hypotheses, may also support entirely different assumptions or causes, or fail to recognize alternative hypotheses. He suggests that the design and methodology of attachment research may actually bias results in a manner that supports the attachment hypotheses. He notes also that patterns of parent–child interactions measured by the strange situation may be stable over time, not *because* of security established by the early attachment relationship, but due to other factors. For instance, perhaps stability is due to an inherent factor in the child, in the child's response to a particular character-istic in the parent, or because the parent–child relationship *itself* is stable over time, hence reflecting an element of the *relationship* and not a pattern of attachment in the child.

Although attachment theorists acknowledge the impact of the environment on the child's behavior (see Sroufe, 1995, for instance), Lamb (1987) criticizes the focus of attachment theory on characteristics believed to reside within the child rather than on the child's inter-action with the environment, or factors within the environment itself. Similarly, Dunn (1993) considers children's relationships to be multidimensional, involving far more than suggested by a typology of attachment security that assigns children to one of three or four groups. She asserts that the framework for understanding relationships over time and the maturity of the individual should focus on developmental change, rather than presumed stability of attachment dimensions over time. As a theorist of individual differences (innate temperament, for instance), Dunn further considers that *both* partners in a relationship con-tribute, and not just the caregiver, and we must therefore consider the contribution of indi-vidual differences in children that partially account for the quality of their relationships. Of this, Kagan (1979) writes that "babies act on their caretakers" (p. 19), meaning that parents respond to the behavior of their children and the relationship that ensues is the result of a two-way interaction, rather than the one-way caregiving relationship implicit in attachment theory.

REFRAMING ATTACHMENT THEORY

These are fair and important criticisms of attachment theory. Although offering a power-ful way to understand and critique human development, attachment theory does have the appearance of assuming a single approach to understanding development, and is also con-fusing, contradictory, and sometimes vague in its formulations. For example, although con-ceptualized as stable over a lifetime, attachment is also considered to be subject to change and redirection and, thus, not stable.

Another contradiction may be found in the application of attachment theory to child rearing and sexual relationships, despite attachment theory itself being quite clear that these are discrete and separate behavioral systems, as Rutter (1997) has pointed out. It is also not clear what it means when we say that a child has an insecure relationship with one parent, but a secure relationship with another; is that child, then, securely or inse-curely attached? Finally, attachment theory seems to be unsure of whether it considers insecure attachment as simply an *adaptive* variant of the attachment process, or a mal-adaptation. Crittenden (2000c) explicitly admonishes that "even the term *quality of attach-ment* carries implicitly the notion of good and bad qualities" and that "attachment terminology should carry no implication of evaluation" (p. 2), and Goldberg (2000b) refers to the "undeserved negative connotations" of insecure attachment (p. 22). On the other hand, it is clear that insecure attachment does, indeed, carry the connotation of mal-adaptation and the development of functional difficulties; Holmes (2001), for instance, directly equates "normal and abnormal" with "secure and insecure" developmental pathways (p. 29).

However, contradictions aside, we are reminded by Atkinson and Goldberg (2004) that a basic tenet of attachment theory is that relationships take place in a broad context, in which attachment is just one aspect of a network of influences involved in child development, and in which the individual is conceptualized as both agent and object. They write that "the diversity of human functioning and the probabilistic (as opposed to deterministic) nature of development can only be understood . . . within this matrix" (p. 15). That is, psychopathology and normative functioning are "dynamic multidetermined processes" influenced by the interaction of many parts during the course of development (Egeland & Carlson, 2004, p. 27). Similarly, Belsky and Nezworski (1988) conclude that while attachment theory recognizes the likelihood of certain developmental pathways, such trajectories are not set in stone and may be altered by life circumstances of all kinds.

Responding to (one of) Kagan's concerns, attachment theory does not, in fact, assert that the mother is responsible for the imparting of well-being and healthy character. Instead, she is described as the facilitator of and active participant in the holding environment and the relationship through which emotional guidance is provided and self-regulation is learned. The primary caregiver, then, does not *transmit* selfhood, but instead enables the facilitative process through which selfhood is discovered and developed. As attachment theory struggles to have relevance to the life course, rather than just the first few years of development, Belsky and Nezworski (1988) tell us that the basic assumption guiding attachment research is not focused on the inevitable effect of the mother–child relationship on all later relationships. Instead, the focus is on the effect that this early relationship will have on the child's experience of and expectations about others and self, and on the development of internal self-regulation and external social skills. Current attachment theory, from their perspective, does not see the child as a passive recipient of experience, but instead as an "active constructor of reality who both creates experiences and differentially attends to diverse information in his/her social world" (p. 6).

With respect to the internal working model, despite its global and unfathomable qualities, it is no less observable than the mind itself, or the mental map that carries the bumblebee from hive to the same flower bed time and time again, and allows it to transmit this same information to other bees from the colony. Even if we can't fully explain it, the existence of such an internal map of the external world is as obvious as the idea of consciousness itself: "If you are conscious, that is it. If you are not, then definition is futile" (Blatz, 1966, p. 17).

On a final note, Rutter (1997) describes "the problem in the wish of many adult attachment theorists to extend attachment concepts to sexual relationships and to parents' relationships with their young children" (p. 25). This problem is of particular importance as we review and discuss ideas of theorists who postulate that early attachment experiences and patterns are significantly connected to the development of sexually abusive behavior. Following Rutter's criticism, we must raise the possibility that a similar process is occurring within the field of sex offender specific research or, to paraphrase Rutter, the wish of many sexual offender theorists to extend attachment concepts to sexually coercive and abusive relationships and to adult sexual molestation of children. We risk not only blending concepts, but also risk weak, ambiguous, and biased research designs that *prove*, rather than *test*, theoretically attractive hypotheses, and hence yield data that, despite the appearance of empirical "fact," are more speculative than certain.

CHAPTER 5

An Attachment Framework

Attachment is about security, imbued through early experience, captured and defined in internal representations, and recapitulated through scripts, plans, and automatic thought and expectations. However, early experience defines but doesn't set in stone the foundations of personality. Werner and Smith's (1992) study of high-risk children offers a powerful example of the ability to "earn" security, despite difficult or suboptimal early experience. In their study of 505 children tracked over a 30-year period, approximately one-third of the original cohort (N = 698) were born into conditions defined by Werner and Smith as high risk. Yet by age 18 one-third of this high-risk group was functioning well despite the odds against them, and by their early 30s almost all of the group of 201 high-risk individuals tracked by Werner and Smith "had staged a recovery of sorts" (p. 193).

Nevertheless, early attachment processes may be understood as the platform upon which personality and the capacity for self-recognition is built, serving as the source of both self-image and human connection. Internalized representations of early attachment experiences contain mentalized conceptions of relationships and what one can expect from them, or, more to the point, what one can expect from other people. They also provide the basis for critical social behaviors that include goal establishment and accomplishment, focus and self-regulation, and social interactions and relationship building. As we consider attachment theory and all it has to offer as a model of human development, flaws included, it is useful to apply it as both a *framework* by which to understand the structure upon which human emotion, thought, and behavior is built, and as a *lens* through which to examine emotion, thought, and behavior in action.

AN ATTACHMENT FRAMEWORK

Attachment theory proposes that images of self and others are forged through the infant–mother system, thus setting the path for relationships that follow. It considers that behind behavior lie emotional and cognitive schemata embedded into a mental map which itself is neurologically configured and hard wired, activated by biologically established and instinctual drives. Whereas attachment theory provides an evolutionary and neurobiological base for understanding human experience and behavior, the operationalization of attachment theory provides a structure by which to develop insight and understanding into the cognitive and emotional psychology of both development and everyday life.

In this regard, an attachment *framework* seeks causes and explanations for current behavior. It is therefore both psychodynamic and cognitive in its exploration of the interactions between the internal (mental) and external (physical) world and social relationships, and in its explanations for the development and role of cognitive schemata. In applying an attachment framework to understanding developmental and functional difficulties in older children, adolescents, and adults it becomes a psychology of emotional and cognitive deficits or, as noted by Sroufe et al. (1999), a theory of psychopathology in which ideas about attachment are also used to understand the cause and development of functional deficits and to define treatment interventions.

The Attachment Lens

Attachment theory may thus be considered as a means by which to make sense of human behavior, seeing and evaluating it in a way that might shed light on behaviors that otherwise make little sense. Consider the attachment *lens* as a way of seeing things otherwise invisible or that may appear to be different when viewed through a different lens, just as an infrared lens reveals aspects of phenomena undetected in ordinary visible light. Through the attachment lens, loud and even out of control behavior in children can instead be seen as the activation of attachment behaviors triggered under conditions that present emotional uncertainty for the child. "Attention-seeking" behavior in troubled children can be understood as "*attachment*-seeking" behaviors designed to ensure proximity, accompanied by signaling behaviors activated to ensure that the child is seen, recognized, and attended to.

Through an attachment lens, agitated and exaggerated behavior in children can be seen as the failure of the child to self soothe in stressful circumstances; the failure to demonstrate self-regulation can be seen as a failure of the early child–caregiver system and the ability of the caregiver to demonstrate and impart self-regulatory skills to the developing child. Detached and even depressed behavior may be understood as the child's intrinsic belief in the inevitable or irretrievable loss of an attachment figure, or all attachment figures. Anxiety can be re-interpreted as the long-term sequelae of early experiences in which responses to the child's signaled needs were perceived by the child as inaccurate or insensitive, unresponsive, or, worse, abusive and punishing. Difficulty in trusting or acquiescing to authority may be recognized as uncertainty about adult figures, perhaps the long-term response to inadequate, incompetent, neglectful, or abusive parents or alternative early caregivers.

Seen through an attachment-informed lens, the inability to tolerate ambiguity can be revealed as evidence of an uncertain sense of self, or failure to see self as worthy of attention, support, or love. Lack of empathy or concern for, or even awareness of, others can be seen as a lack of theory of mind (metacognition), rather than callousness or psychopathy, per se. Finally, easily triggered behaviors or behaviors that appear completely out of synch with the current situation, out of proportion to current stressors, or out of touch with what is actually happening may be the result of the kindling of neural circuits primed to respond in a particular fashion, perhaps the result of repeated early experience or adaptation to early conditions drilled into neural circuits.[1]

Therefore, an attachment lens driven by an attachment framework can help us to make sense of some behavior that otherwise challenges understanding and in other cases adds an additional perspective to already existing ideas about behavior. This lens can allow us to see patterns that we might otherwise miss, recognize appropriate treatment interventions, and suggest a framework for treatment. That is, an attachment perspective can help to define the treatment relationship between clinician and patient, as well as the actual modes, techniques, and interventions of treatment.

DYSFUNCTIONAL BEHAVIOR: THE SOCIAL SELF DRIVEN BY ANXIETY

From an attachment point of view, a sense of both self and self-and-others is central in understanding social behavior and human connection: "How we experience ourselves in relation to others provides a basic organizing perspective for all interpersonal events" (Stern, 1985/2000, p. 6). Accordingly, as we attempt to define a framework for recognizing and understanding the impact or driving quality of attachment[2] on behavior, it is necessary to understand important components of the process by which attachment is translated into selfhood, and consequently into behavior and later relationships. In Chapter 4, we described a model of the self formed by the interaction of selfhood and social forces, resulting in the formation of "self-in-society"—the dynamic self produced by interactions between internal and external forces. Here, as we create a framework to better or differently understand behavior, we recognize that the person producing the behavior is him/herself a complex product of internal psychic and external social forces, including his or her relationship to others.

But, although this model of social self may help us to better understand the individual, including the development of self through the attachment experience, it is not enough to always help us to understand the behaviors produced by those individuals, and particularly when those behaviors are dysfunctional, antisocial, or pathological, and especially how such behaviors may be driven by attachment anxiety. The attachment lens must reveal to us those attachment elements that drive and explain behavior, or it is hardly worth mentioning.

---

[1] In effect, *kindling* and *priming* are akin to wood kindling which is easily sparked into fire and a water pump primed to readily and quickly pump water. Kindling is a process whereby areas of the brain can be easily activated, even by low stimulation. Most typically associated with epilepsy, repeated seizure activity is believed to "kindle" affected areas of the brain by causing damage that results in easy reactivation of the same process (for instance, repeated seizures). The limbic system of the brain is considered especially susceptible to kindling, including the amygdala and hippocampus, both considered centers of emotion and memory, as discussed in Chapter 15. The threshold of that area of the brain to excitement is lowered as a result of repeated stimulation making it susceptible to excitement, thus becoming *primed* to recall and reconstruct frequently repeated events and experiences embedded in implicit memory. As implicit memory stores non-conscious procedural memories, primed memory often involves "automatic" behaviors easily evoked by the priming process. Priming, therefore, results in increased response due to prior exposure to the primed experience, without intent or task-motivated behavior. In effect, kindling is a physical process that establishes the basis for priming.

[2] Remember, we are using the term "attachment" to describe the internalization of early attachment experiences, as well as the process of being and feeling attached, even at the implicit level.

Just as self-in-society is a construct formed by a constellation of interacting elements (Figure 4.2, Chapter 4), so too is there a constellation of elements that coalesce to produce behaviors driven by the need for security, or rather driven by the experience of attachment insecurity. Figure 5.1 illustrates this model of security-driven behavior, simply illustrating the sort of elements that are related to the attachment behavioral system, focusing on internal/emotional states that might activate attachment behavior. The more elements that are activated, the greater the display of attachment behaviors, and combined they produce a powerful constellation of security-driven behaviors.

Although the model shown in Figure 5.1 may illustrate the drive to achieve security, like the model of self-in-society, it cannot in itself be used to explain the sometimes erratic behavior seen in dysfunctional individuals, or functional individuals for that matter who nevertheless sometimes engage in dysfunctional behaviors.

If we partially overlap the model of self-in-society with the model of security-driven behavior, we see a shared area in which aspects of social self and security-driven behaviors come together, interact, and potentiate one another. This fusion produces behaviors idiosyncratic to each particular individual, based in part on his or her psychological attributes, socialization experiences, and quality of attachment, and conditions that evoke or subdue anxiety in that individual. Further, the interaction and potentiation of specific elements are not defined only by the individual's sense of self and security of attachment, but also by the particular situation under which sense of self and experienced attachment needs come together. Such current circumstances actively influence and define how self

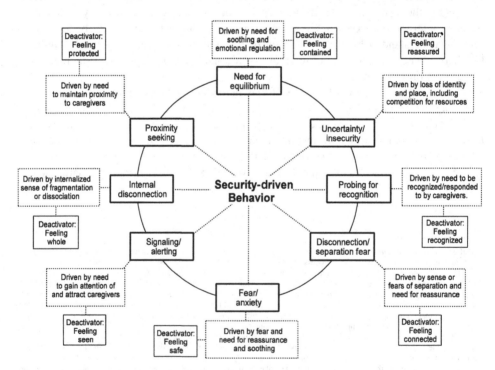

Figure 5.1   Security-driven behavior: Constellation of elements

and security interact in those particular circumstances, which in turn are shaped by prior history and the availability of security solutions. This highly dynamic zone of attachment-driven behavior is shown in Figure 5.2, with behaviors in the shaded zone produced by the interaction between self, insecurity, and current circumstances.

Nevertheless, despite the uniqueness of the zone for each individual and the variation in circumstances that influence zone behavior in a single individual, components of this complex interactional process remain stable. Elements of self and attachment security, for instance, do not change from day to day, or month to month. These dimensions that underlie specific/idiosyncratic behavior are relatively invariant in the short and moderate run. There is thus a predictable pattern to the *sort* of behavior we can expect in any given individual, even if we cannot always understand the behavior itself.

However, the goal of such a model is to help us to recognize the nature, source, and purpose of the behavior, and thus demystify it. If psychology, and psychotherapy in particular, always has as its goal the demystification of behavior, both functional and

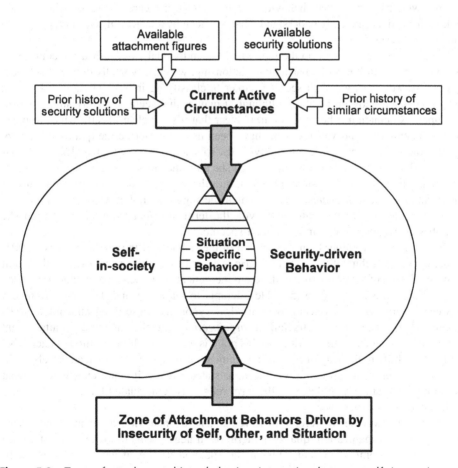

Figure 5.2 Zone of attachment-driven behavior: Interaction between self, insecurity, and circumstance

dysfunctional, pathological and non-pathological, then an attachment-informed framework is simply one more tool to accomplish the resolution of sources of impairment and the improvement of emotional well-being and behavioral functionality.

Using a lens through which our observations of behavior are informed by attachment theory, we can begin to understand many types of behavior as the result of experiences and representations embedded into the mental map, triggered into activity by particular circumstances, and, despite fluctuations in the activating events, resting upon attributes of self and patterns of behavior that are relatively stable during any given stage in life. The goal, then, is clear—seeing the root and route of behavior, and especially behavioral disturbance.

AN EXPLOSION OF TERMS: PATTERNS OF ATTACHMENT

To more fully develop an attachment-informed framework or an attachment-informed lens through which to understand behavior, we must form a clearer sense of what we are looking for and more clearly understand what we mean by attachment. We start, then, with attachment "types."

As we describe attachment in the individual, the individual's typical way of connecting to others, or the attributes of a particular relationship, we most typically define attachment "types." However, as we shall see in Chapter 6, classifying individuals into assessment categories is a muddy proposition, although it may at first seem relatively simple. Actually, upon examination it becomes entirely clear that it's *not* clear exactly what we mean by attachment type, and various terms have been used to describe the quality or content of the experience of attachment in individuals. Johnson (2003), who has described confusion in the use of attachment terms, which she attributes to the "richness" of the literature (rather than actual confusion), also identifies the synonymous and overlapping use of terms. She notes that *attachment styles*, which she suggests implies an individual characteristic, is often used interchangeably with the term *attachment strategies*, which she describes as behavior that is more context-specific.

More to the point, rather than a reflection of the richness of the literature, Ross (2004) points out that attachment theorists use various descriptive terms inconsistently, the result of an "explosion of terms relating to different theoretical constructs of attachment . . . used in a rather confusing way" (p. 57). He attempts to tease out and describe differences between several terms that seem to be used as synonyms, describing attachment *style*, attachment *representations*, attachment *organization*, attachment *quality*, attachment *status*, and attachment *pattern*. Although his point is well made, his definition of each label really offers little in the way of resolving significant differences, and instead largely highlights the confusion in terminology. Indeed, as stated already, it is not exactly clear what we do mean by attachment because the term reflects several related but discrete aspects of the attachment experience.

Nevertheless, whether we refer to observed attachment behaviors as an attachment type, style, approach, organization, quality, pattern, or strategy seems to make little difference to the idea that is embodied in attachment classification. That is, when we classify attachment into categories we are identifying a pattern of behaviors or ideas, both or either of which are considered to reflect enduring aspects of the attachment experience in the individuals who exhibit such behaviors or ideas. Classification labels define not only a psychological phenomenon experienced *by* the individual, but also a pattern observable *in* the individual by others, through the behaviors of the individual (as in the strange situation), through the coherence and consistency of their memories of attachment (as in the adult attachment interview), or through their description of ideas or attitudes about relationships (through various paper-and-pencil attachment inventories and self-reports).

The Ambiguity of Attachment

Although we can describe attachment, as in attachment theory, it's not necessarily clear how to definitively operationalize the ideas, measure the content of the attachment experience, or classify the behaviors. Actually, as we have discussed, it is not even clear what we are exactly referring to when we say that someone is attached, securely or insecurely. Attachment classifications, on the one hand, seem to refer to the state of the *individual* as attached or unattached, but, on the other hand, appear to reflect the quality of the individual's *relationships* as attached or unattached. Actually, as in attachment theory it is so rare to be *un*attached, using standard and widely accepted attachment terminology, we generally mean *securely* or *insecurely* attached (rather than attached or unattached[3]), or *organized* or *disorganized* in the use of strategies for developing and maintaining attachment in relationships. But are we talking about attachment as: (i) a thing that exists inside an individual, (ii) the quality of a particular type of relationship (which, according to attachment theory, must contain the asymmetrical but complementary qualities of dependence in one party and caregiving in the other), (iii) qualities present in the way that an individual operates within all dependent relationships (that is, relationships with all caregivers), or (iv) qualities within the individual and patterns of behavior and experience at play within all subsequent relationships? That is, is an individual securely attached as a *person*, securely attached in his or her *relationships*, or *differently* attached in different relationships? Only in the first case can we legitimately think of the attachment classification of the individual as an enduring quality that resides within the individual.

Also bear in mind, the nature of *attached* relationships, again a source of potential confusion and paradox. In attachment theory, "attachment" refers *only* to affectional relationships with *significant* and *specific* individuals, namely caregivers. According to Ainsworth (1969), attachment forms discriminately with only specific individuals and does not apply to transitory relationships, or even affectionate relationships that are enduring but do not reach the tripartite watershed of *dependence, responsiveness*, and *attunement* that marks the attachment relationship. Here, again, we get into confusing waters because attachment theorists, from Bowlby and Ainsworth onward, have defined attachment both as the product of an instinctual behavioral system that is present and activated in young children with particular regard to caregivers *and* as a psychological construct that grows out of this early relationship and is later directed to significant others who are *not* caregivers. Indeed, we have already noted Rutter's (1997) criticism of attachment theorists who extend the relatively obvious and easily observed notions of attachment

---

[3] Although attachment theory does recognize *de*tachment, this is considered an aspect of insecure attachment or a deactivation of the attachment behavioral system, in response to insecure attachment.

relationships in children to the romantic, sexual, partnered, family, and parental relationships of adults.

Attachment in Childhood and Adulthood

Although we recognize the relationship of children to their parents as attached—especially
in infancy and through mid-childhood—and we can continue to extend the concept of
parents as "caregivers" through adolescence, it is certainly not true that older children or
adolescents depend on their parents for survival and often, far from seeking proximity,
seek distance and independence. Beyond adolescence, of course, adult relationships do not
involve a relationship in which one individual depends upon the other for caregiving and
survival, and healthy adult relationships do not, in the least, resemble the relationship
between a dependent child and a parent. Although it is true that in infancy and early childhood the reciprocal and complementary behavioral systems in play represent attachment
for the child and caregiving for the parent, this is obviously not true in adult relationships
and considerable change is also obvious in the relationship between adolescents and their
parents.

The relationship dependency that exists in childhood and the controlling nurturance of
the parent is considered smothering in parent–adolescent relationships and unhealthy in
adult relationships. A highly developed attunement in infant–mother relationships might
be considered to be enmeshment in an adolescent–parent relationship, and between adults
might be considered to be co-dependent. Healthy, close adult relationships are either *affectionate and affiliative* or *affectionate, affiliative, and romantic* and do not include either
dependency or caregiving, although such relationships are marked by mutual and equal
*inter*dependence. By adulthood, the attunement and intimacy of childhood attachment has
evolved into the attunement and intimacy of enduring affectional relationships between
equal partners, transformed during late childhood and adolescence from one into the other.

Frankly, the word "attachment," as described in Chapter 1, is an appropriate term to
describe these increasingly equal partner relationships of adolescence and adulthood.
Indeed, attachment describes the idealized connections we seek between people in general,
as well as between individuals and society, and this is how the term is generally used and,
from my perspective, *best* used. This is what we are actually describing when we ask if
someone is "attached"—that is, socially connected to others—and this is almost certainly
the phenomenon in which we are most interested when we discuss attachment in the
context of antisocial, criminal, and sexually abusive behavior. However, attachment theory
continues to describe attachment across the life span in terms of its appearance and function in early childhood, based on security and secure base behavior; this requires that,
throughout the life span, attachment partners are considered to essentially serve the same
role as the early primary caregiver. This clearly makes it difficult to understand, measure,
or describe attachment in adolescents and adults, and is a serious flaw in attachment
theory's ability to operationalize its ideas.

In adolescent and adult functioning, we are interested in what childhood attachment has
transformed into, not childhood attachment per se. In older children, adolescents, and
adults, we are interested in the experience of self-worth, the placement of trust and value

in others, and ultimately the capacity to engage in relationships that are mutually healthy to all parties. And lest we find the term "healthy" too loose, let's explain it as something we *know* when we see it. Actually, the very way in which we would express health in a relationship is the way in which we describe secure attachment: an attribute or quality in a relationship that offers the individuals in the relationship a sense of personal and interpersonal security; something that aids and bolsters growth and the capacity for efficacious self-agency, rather than something that impedes or damages growth and self-esteem.

The Quality of Attachment: Where Does It Reside?

There also remains an unanswered and central question of whether attachment theory is measuring a quality of attachment in the *individual* or a quality of attachment in the *relationship*. Goldberg (2000a) notes that some writers assert that attachment is both a trait *and* a characteristic of dyadic relationships. As a trait, attachment resides within the individual as an enduring quality that is characteristic of the individual and is relatively unchanging across relationships. As a characteristic of a particular relationship, the attachment experience will change from relationship to relationship. However, Goldberg goes on to suggest that there is little empirical support for the trait concept, leaving us to believe that attachment is thus about relationships and not the individual within the relationship. Nevertheless, the idea that "attachment" is a quality belonging to a relationship, rather than the individual within the relationship, makes little sense and is impractical as a means for assessing the internalization of attachment within the individual or for organizing future attachment experiences. The idea that attachment is relationship-based has little value other than providing a means of assessing specific relationships, rather than relationships in general, and is contra-indicated (contradicted) by both Bowlby (1988) and Ainsworth (1969) who describe attachment as an enduring characteristic that lies within the individual, imprinted and serving as a template within the internal working model.

In addressing the trait/relationship duality, Michael Rutter (1997) is critical of the idea that attachment is a trait of the individual. He sees attachment, as measured by the Adult Attachment Interview for instance, as a measure of the relationship and not the individual. He notes that the same person has different relationships with different people, the same parents have different relationships with each of their children, and children have different relationships with each of their parents. However, this view of attachment as *relationship*-resident, rather than residing within the individual, not only conflicts with the internal working model perspective of attachment theory, but also requires us to consider attachment as transitory, shifting from relationship to relationship.

Conversely, in his critique of attachment theory, Lewis (1997) asserts that the attachment model does postulate the idea that early attachment experiences create in the child "a kind of trait or characterization, which in turn determines the child's subsequent relationships" (p. 138). Similarly, Ainsworth (1969) writes that attachment relates to something inside the person, distinguished from the behaviors that mediate and bring attachment to life. In this conceptualization, which we adopt here, attachment resides within the *individual*, and not the relationship. Over time the experiences of early attachment transform and mature, but as they do they leave indelible shadows, imprinted into the mental map, shaping self and later relationships.[4]

Characterized by interactions, transactions, and relationships, self-in-society is revealed through the patterns, styles, and experiences of attachment demonstrated in the individual, rather than a particular relationship. Attached and other relationships, then, reflect the traces, not of the relationship itself, but of the individuals within the relationship and the self-in-society they each bring to the relationship. It is this sense of self, I think, in which we are most interested as we struggle to understand sexually abusive behavior.

This again appears to reflect construct and definitional difficulties with attachment as a concept. It reflects the kaleidoscope-like qualities attributed to attachment and the ambiguity of the term, and is as much about semantics as construct. Again, we are reminded that "attachment" has several meanings: (i) reflecting attached relationships, (ii) strategies for forming and maintaining attached relationships, and (iii) the experience of attachment as either a satisfying or in some way anxiety-provoking experience. In the first instance, we can see that "attachment" does lie within the relationship, but in the latter two cases resides within the individual, where, over time, it comes to form a trait-like quality. Attached relationships, of course, do differ from dyad to dyad but we must consider the template, from which is derived the ability to form attachments and feel attached, to reside within the individual or we have nothing of value to help us to understand the functioning of the individuals who exist within and outside of relationships.

MUDDY CONCEPTS

Attachment theory fails to remain consistent or coherent, reflecting Karen's (1994) comment that the theory is flawed and leaves "huge unanswered questions" (p. 437) and Bolen's (2000) report that attachment theory has many problems to resolve in its theory and proof. This makes it problematic to classify individuals into meaningful categories of attachment that describe their patterns, style, or experience of attachment, or provide insight into internal experience and behavior. As they exist now, attachment classifications are weak and far from complete descriptions of either the individual or the individual's experience of attachment. To say that a person is securely or insecurely attached has little concrete meaning, as it is not clear to what we are actually referring.

Recall also, from Chapter 3, that in current attachment theory there is no clear consensus about what attachment theory is actually theorizing (i.e., describing). For Schore (1999), attachment theory is a theory of *self-regulation*, but for Lyons-Ruth et al. (2004) it is a theory of *conflict and defense*. Johnson (2003) defines attachment theory as a *trauma* theory, but Sroufe et al. (1999) define it as a theory of *psychopathology*, and Moretti and Holland (2003) describe attachment theory as *self-discrepancy* theory. And, although never using the term, Bowlby describes attachment theory as a theory of *biopsychosocial* development over time.

Johnson (2003) describes attachment theory as so rich that readers may be confused by the use of different terms by different writers to describe the same phenomena. She asserts

---

[4] In the case of childhood trauma, Rasmussen, Burton, and Christopherson (1992) describe such indelible markers as "trauma echoes."

that this is because different theorists are addressing attachment at different points in the life span or using different measures of attachment. Her explanation is only partly true. It reflects the perspective that attachment is quite different at different points in human development and the fact that we have inadequate measurement tools. However, a larger issue is that attachment theory is not coherent or consistent in either its definition, approach, or operationalization. In many ways, in trying to develop *specificity* in terms and concepts, attachment theory sacrifices *sensitivity*, and succeeds in confusing matters and muddying up concepts—that is, in trying to narrowly define terms and concepts (specificity) it loses the ability to explain or maintain consistency across broad phenomena (sensitivity). To this end, Lewis (1997) writes that attachment theory "tries to explain too much and, in doing so, explains little" (p. 162).

Actually, the idea of attachment theory is simple enough. It's the application of the theory throughout the life span that makes it problematic, in large part because it is not a stage model and therefore does not move towards conceptually greater complexity. Recall that unlike a stage model in which one stage unfolds and prepares the groundwork for and is subsumed by the following more advanced stage, attachment theory is static. That is, although there are phases through which young children pass as they become attached, this process occurs fully before age 4, and after that, and actually largely by age 1, attachment is most typically considered categorical and relatively stable throughout life. Consequently, poorly understood and defined, in attachment theory adolescent and adult attachment is considered simply a variant and a later development of the attachment experience and patterning formed during infancy and early childhood.

In developing an attachment-informed framework, however, it is important to clear up such confusion and create a firm ground upon which to build attachment-informed practice. Accordingly, it is perhaps most useful and simple to conceive attachment as a basic biopsychosocial process. This helps us to understand attachment theory as a means to healthy adult development rather than as a theory of trauma, pathology, relationships, self-regulation, or self-image, each of which is a *derivative* of the attachment process rather than a primary process. Above all, attachment theory is a model of human development, from which we can develop secondary theories of this-or-that. Following Crittenden (2000a, 2001), we can add the further dimension of chronological development in the form of maturing biological systems (physiology, cognition, and emotion) and the acquisition of experience over time. It is a theory of human development stemming from the interaction of animal biology and human consciousness in the social environment.

Beyond Childhood: The Changing Nature of Attachment

Ainsworth (1989) writes that in adolescents the nature of attachment changes dramatically, "occasioned by hormonal, neurophysiological, and cognitive changes and not merely by socioemotional experience" (p. 710). This clearly suggests that attachment is not *only* related to the dependant–caregiver dyad. If adolescent and adult attachment is a result of a romantic partnership that involves the reproductive and caregiving systems *as well* as the attachment system, as Ainsworth clearly states, then this creates interesting problems for attachment theory and our understanding of attachment. Either adolescent and adult attachment is actually a synthesis of three or more *different* behavioral systems, and not "attachment" at all as defined by the biological and ethological bases of attachment theory, or it is the development and outgrowth of, and *more than* and *significantly different* from, attachment of early childhood. As described, this results in an expanded definition of attachment that approximates our real-life understanding and use of the concept.

This further requires that attachment theory explicitly recognize that what is currently described in attachment theory as "attachment" be defined as "attachment of infancy and early childhood" and conceptual and operational definitions of adolescent and adult attachment be developed. These will describe transformations in attachment through the accumulated experiences of attached relationships, changes in cognitive and emotional development, the development and implementation of behavioral strategies, and environment feedback (or cause-and-effect) from childhood through adolescence and into adulthood. In addition to allowing attachment theory to have application and meaning throughout the life span as a biological and psychological imperative, recognizing and defining the transformation of *childhood* attachment into *adolescent and adult* attachment will allow for more accurate means to conceptualize and measure such concepts.

A simple illustration of such changes is provided in Figure 5.3, showing the increasing level and complexity of bases that underlie attachment at different development stages. Each developmental epoch of attachment builds upon and subsumes earlier bases of attachment, with infant and childhood attachment most simply and directly shaped by biologi-

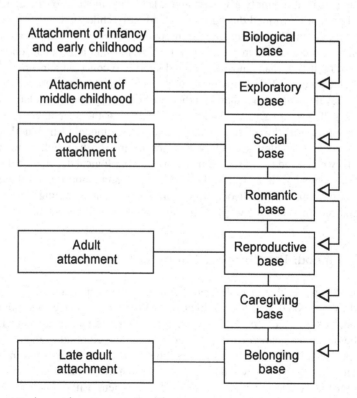

Figure 5.3 Attachment bases across the life span

cal drive. In this simple model, middle childhood attachment continues to be driven by biology, but more complex and sophisticated exploratory drives are at play as new attachments form and move towards adolescence. During adolescence and into adulthood, attachment is increasingly driven by social affiliation and then, for many, romance and eventually the drive for reproduction (rather than just sexual intercourse) and caregiving. Following Erikson's (1959/1980) model of human development through the life span, the model proposes that attachment in later years is belonging based, in which the experience of attachment is largely based on remaining connected to family, friends, and society. Although simple and not intended to convey the complexity of attachment as it transforms and develops across the life span, the model illustrates not simply changes in attachment, but the idea that attachment is transformed and develops in stage-like fashion.

The Transformation of Attachment

Bowlby's description of attachment does not recognize attachment transforming over time. Instead, it considers attachment passing through phases that simply deepen the initial attachment structure and the further development of already established organizational strategies for maintaining proximity to caregivers.

However, the attachment process is more complex than can be described without conceptualizing attachment as forming in developmental stages, or at least as a continuous process marked by recognizable changes in attachment purpose and content, roughly broken into stages that fall between childhood and adulthood. The result is that we get stuck with definitions of attachment in adolescence and adulthood based on the same criteria that we use for understanding attachment in infants. However, it is inconceivable that attachment in adults is essentially driven by the need for proximity and fears of separation, as it is in childhood. Rather than reaching its final point of development somewhere around age 4 or 5 years and then remaining stable as a biopsychological structure, it is far more likely that attachment continues to change with each developmental epoch (middle childhood, adolescence, adulthood, and later adulthood) in order to meet and prepare the individual to address different needs. Attachment is thus transformed through the life span, as shown in Figure 5.3.

In fact, the attachment experience in adults *must* be different from that in children. Indeed, West, Rose, Spring, Sheldon-Keller, and Adam (1998) write that a major reorganization in childhood relationships occurs during adolescence as parent–child relationships are relinquished and replaced by new affectional ties to peers. At that point, attachment relationships to parents change, described by Weiss (1982) as relatively continuous until that time and demonstrated by clear displays of attachment behavior. Adolescents, however, begin to establish, demonstrate, and experience independence from parents—a trend which, of course, continues into adulthood, entirely transforming the attachment relationship. Despite this, one of the weaknesses of mainstream attachment theory lies in its use of childhood patterns of attachment to frame, understand, and define attachment in adolescence and adulthood. Accordingly, it is important that we define a model that recognizes changes in the construction, meaning, and experience of attachment over the course of human development, in which not only do attachment roles and functions change, but so too do the needs they fill and the persons who fill those roles.

THE NEED FOR A NEW CONCEPTION OF ATTACHMENT

Although, on the one hand, the literature recognizes attachment as a changing developmental construct, on the other its focus on an unchanging view of attached relationships is epitomized by Hinde (1982) who emphasizes that "attachment is limited to ties with an individual perceived as stronger and/or wiser" (p. 65). This, of course, is clearly not true in either adolescent or adult relationships with peers or romantic partners. In fact, we would typically consider such a relationship unequal, and in many cases emotionally unhealthy for one or both partners.

As recently as 2004, Atkinson and Goldberg asserted that attachment serves a protective function (p. 16) and throughout life continues to trigger related distress-regulating (attachment) behaviors. Lyons-Ruth et al. (2004) recognize the underlying nature of attachment as a system that develops for the *primary* purposes of maintaining a sense of security (rather, for instance, than maintaining proximity, per se). Nevertheless, they also consider the attachment behavioral system to be the pre-eminent behavioral system *at all ages*, overriding all other motivational systems when activated, driving the individual away from all other activities and towards the "security-providing responses of others" (p. 68). This maintains the idea that attachment is about a sense of security derived *through* the other/caregiver, rather than contained in the self. This drives home the troubling notion that *all* attached relationships, at *any* age, rather than involving self-regulation and interdependency, are driven by dependency and anxiety-triggered proximity-seeking behavior in which the other is always seen as the "stronger and/or wiser" individual described by Hinde. Similarly, Hilburn-Cobb (2004) writes that attachment may be understood as a means to achieve emotional and cognitive regulation by "eliciting care from a unique relationship" (p. 100). This, too, supports the view that at any age, under stress, attachment is essentially about being cared *for*, and security is derived through an *external* source of regulation (the other/caregiver) rather than the internalized experience of security derived from early attachment experiences. This is hardly the interdependent and independent relationship that attachment theory holds as the ideal in secure attachment.

In this view, in order to consider a relationship at any point throughout the life span as an attached relationship, the other must serve the role of stronger and wiser caregiver rather than that of an equal partner (whether friend or lover). Thus, in the attachment model, attachment is a relatively invariant construct, more-or-less fully defined by age 4 or 5. Presumably, according to attachment theory's narrow definition of an attachment relationship, both partners in an adolescent or adult relationship seek in one another a wiser and stronger caregiver, and both are thus mutually dependent on the other rather than mutually interdependent. This would, however, create what we would consider a co-dependent relationship, rather than the independent and mutually interdependent relationship that we consider healthy between adults.

Despite its assertions, then, that attachment is not about dependence, the attachment model proposes that, in effect, adults will always require a mother figure, needing to turn to their partners in time of stress for a form of caregiving. Hence, from an attachment theory perspective, *only* partners who can be psychologically turned by the individual into a mother figure may be considered as attachment figures. In this model, we cannot even consider ourselves to be attached to our own children, as the attachment bond is one way—dependent child to caregiving parent. However, this is a view that cannot be supported, particularly when we recognize that healthy close adult relationships include neither dependency nor caregiving. As described, ideal adult relationships are either *affectionate and affiliative* among close friends, or *affectionate, affiliative, and romantic*, in both cases marked by both mutual interdependence and independence.

I reiterate, then, that the purpose and experience of attachment in adolescents and adults must be different from its purpose and experience in children. The inability of attachment theory to recognize the *entire* transformation of attachment from late childhood on has weakened its ability to fully conceptualize attachment as it changes and meets different needs, as well as confusing terminology and ideas. It is as if the attachment process does not develop beyond the fourth phase of goal-corrected partnership, simply adjusting to adolescent and adult life circumstances but never really changing in function, character, or experience. The result is that attachment theory expends a great deal of effort in trying to "fit" *adult* attachment into a model of *childhood* attachment. It is important that we do not apply the same error as we work to fit attachment theory with explanations and theories of sexually abusive behavior.

Stages of Attachment

During adolescence and into adulthood, attachment is increasingly driven by social affiliation and then, for many, romance and eventually the drive for reproduction (rather than just sexual intercourse) and caregiving. As shown in Figure 5.3, this perspective, following Erikson's (1959/1980) model of human development through the life span, proposes that attachment passes from a dependent and security-driven attachment, through adolescent and adult variants, to a belonging-based attachment in later adult years in which the experience of attachment rests largely on maintaining existing connections to family, friends, and society. Although simple and not intended to convey the complexity of attachment as it transforms and develops across the life span, the model illustrates not simply changes in attachment, but the idea that attachment is transformed and develops in stage-like fashion.

If we can conceive of attachment undergoing metamorphosis, then we can recognize early attachment as the prototype from which later transformations emerge; the natural product of cognitive, emotional, and physical changes, accompanied by changes in social relationships, self-identity, and developmentally related personal needs. As with any stage model, subsequent transformations are evolutionary rather than revolutionary; earlier variants of attachment are not discarded, but produce the material from which transformation emerges. Hence, earlier experience is embedded as the molecular structure and material of later transformations (the genotype), fully incorporated and woven into the new attachment (the phenotype). As in any stage model, earlier stages are incorporated into and nesting within later stages, as shown in Figure 5.4.

If it was true that attachment did not develop in stages, then the only kind of attachment and the only kind of attachment bonds that could exist at any age would be those with caregivers, or caregiver substitutes. Nevertheless, although equivocal on this point, this idea remains at the heart of current attachment theory. Thus, peers and romantic partners have to be "squeezed" into the role of substitute caregiver in order for the concept of attachment to be considered relevant at points from late childhood onwards. However, considering adolescent or adult partners as "caregivers," rather than equal partners, suggests psychological regression or developmentally immature dependency, and not mature and independent relationship skills. On the other hand, a stage model recognizes that attachment transforms with development, and that non-caregiver social affiliations can therefore become attachment relationships in their own right. This allows adolescent and adult partners to be considered attachment figures without filling a care- or security-giving role.

The Seat of Attachment

In its conceptualization of the internal working model, attachment theory already has the capacity and provides the base for embracing and explaining the evolving and dynamic

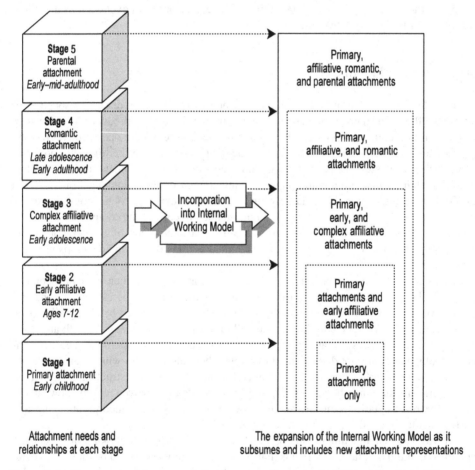

Figure 5.4 Developmental stages of attachment and attached relationships, from infancy to adulthood, with concurrent and resulting changes in an internal working model that expands to subsume and incorporate changes and additions to attachment, and within which earlier primary attached relationships are nested and remain active

transformation of attachment over time. The internal working model is already conceived as the embodiment of exactly such accumulated experiences, both the product and driver of experience. It is the engine of the self-in-society. And although far easier to recognize, measure, and predict observable behavior, thus rendering it accessible to empirical practice, we are nevertheless already trying to "measure" aspects of our internalized mental maps. Measures such as the adult attachment interview and other interviews and self-reports are designed to reveal recollections, impressions, attitudes, beliefs, and other aspects of the mind not necessarily available or too difficult to recognize or quantify through direct observation.

Of course, attachment in young children, and infants especially, is a much simpler phenomenon to recognize, conceptualize, and understand than its adolescent and adult equivalents. In fact, classification of attachment in children at age 12 to 18 months is based strictly on observed behavior, rather than attitude, mindset, or metacognition, or anything other than behavior. Mental maps and the experiences of attachment are inferred from such observation, but actual assignment to attachment categories is based upon behavior. This is because in young children the attachment process is emotionally, cognitively, and, philosophically simple. It is far easier to recognize and categorize because it is uncluttered and elementary, compared to attachment at older ages. Babies, for instance, are not capable of empathy, intimacy (as we understand it), perspective taking, moral reasoning, or any of the other qualities that we think of as central in an attachment model that includes dimensions such as self-image and mental representations of others. This means that the young child's experience of attachment is far more primitive and more like that conceptualized by Bowlby and Ainsworth as protection and secure base seeking, thus simplifying the process of classifying attachment behaviors into dichotomous "secure" and "insecure," "organized" and "disorganized" categories. It is the emergence and growth of cognitive, emotional, behavioral, and autobiographical repertoires, skills, and capacities that start to weaken the definitional, descriptive, and operational aspects of attachment theory.

Despite the weaknesses in theory and construct definition, we can more fully appreciate the work of Mary Ainsworth and others who have not only categorized attachment, but through longitudinal, prospective, and retrospective studies have both suggested and demonstrated that patterns of attachment—not only in *individual* relationships, but across all relationships—are relatively persistent. That is, although the attachment style or experience implied by assignment to an "attachment category" can change during the course of development from childhood to adulthood, patterns of attachment seem to generally remain stable, showing up in adult representations of attachment that match childhood patterns in the same individuals. As Ainsworth says, although borne of a particular relationship—that is, with the caregiver—a quality comes to exist within the individual that far outlives the original relationship. Accordingly, attachment classifications appear to represent more than simply the experience of attachment within a *single* relationship but rather an expression of social connectedness across relationships, presumably because such representations are established within a dynamic model of self-in-society, driven by the internal working model.

One must conclude, therefore, that "attachment" is *not* about the relationship but is a quality that forms within the individual as a result of the early attachment experience, the product or shadow of that early experience. That quality, reflected in the dynamic interaction of any given relationship, is really resident within the individual. Thus, the seat of attachment must lie within the individual, and is appropriately the subject of interest in understanding the relationship between social connectedness and the development of sexually abusive behavior in children and adolescents. As sexually abusive relationships are, in most cases, *relationships*, as described in Chapter 15, and not simply arelational and faceless crimes, sexual abuse implies social connection and the drive for relationships gone wrong.

Seeing Through the Attachment Lens

Holmes (2001) describes attachment theory offering an integrative approach to therapeutic practice, and suggests that the overarching goals of social behavior involve the search for *intimacy* and *autonomy*. He writes that the capacity for intimacy results from attunement, not only in early life but throughout life, including the processes experienced during psychotherapy.

However, like Slade (1999), who writes that understanding the nature and dynamics of attachment *informs* rather than *defines* clinical thinking, Holmes cautions that we should not assume that defined attachment styles of patterns, such as anxious (ambivalent) or avoidant attachment, can be simply superimposed onto clinical phenomena. He writes that "many of the patients seen in clinical practice show both avoidant and ambivalent patterns at different times and in different circumstances" (2001, p. 29). Slade, too, warns that it "simply does not make sense to think of patients in terms of single, mutually exclusive attachment classifications that presumably remain stable within the clinical situation" (p. 585).

Recognizing that there are many valid and important ways to conceptualize and understand human behavior and motivation, and that attachment organization does not define all aspects of human experience, Slade (1999) writes that attachment theory offers a broad view of human functioning that can change the way clinicians think about and respond to their patients. She asserts that in "the same way that diagnosis serves as a guide (but not a recipe) in the treatment situation, notions of attachment organization provide a therapist with metaphors for thinking about early patterns of affect regulation and defense" (p. 585), and suggests it can add to the way that clinicians listen to the stories of their patients and understand their behaviors.

CONCLUSION: ATTACHMENT AND SECURITY

We can now say there are three interactive processes at play in the formation of this elusive quality of attachment: (1) the attachment behavioral system through which attachment behaviors are activated and employed to seek physical and eventually psychological safety, (2) the attachment experience itself, which fulfills or fails to fulfill the physical, emotional, and cognitive needs of the growing child and emerging self, and (3) the trait-like quality of attachment which forms within the psyche of the individual, embedded within the internal working model and thus carried forward into self-image, model of others, personality, and future relationships.

To this end, as described in Chapter 1, attachment is a process, an organized set of procedures, *and* a state of being. The attachment concept, then, is operationalized as a subjective experience, a style or pattern, and an approach or strategy. It is initially, and for many years, dependent upon a caregiving adult, and transformed through attunement and interactivity into an eventually mutually affectionate and important affiliation between coequal relational partners. "Attachment" represents both a sense of connection with others and the sense of selfhood and respect for other that resides within the individual. It is impossible to experience the attached relationship without the sense of self and others that drives the ability to have the experience.

Attachment, although perhaps not sufficient in and of itself, is nonetheless a necessary element in the development of personal identity. Accordingly, the attachment experience provides a foundation upon which identity is built and internalized. It either contributes to secure attachment and resiliency, serving as a protective factor against negative or hostile life circumstances, or as a developmental vulnerability in which insecure attachment not only fails to protect but under adverse conditions, and particularly when combined with other risk factors, is quite possibly a risk factor in its own right. In this model, only secure identity leads to a coherent and self-efficacious personality, whereas insecure and disorganized identities (in all their variances and forms) are linked to incoherent and ineffective personalities. As we conclude this chapter, it is reasonable for us to think that attachment is, in fact, a measure of security in self, others, and resulting relationships.

CHAPTER 6

Patterns of Attachment

Although we recognize that each mental model is unique to the individual within whose brain it resides, we also believe that the underlying biology and psychology that makes us human allows us to understand the experiences of individuals as common to and reflections of the larger human experience. Attachment, therefore, although an experience unique to each individual, is thought to follow a predictable pattern for all people, and can accordingly be described as an aspect and process common to the human experience of socialization. In order to better understand that experience, we explore how we become attached and what it means to be attached, as well as the outcomes of attachment. In the process, we find ways to observe and interpret thoughts, emotions, and behaviors that we believe are related to and reflect the attachment experience.

UNIVERSAL PRINCIPLES

In their critique of attachment theory, Rothbaum, Weisz, Pott, Miyake, and Morelli (2000) describe a universalist perspective held by attachment theorists to apply in all cases, comprising three central hypotheses. The *sensitivity hypothesis* holds that the process of attuned and accurate mother–child communication mediates optimal attachment in the infant. The *competence hypothesis* considers social competence to be an outcome of optimal attachment. The *secure base hypothesis* presumes that security is reflected in the use of the parent as a safe haven, in which exploration and the development of autonomy is sparked only when the child feels adequately protected and comforted by the parent.

Indeed, some principles are considered to be central to attachment theory, and virtually universal in application. Reporting that Ainsworth's three childhood attachment patterns have been found in all cultures in which attachment has been studied, van Ijzendoorn and Sagi (1999) derive four propositions that they believe exemplify the process of attachment, to which Holmes (2001) has specifically added three more. To these, we add the tenet that attachment is adaptive to the environment in which the child is reared, and the typical belief that attachment develops in a dynamic manner over time, influenced by multiple factors in the environment. We can thus identify nine principles, including those of Rothbaum et al. (2000), which indeed appear central and universal to attachment theory.

- *Universality of attachment.* All normatively developing infants become attached to one or more specific caregivers.
- *Normativeness of secure attachment.* The majority of infants are securely attached, regardless of culture.
- *Continuity of attachment.* Childhood attachment patterns affect relationship skills, experiences, and internal representations of relationship throughout the life span.
- *Adaptiveness of attachment.* In most cases, patterns of attachment form in response to the child-rearing environment and the behaviors of caregivers, and are most appropriately considered to be adaptive strategies rather than functional or dysfunctional modes of attachment.
- *Sensitivity-contingent attachment.* The basis for attachment security is contingent on the child-rearing environment, with particular respect to accurate and prompt caregiver response to the attachment signals of the child.
- *Attachment develops dynamically.* Attachment patterns, although intrinsically stable, are also influenced by multiple factors within the environment, as well as by characteristics that reside or come to reside within the child.
- *Attachment-contingent social competence.* The emergence of social competence, including self-regulation, relationship skills, and the development of cognitive and metacognitive skills, is directly related to security of attachment.
- *Attachment-contingent metacognition.* The capacity to accurately recognize and reflect upon the minds of self and others is built upon and leads to secure attachment, resulting in increased capacity for mentalization over time.
- *Attachment-reflected narrative competence.* Secure childhood attachment is reflected in adults through coherent and cohesive recollection, construction, and description of their current lives, history, and prior important relationships.

However, despite defining attachment theory to a large degree, these nine principles reflect ideas that are far from certain, and continue to be debated. In fact, attachment theory itself is equivocal about these principles, filled with inconsistent ideas that often modify, and sometimes contradict, the ideas and beliefs contained within the principles. In reviewing the validity of attachment theory, Bolen (2000) describes empirical support to be equivocal and partial, largely due to contradictions and inconsistencies of the theory, writing that many problems require resolution.

Universality

Although non-attachment has been described in infants and young children (Lieberman & Pawl, 1990; Zeanah, 1996; Zeanah, Mammen, & Lieberman, 1993), for the most part, attachment is considered to form in virtually every case, and in a manner that is usually adaptive to the environment in which the child is reared. Kim Chisholm (2000) writes that even children institutionally reared for the first three or four years of their lives are able to form attached relationships, once removed from the sterile environment.

In fact, with possible exceptions, there seems little doubt that attachment always occurs in some form, falling into one of several categories, usually described as secure or insecure. Attachment patterns that are difficult to understand or categorize are typically classified as disorganized or not classifiable, hence treating virtually all social behaviors as demonstrating some version of an attachment pattern. Moreover, it is widely held that most children and adults, in most cultures, are attachment secure, reflected in the tenet that ideal psychological and social fitness is mediated by secure attachment. However, although there is much support for the universality of attachment, discussed later in this chapter, the distribution of attachment types may reflect cultural influence, rather than universal patterns of attachment.

Adaptivity

Goldberg (2000a, 2000b), Crittenden (2000c), and others (Bates & Bayles, 1988; Greenberg, 1999; Greenberg, DeKlyen, Speltz, & Endriga, 1997; Greenberg & Speltz, 1998) argue that attachment strategies represent healthy adaptations to social context, rather than *good* or *deficient* forms of attachment. In fact, Crittenden and Goldberg consider the very terms "secure" and "insecure" to have pejorative meaning, implying health or pathology rather than environmental adaptation. Consequently, the terms "optimal" and "suboptimal" or "nonoptimal" are often used to describe the two poles; nevertheless, even these suggest the idea, not of adaptation, but of maladaptation or undesirability.

Rather than just semantic idealizations, ideas about adaptation are central to our conceptualizations about how attachment develops, the function it plays, and how it works to shape thinking, emotion, and behavior. James Chisholm (1996) writes that attachment patterns are facultative adaptations to the environment; children thus have the ability to survive in various environments by developing responses (in this case attachment patterns) that are tuned and appropriate to the environment. The "facultative" process allows certain characteristics (including aspects of social relatedness) to be shown or not shown, making it possible to live under a variety of social conditions, even without full social support. Pat Crittenden considers virtually every attachment pattern to be facultative or adapted. For her, the exceptions are those attachment patterns that are out of synch with the environment and are thus *temporarily* maladapted, disorganized, or otherwise disabled. If not reoriented back towards adaptation, it is these maladapted patterns that contribute to mental health problems because of the individual's inability to align them with environmental conditions. In other words, it is the adoption and internalization of an attachment pattern that does not match the environment that makes it unhealthy. She reminds us that "attachment is not a theory about happiness; it is about protection . . . happiness is desirable, but it is not essential to these ends; moreover, it can limit adaptive functioning under some conditions" (1997, p. 86).

From a neurobiological perspective, we can also see how attachment styles reflect adaptation and not maladaptation. In cases of early trauma, Teicher (2000) considers the underdevelopment of the left brain, and the resulting bias towards right brain processes, to be the result of early exposure to unsafe or stressful external environments. However, rather than considering this brain morphology to be the result of maladaptation, damage, or underdevelopment, he considers these physical developments to be successful adaptations to the social environment. Although Teicher (2000) started with the hypothesis that early stress is a toxic agent that damages normative brain development and leads to psychiatric difficulties, he later concluded that the brain is designed to respond to and be shaped by experience (Teicher, 2002). In response to ongoing maltreatment, trauma, or other adverse conditions in the environment, the development of right-hemisphere-dominated brain processing and its rapid, self-protective responses is an appropriate *adaptation* to an adverse environment, rather than evidence of malfunction or damage. In response to the behavior and attunement of the caregiving environment, "stress sculpts the brain to exhibit various antisocial, though adaptive, behaviors" (2002, p. 75).

It is quite likely that early experiences establish both developmental vulnerabilities (internalized risk factors) and characteristic resiliencies (internalized protective factors), setting the pace for that which follows in life. However, although secure attachment is considered to yield the most effectively functioning children and adults, and insecure attachment is believed to place the child at risk for later difficulties, none of these attachment categories are considered to be pathological, or even necessarily related to the development of later pathology. Although there is a far greater incidence of insecure attachment (as opposed to secure) among clinical populations, most individuals with insecure attachment styles do not develop psychopathology. Accordingly, although secure attachment is most associated with healthy and successful adaptation, insecure attachment is not considered to be pathological or otherwise disordered. Each of the organized group labels is considered to be descriptive only, and each attachment type is considered to be an *adaptation* to circumstances, neither positive nor negative.

Nevertheless, despite this theoretical leaning towards understanding all forms of attachment as adaptations rather than disorders, it remains true that secure attachment is considered as the preferred variant and is the attachment category most commonly found among both children and adults in the United States. In defining insecure attachment patterns as suboptimal, attachment theory asserts that when the child is raised in a non-optimal environment there is a price to pay in later development and functional capacity. However, such a conceptualization implies that it is insecure *attachment* that is suboptimal, rather than recognizing that it is the child-rearing *environment* that is suboptimal and which contributes to the development of attachment patterns that are adaptive to that environment (in this case, patterns of insecure attachment and their accompanying behavioral strategies).

Almost immediately, then, we see equivocation in attachment theory. Despite a belief that attachment is adaptive, we also see that *secure* attachment remains the normative ideal. In fact, this is one of those apparent contradictions that run throughout attachment theory, in its inability to clearly, consistently, and without contradiction define its own ideas. Despite asserting that attachment is adaptive, attachment theory in practice also unquestionably believes that suboptimal, or insecure, attachment leads to later functional difficulties, setting into motion the pathway along which significant dysfunctionality may later develop, whereas secure, or optimal, attachment does not. The contradiction is easily resolved, however, when one sees that the issue is social, and not psychological. That is, we must recognize that the dysfunctionality lies within the social environments that lead to insecure attachments rather than within the individual, although the insecurely attached child eventually reflects the dysfunctional environment in which he or she was raised.

CONTINUITY OF ATTACHMENT

As theorized, through internalization, experiences of the external world are mentally recreated and absorbed into enduring mental models that contain representations of the external world. This conceptualization is not limited to psychodynamic theory alone, but is also subscribed to by cognitive psychologists in the form of mental schemata, scripts, plans, and automatic thinking. In a biologically informed model, these are also neurobiological experiences, hard wired into the central nervous system. In such a model, the events and experiences of early life lay the groundwork for anticipating, understanding, and influencing future experience, and forming plans and scripts that will, partially at least, shape present and future automatic and intentional behavior.

There seems to be little doubt that early developmental experiences do, indeed, shape affect, cognition, and behavior, as well as setting the pace for later experiences. In a model of homeorhesis, considerable internal and external pressure keeps the individual on the path started early in life, contributing to the possibility, or even likelihood, of stability over time. Consequently, it is commonly asserted that early attachment patterns remain stable throughout life or, in the jargon of attachment theory, show concordance between childhood and adulthood. However, this is an uncomfortable position for attachment theorists because attachment theory is not intended to be deterministic. Accordingly, attachment theory is equivocal on the subject of enduring attachment patterns, professing that attachment patterns are both stable but can, and do, change over time. This is because attachment theorists are quite focused on describing the dynamic and changeable aspects of attachment, while also asserting the likelihood that childhood attachment patterns, established by 12–18 months of age, are the relatively stable building blocks of all that follows, establishing the first steps along a developmental pathway. The central idea in any such model, described by Belsky and Nezworski (1988), is that there is continuity only when future experiences support directions that have already been established. Change is possible when future experiences are inconsistent with and powerful enough to overcome the current trajectory. This is similar to the idea of inertia, in which things have a tendency to stay on the same track unless acted upon by an outside force. Early attachment experiences set the child along the developmental pathway, and remain stable unless there is outside intervention. However, with respect to the actual evidence of stability in attachment over time, it is, in fact, quite mixed.

Scharfe (2003) provides a excellent overview of research into the stability of attachment patterns, within and across different developmental epochs (such as attachment stability during infancy, and evidence of stability from infancy to young adulthood). She concludes that attachment has been shown to be moderately to highly stable across development, noting, not surprisingly, that variability in attachment status after infancy seems closely linked to environmental change and life style transitions. Lyons-Ruth et al. (1993) found that attachment behaviors at age 7 were predicted by attachment type at age 18 months, and Waters (1978) reported 96% stability in infants across a 6-month interval. Waters, Merrick, Treboux, Crowell, and Albersheim (2000) reported that 72% of 20-year olds who had been assessed at age 1, maintained the same attachment type when assessed as either secure or insecure (rather than using the two variants of insecure attachment) and 64% maintained the same attachment type when using a three-classification model (secure, insecure ambivalent, and insecure avoidant). Similarly, Main and Cassidy (1988) described 84% stability in attachment classification from ages 1 to 6. Solomon and George (1999a) also report high stability of attachment over time, with rates as high as 96% in the short-term reassessment of middle class infants, and 82% stability between the ages of 1 and 5, although they acknowledge lower stability in studies of pre-school children, and greater instability in patterns of insecure attachment. Kerns, Tomich, Aspelmeier, and Contreras

(2000) have also reported moderate to high stability of attachment in their sample of latency age children over a two-year period.

In their study of adults, Benoit and Parker (1994) found stability of 90% across an 18-month period, and Hesse (1999) reports a wide range of support for stable attachment as measured by the Adult Attachment Interview (AAI). In their assessment of adult attachment, Crowell, Treboux, and Waters (2002) found that 78% of their sample remained stable, although only 46% of those with unresolved attachment retained the same classification. They concluded that change was the result of stressful relationships and life experiences. As a variant of stability, with respect to the intergenerational transmission of attachment, Fonagy (1999a, 1999b) reports that several studies, including his own, have demonstrated that in 80% of cases it is possible to predict infant attachment at age 12 months on the basis of adult attachment classification made before the birth of the child.

On the other hand, many studies have found attachment stability to vary and prove inconsistent over time. In their study of 43 infants, Thompson, Lamb, and Estes (1982) found a low stability rate of 53%, which is little better than chance, noting that changes in attachment appeared to be related to changing family circumstances and child-rearing practices. In the longitudinal study conducted by Waters et al. (2000), 36% changed attachment types over the 20-year period to young adulthood, and some moved from a secure to insecure classification. In most cases that involved change from a secure to an insecure attachment category, or from an insecure anxious to an insecure avoidant category, stressful life situations were evident, suggesting that external stress and adversity may be implicated in such changes. Belsky, Campbell, Cohn, and Moore (1996) concluded from their study of 240 subjects that, because rates of stability were so low, ranging from 46 to 55%, stability of attachment cannot be inferred, writing instead that "it now seems *inappropriate* [italics added] to assume that stability rather than instability is the norm when it comes to the measurement of attachment security" (p. 924).

With respect to attachment style in adults, frequently measured by self-report questionnaire, Baldwin and Fehr (1995) reported that approximately 30% of their subjects changed attachment classifications during brief periods of time (1 week to several months), mostly within the insecure categories. They concluded that attachment style measured by self-report questionnaire is more likely to reflect the active relational schema at that moment rather than an enduring internalized disposition. Davila, Burge, and Hammen (1997) found a similar pattern in their study of 155 women, concluding that change in attachment pattern reflected one of several explanatory variables. Again, insecure more than secure individuals were likely to fluctuate in their sense of security partly, the authors speculate, because they lack a clearly coherent personal narrative, because they have a more amorphous sense of self, because they are more likely to have experienced symptoms of psychopathology that may influence perceptions of attachment, and because, they write, experiences of insecurity are tied to disturbances in personality.

Nevertheless, it seems likely that early attachment patterns do remain relatively stable, serving as the base for the developmental pathway, canalized by homeorhesis. However, coupling a developmental pathway model (changes are always possible, but they become increasingly difficult over time) with the ideas demonstrated in the work of Werner and Smith (with help, individuals can overcome great difficulty [1992, 2001]), we can understand both the stable/relatively deterministic branch of attachment and the shifting and adaptive/dynamic branch. In reviewing studies, we also see that secure attachment, once laid down in early life, is less likely than insecure attachment to change or erode over the life span. The good news is that, although insecure attachments are more unstable, they are consequently always able to, and sometimes do, move towards security and autonomy, or "earned" security.

NORMATIVENESS

It is widely accepted that secure attachment is the pattern displayed by most adults and children. Most typically about two-thirds of the population, based on the measurement of young children and adults (rather than adolescents), appear to experience secure attachment, with most of the remaining 33% experiencing a variant of insecure attachment (Goldberg, 1997; Levy & Orlans, 1998). Karen (1994) and Goldberg (1997) report that 10–14% of US infants and children are ambivalently attached, and 20–25% show patterns of avoidant attachment. Both Goldberg (2000a) and van Ijzendoorn and Sagi (1999) describe the majority of infants in all cultures studied as secure, and van Ijzendoorn and Sagi describe secure attachment ranging (in cultures studied) between 56–80% in Israel and 67% in the United States, with a mean average of almost 67% of children classified as securely attached.

That said, although insecure attachment appears to be experienced by approximately 33% of the general population, including both young children and adults, we can not presume that this includes adolescents as well. In fact, it may be that insecure attachment may be more common during adolescence, if only as a feature of adolescence itself, becoming secure once again in adulthood. That is, attachment research with non-clinical adolescents is relatively rare, but studies that have explored attachment and mental health in adolescents and young adults suggest that adolescent insecure attachment in the non-clinical population may be more like 40–45% rather than the 33% considered the norm for children and adults.

Regardless of the quality of normative adolescent attachment, Crittenden (1997) asks why, if secure attachment is optimal, the evolutionary process has not hard wired it into our brains? She describes the reason as both functional and contextual: cognitive, emotional, and behavioral strategies associated with secure attachment are not only defined by social and cultural conditions, but may be a disadvantage, and even dangerous, in adverse circumstances. That is, in a hostile environment, it may be strategically advantageous to be insecurely attached and thus more likely to survive such an environment. Nevertheless, the assumption of secure attachment remains the normative ideal, believed to reflect the attachment experiences of most children and adults.

Attachment from a Cultural Perspective

The idea that attachment patterns are actually adaptations to the social environment stands in contrast to the implication that secure and insecure attachment classifications actually reflect preferred and non-preferred (ideal and less-than-ideal) poles. From the contextual point of view, attachment is only suboptimal or maladaptive when attachment behavior does not fit with or promote adaptation to the social context. From the universal fitness perspective, attachment is *only* optimal when secure. However, *both* perspectives (attachment as healthy/unhealthy versus attachment as adaptive) are held true by attachment theory, representing one of those paradoxical problems inherent in attachment theory. It is of specific importance when, within different cultural contexts, attachment styles are assessed as optimal or suboptimal.

In fact, it is unclear whether the apparent normativeness of secure attachment is culturally influenced. As noted, in attachment theory the majority of infants and adults in all cultures studied are considered secure. However, Crittenden (2000a) reports that when non-middle-class and non-American children are included in studies, as well as children assessed as disorganized in their attachment, fewer than 66% of infants and young children are classified as secure, and this number decreases when attachment is assessed in older children. She and others note that several studies suggest that distributions of attachment patterns vary by culture, including both the avoidant and anxious ambivalent patterns as the predominant pattern in other countries (Germany, Israel, and Japan, reported in several well-known studies). Indeed, LeVine and Miller (1990) consider that the assessment of attachment in young children is based entirely on cultural conditions, with no utility outside the US middle-class family. LeVine (2002) goes further, and generally rejects attachment theory altogether, characterizing it as perpetrating pop psychology in which mental health risk is created out of normal individual differences. He considers the attachment model entirely grounded in western cultural ideology, rather than anything resembling universality.

Goldberg (2000a) recognizes that patterns and expectations associated with optimal attachment shift with respect to the culture within which attachment is observed and evaluated as optimal or suboptimal. She acknowledges that, although secure attachment has been considered optimal in middle-class America, "different patterns of parental behavior and accompanying patterns of organized attachment can be optimal under other cultural conditions" (p. 206). Hinde (1982) also notes the possibility of a cultural bias, not necessarily in the measurement of attachment, but in how attachment patterns are developed. He describes overwhelming evidence that the secure attachment pattern is clearly preferable in US society, but recognizes that in other cultures a different attachment pattern may be modal or even preferable, reflecting a different child-rearing style. This was highlighted by Grossmann and Grossmann (1981) in their study of German children in which they classified two-thirds of the children as insecure avoidant. They described a troubling and intriguing problem in this finding, asking which pattern (secure or avoidant) "should be considered species-adaptive" when two cultures (US and German) show distinctly different patterns of attachment in their children (p. 697).

Rothbaum et al. (2000) are critical of what they consider cultural bias in attachment theory. They describe attachment theory as ethnocentric and assert that, despite acknowledging cultural differences, attachment theory nonetheless maintains that such differences are relatively minor. In summary, they consider that attachment theory has adopted a universalist perspective that blurs and downplays cultural differences, "infused with cultural assumptions, leading to misguided interpretation" (p. 1102). As we have seen, van Ijzendoorn and Sagi (1999) and Holmes (2001) have, indeed, adopted such core ideas in their description of beliefs about attachment that they consider universal.

However, Chao (2001) considers it impossible and disastrous theoretical thinking to consider culture *before* attachment, as it would eliminate the possibility of any clear theory of attachment. She writes that this would require an attachment theory specific to each culture throughout the world, with a resulting indefinite and unmanageable number of mini-theories.[1] She considers that attachment theory must be enriched, but not overwhelmed, by culturally-driven categorical and methodological structures and an awareness of cultural specifics. In a similar vein, Karen Grossmann (2000) sets attachment pattern before cultural influence, writing that the nature of the attachment experience provides the basis for how cultural influences ultimately affect the developing child. "Viewed properly," she writes, "attachment is the very foundation for a child's ability to understand and participate in the extended social and cultural world" (pp. 92–93). In describing cultural influences on child rearing, Grossmann and Grossmann (2000) describe the parental task in all cultures as that of taking care of and enculturating their children. In so doing, parents prepare their children for the sort of situations they are likely to encounter in their culture and the social behaviors they are expected to master and demonstrate in coping with such circumstances, in order to "survive and thrive."

There may then be a cultural bias towards different attachment styles. That is, although attachment itself may be a biological imperative, the form it takes may not be. Nevertheless, rather than dismissing attachment theory as culturally irrelevant and impossible to apply across cultures, insisting that we be aware of culture and cultural bias in how we see and measure attachment, Crittenden (2000c) states nicely that "culture is the ground we walk on, but because it is always there and invariant, we rarely see it" (p. 5). In fact, if we were to adopt the culturally relevant perspective, we would not be able to make inferences about any human behavior or define human psychology, short of the indefinite number of mini-theories described by Chao. Crittenden's (2000a) perspective instead is that attachment patterns vary partly because they are adaptive to circumstances and culture, but also because they reflect a dynamic interplay among current circumstances, including individual experiences and characteristics that include maturation over time, thus allowing a wide range of possible strategies.

Attachment and Mental Health: Psychological, Social, and Pathological Functioning

On the face of it, regardless of cultural influence or terminology, high percentages of secure attachment in the general population suggest either that attachment is not a very strong indicator of emotional or behavioral disturbance, or that mental health problems exist largely *only* among insecurely attached individuals. This is because, despite relatively high levels of secure attachment, mental health problems are relatively widespread in American society. The US Surgeon General's report on mental health (US Department of Health and Human Services, 1999) estimates that 20% of Americans experience a mental disorder during the course of a single year, and Regier et al. (1988) reports that 15% of Americans adults meet the criteria for at least one substance abuse or mental health disorder. The Surgeon General's office also report that almost 21% of all children aged 9–17 show

---

[1] Van Ijzendoorn and Sagi (2001) write that with at least 1,200 different cultures and at least 186 different cultural areas, claims for the cross-cultural validity of *any* theory can only be made tentatively.

symptoms of a psychiatric disorder, with 11% demonstrating significant impairment and 5% experiencing extreme functional impairment during the course of any given year. Similarly, Levin, Hanson, Coe, and Taylor (1998) report broad mental health disorders in 12–20% and serious emotional disturbance in 9–13% of children and adolescents in the United States.

Of note, most of the reported patterns of secure attachment are based on measurement of the normative—or non-clinical—population, often in families somewhere in the middle-class range of socioeconomic status. However, when it comes to assessing the patterns of troubled children, adolescents, and adults a different pattern appears, in which secure attachment is far more limited, and insecure and disorganized attachments are more the norm. Studies consistently reflect a far higher proportion of insecure or disorganized attachments among adolescents and adults experiencing psychiatric difficulties, and a reduced and relatively low frequency of secure attachment compared to the general population.

In studying the sequelae of psychiatrically disturbed adolescence, Allen, Hauser, and Borman-Spurrell (1996) found that, when re-interviewed after 11 years, only 8% of 25-year-old adults who had been psychiatrically hospitalized at age 14 could be classified as securely attached, compared to 45% of a non-clinical cohort. Similarly, Fonagy et al. (1996) found that only 11% of the 82 emotionally disturbed young adults in their study could be classified as secure, compared to 59% of a non-clinical control group. In their study of 133 adolescents in outpatient and residential treatment, Adam, Sheldon-Keller, and West (2000) reported that only 16% could be classified as secure-autonomous. As nearly half the sample had disorganized attachment patterns connected to unresolved trauma, their conclusions showed support for the idea that early traumatic experiences are linked to later psychiatric disorders. Moretti and Holland (2003) studied 170 adolescents referred for assessment and treatment due to severe behavioral disturbances, classifying only 7% as secure. In her study of 127 behaviorally and emotionally disordered adolescents aged 10–17, Scharfe (2003) similarly reported that 94% of the adolescents were insecurely attached. Hesse (1999) reports similarly high percentages of suboptimal and disorganized attachment classifications among clinical populations measured by the Adult Attachment Interview (AAI), compared to the relatively low incidence of insecure attachment classifications in non-clinical populations.

In a study of 62 low income families, Lyons-Ruth, Alpern, and Repacholi (1993) classified 71% of aggressive 5-year-old children as disorganized. In a later study of fifty 7-year-old children (Lyons-Ruth, Easterbrooks, & Cibelli, 1997), 42% were classified as secure, but of the children identified by teachers as highly externalizing and aggressive, 83% were classified as disorganized. Further, in these children, externalizing behaviors at age 7 were predicted by attachment-related assessments made at age 18 months, suggesting the stability of assessment patterns over time. With particular regard to disorganized attachment, Solomon and George (1999b) state that whereas disorganized attachment may be found in approximately 15% of infants in non-clinical middle-class samples, disorganized attachments are to be found among approximately 80% of maltreated children.

There is certainly support, then, for the idea that emotionally and behaviorally disturbed children are, or become, less secure in their patterns of attachment. We also see that severe disruptions in childhood attachment can be correlated with serious adolescent and adult psychopathology, including dissociation, depression, anxiety, and other primary mental health disorders; personality disorders; substance abuse; and aggression; and, described below, sexually abusive behavior. Levy and Orlans (1998) conclude that children with a history of severe attachment difficulties develop aggressive, controlling, and conduct-disordered behaviors, contributing to the development of antisocial personality. They describe these children, often by mid-childhood, demonstrating antisocial behaviors that exemplify self-gratification with blatant disregard for family and social rules and standards.

However, the reader is cautioned to remember that correlation is not causation. That is, there may be a common link between insecure and disorganized attachment patterns and psychopathology, or it may be that underlying causes of psychopathology or the pathology itself precedes (and perhaps determines) insecure attachment rather than vice versa. We do recognize, however, that suboptimal attachment and suboptimal psychological functioning commonly appear together. We also see a level of general disturbance, not in itself considered pathological, reflected in emotional, behavioral, and relationship difficulties in later childhood and into adolescence. For instance, Allen et al. (2002) studied 117 moderately at-risk adolescents at ages 16 and 18, assessing attachment organization and autonomy at age 16. Earlier attachment security predicted relative increases in social skills from age 16 to 18, whereas insecure attachment predicted increasing delinquency during this period. Increases of this sort, in social competency or in social difficulty, are considered closely related to and predicted by earlier attachment patterns.

In fact, evidence consistently suggests that the emotional and neural sequelae of insecure attachment, and particularly when attached to neglect, abuse, or other forms of overt maltreatment, contribute to psychological and neurobiological vulnerabilities. If we consider attachment "disorders" to be disturbances in internal working models, we're describing the quality and internalization of the attached relationship as the starting point and ongoing shaper of the development of mind (and selfhood). When insecurely developed, the internal working model subsequently leads to disturbances in emotional regulation, thinking and cognitive processes, behaviors, and social relationships.

Nevertheless, as noted, there is little evidence to support the idea that *any* of the organized attachment classifications are directly related to psychopathology. However, it appears that troubled children and adults are more likely to emerge from the population of insecurely attached children than from the securely attached population. "It is . . . clear that insecure attachment is not itself a measure of psychopathology, but may set a trajectory that, along with other risk factors, may increase the risk for . . . psychopathology" (Greenberg, 1999, p. 482). In fact, if pathology does later emerge, it is most likely to be linked with *disorganized* attachment.

EARLY ATTACHMENT AND LATER SOCIAL FUNCTIONING

Levy (2000) has written that beyond the basic function of secure attachment, attachment and its reciprocal relationship to exploration and ultimately self-regulation contributes to other developmental functions that children must accomplish:

- Learning basic trust and reciprocity, serving as a template for future emotional relationships.

- Exploring the environment with a feeling of safety and security, leading to healthy cognitive and social development.
- Developing the ability to self-regulate, resulting in effective management of impulses and emotions.
- Creating a foundation for the formation of identity, including a sense of competency, self-worth, and balance between dependence and autonomy.
- Establishing a prosocial and moral framework, involving empathy, compassion, and conscience.
- Generating a core belief system, which comprises cognitive appraisals of self, caregivers, others, and life in general.
- Developing a defense against stress and trauma, incorporating resourcefulness and resilience.

Levy writes that children who begin their lives with secure attachment fare better in all aspects of their later capacity to function well, a finding much reported in the literature of attachment theory. Similarly, Siegel (1999) writes that emotional regulation lies "at the core of the self" (p. 274), and asserts that the development of self-regulatory skills emerges from early dyadic (caregiver–child) attachment experiences. In fact, there is a consistent belief that later social functioning, in childhood, adolescence, and adulthood, is built upon earlier attachment experiences. Greenberg (1999), for instance, reports substantial evidence that secure attachment within the first two years of life is related to later higher sociability with other adults and children, greater compliance with parents, and more effective emotional regulation. Conversely, he reports that insecure attachment prior to age 2 is related to lower sociability, poorer peer relations, symptoms of anger, and poorer behavioral self-control during the pre-school years and beyond. Already described is MacDonald's (1985) conclusion that children who have not formed secure attachment by age 2 are likely to have later behavioral and emotional difficulties. Sroufe (1988), too, writes that securely attached children are later more self-reliant, more cooperative with adults, and more empathic and less hostile with peers than insecurely attached children.

Perry, Perry, and Kennedy (1992) report that insecurely attached children believe that they cannot depend on others and that they will be treated unfairly. They thus become more disposed than securely attached children towards conflict and oppositional defiance as strategies initially designed to gain the attention and response of caregivers. Greenberg and Speltz (1988), likewise, write that insecurely attached young children are likely to show behavioral problems that, in many cases "can be viewed as strategies for gaining the attention or proximity of caregivers who are unresponsive to the child's other signals" (p. 206). However, such children succeed in behaving in ways that annoy and alienate supporters. Consequently, they become and are experienced by others as negative, attention seeking, and sometimes needy, engaging in the development of self-fulfilling developmental pathways in which they sadly contribute to their inability to get needs met, thus strengthening negative and insecurely driven behavior. Indeed, Egeland and Carlson (2004) describe insecure children as more likely than secure children to experience others as negative in social situations, and in pre- and elementary school are likely to be and are experienced by others as dependent on teachers and less confident and assertive. They and others (for instance, Greenberg, 1999; Thompson, 1999) describe clear patterns of social functioning emerging by age 9 or 10 that are predicted by earlier attachment patterns, with securely attached children showing greater social competency, doing better on social tasks, and engaging in healthier and more fulfilling social relationships than insecure children.

Moretti and Holland (2003) conclude from their studies that secure attachment is linked with adaptive functioning in adolescence, while insecure attachment predicts poor psychological outcomes. Greenberg et al. (1997) concur, writing that data from the Minnesota High Risk Project link insecure attachments in early childhood to later behavioral and social problems. This supports the idea that although insecurity is not viewed as synonymous with disorder, it does serve as a risk factor that interacts with and is potentiated by other development vulnerabilities experienced by children: "We believe that attachment process may be an important risk factor but neither a necessary nor a sufficient cause for later externalizing problems" (p. 199). Similarly, Bates and Bayles (1988) write that there is insufficient justification to consider attachment insecurity alone as a clinical problem. Nevertheless, although they assert that there is no justification for using early attachment classification as a screening tool for intervention, they note that we must pay attention to the manner in which attachment difficulties intersect with and potentiate other risk variables.

Although Thompson (1999) reports similar findings with respect to early attachment and later functional social behavior, he also writes that outcomes are diverse and multi-determined, making their relation to early attachment security complex and contingent. His point is that the theorized relationship between early attachment and later psychological functioning is neither clear nor straightforward. He writes, "two decades of inquiry into the sequelae of early attachments yield this confident conclusion: Sometimes attachment in infancy predicts later psychosocial functioning, and sometimes it does not" (p. 274).

RECOGNIZING RESILIENCY

Michael Rutter (1987) describes resilience in terms of individual variations in risk response: where some people are overwhelmed by pressure and adversity, others resist stress and overcome obstacles. Indeed, some children are so resilient that they appear "psychologically invulnerable" to use Anthony's (1987) term, apparently able to weather earlier and ongoing difficulties and still establish themselves as capable and competent, including children born into and raised under high-risk conditions. As described briefly in Chapter 5, in a 30-plus year study of 505 Hawaiians born on Kauai in 1955, Werner and Smith (1992) assessed that approximately one-third were born "with the odds against successful development" (p. 2).

They described the high-risk children in their study experiencing significant degrees of perinatal stress, growing up in chronic poverty, reared by parents with little education, and in many cases living in disorganized families. "Their homes were troubled by discord, desertion, or divorce or marred by parental alcoholism or mental illness" (p. 2), some of the very problems and factors considered to give rise to insecure and/or disorganized patterns of attachment. By age 10, two-thirds of these children had developed serious learning or behavioral problems, and by age 18 had delinquency records, mental health problems, or pregnancies. However, Werner and Smith report that by age 18, one-third of the 201 high-risk children had "developed into a competent, confident, and caring young adult" (p. 2), growing "into competent young adults who loved well, worked well, played well, and expected well" (p. 192). By age 31/32 they report that not only had most of the delinquent adolescents in this group *not* continued into adult criminal careers, but most of these high-risk youths, including those who had shown serious coping problems in adolescence, "had staged a recovery of sorts by the time they reached their early 30s" (p. 193). In their 40-year follow up, Werner and Smith (2001), having tracked 70% of all individuals born on Kauai in 1955, noted that only 16% of the original cohort were doing poorly, despite an original 33% assessed as high risk during early life, and at age 40 most of the high-risk group had staged a functional recovery.

Werner and Smith describe the balance that exists at each developmental stage in the individual's life, from childhood through adulthood, between stressful life events and risk factors that exacerbate vulnerability and protective factors that enhance resilience. In addition to parental competence and caregiving styles that were described by Werner and Smith as protective buffers in the lives of high-risk children, other protective factors included temperamental attributes that brought positive response from adults, affectional ties with parents and other family members, and an external, non-family support system. Self-esteem and self-efficacy are described as central in the healthy and resilient development of these children into competent adolescents and adults, facilitated through supportive adult relationships: "the resilient youngsters in our study all had at least one person in their lives who accepted them unconditionally" (p. 205).

Of particular interest here, by young adulthood some of the resilient children had developed attachment styles that detached them from their parents and siblings whose own difficulties threatened the well-being of the resilient children. Based on this brief description, these young adults may well be assessed through the Adult Attachment Interview as dismissing in their attachment style, the more-or-less adult equivalent of the insecure avoidant pattern in childhood, but in these resilient adolescents and young adults this suggests and supports the idea that attachment patterns reflect *adaptation* rather than maladaptation, even if resulting in a distant and perhaps avoidant or dismissing pattern of attachment. Slade (1999) perhaps addresses this very issue when she writes that attachment represents only one aspect of human functioning, and "although attachment processes define an aspect of human experience, they do not *define* an individual in all his or her complexity" (p. 590).

Risk and Protection

One may argue that resiliency is based upon the presence and action of protective factors, or those elements that mediate, negate, or buffer against the effects of stress or allow individuals to successfully engage with and overcome adverse conditions. Rutter (1987) describes both risk and protective factors as most relevant at key turning points in life, because the power of each is most critical at this juncture. This is because what follows may be substantially altered by the effect of the factor, strengthening, weakening, or otherwise altering the previous trajectory. Although Rutter describes risk and protective factors as instrumental and most significant at turning points, he seems to be describing such factors in terms of their dynamic qualities. It is clear also that other risk and protective factors exist that are static in nature, and exist all along, affecting and shaping life in ways far less dramatic than those risk and protective factors described by Rutter. These static factors act on trajectory, not simply at critical life junctures, but throughout, and are instrumental in the very process of shaping trajectories—one might argue, even before they become trajectories, in part determining what trajectories our lives take.

Attachment is somewhat unique in this regard, because, as described in Chapter 5, we can think of attachment as both a risk factor *and* a protective factor. That is, insecure attachment lends itself to difficulties during the course of ongoing development. Alone, insecure attachment is not a strong enough factor to create or ensure problems, but a lack of secure organized attachment is a risk factor that may become heightened as it interacts with other risk factors, contributing or leading directly to social and/or emotional problems.

Sroufe (1988) describes insecure attachment as a marker or risk factor, suggesting a developmental pathway that may be related to later problems. Although not a causative factor, insecure attachment may place individuals at greater risk for pathology. He describes secure attachment as the other side of the equation, noting that securely attached individuals are more able to develop, seek, use, and benefit from social support when needed; a history of secure attachment is an "important factor in buffering individuals with respect to stress and their ability to cope with stress" (p. 29). Whereas insecure attachment may be a risk factor, secure attachment serves as a protective factor. It strengthens the individual, buffering against adverse social conditions and neutralizing or weakening internalized factors that may otherwise increase risk.

CONCLUSION: EARLY EXPERIENCE IN JUVENILE SEXUAL OFFENDERS

Insecure attachment is considered to develop in part due to either insensitive or adverse early developmental condition. However, because of extremely limited studies of attachment patterns in sexually abusive children and adolescents, we cannot describe the distribution of attachment types among these juveniles. However, without question, juvenile sexual offenders fall into the category of children raised under adverse conditions.

Ryan (1999a) writes that when physical violence, sexual abuse, and parental neglect are included as maltreatment factors, "almost the whole population (of juvenile sexual offenders) can be seen to have experienced some type of maltreatment" (p. 134). In their wide ranging review of the professional literature on juvenile sexual offending, Righthand and Welch (2001) agree, suggesting that childhood experiences of physical abuse and family violence are both common and seem associated with sexual offending, and Bailey (2000) writes that "juvenile sexual offenders often come from disadvantaged backgrounds with a history of victimization" (p. 206). Similarly, Weinrott (1996) writes that "however flawed the measures of personal victimization, it seems pretty clear that juvenile sexual offenders are likely to have encountered some form of abuse or parental neglect" (p. 23). Pithers, Gray, Busconi, and Houchens (1998) suggest that an important link to the development of adolescent offending of all types may in part be due to the insecure and damaged attachment that develops between children and parents as a result of neglect and maltreatment, and Bailey writes that physically abused and neglected infants typically develop insecure attachments with care givers. Lee, Jackson, Pattison, and Ward

(2002) agree, stating that family dysfunction often goes hand in hand with childhood difficulties among sexual offenders, concluding that childhood sexual, physical, and emotional abuse and family dysfunction are general developmental risk factors.

Lewis, Shanok, and Pincus (1981) report that 79% of the incarcerated juvenile sexual offenders in their study were witnesses to domestic violence. Print and Morrison (2000) conclude that "adolescents who sexually abuse others often have major care deficits and frequently grow up in families in which they experience and/or witness violence, lack of empathy and a lack of sexual boundaries" (p. 296). Experiences such as these certainly make it likely that sexually reactive children and juvenile sexual offenders will be classified as insecurely attached, and help to explain the usually exhibited suboptimal functioning. Nevertheless, it is absolutely clear that childhood maltreatment alone does not make it likely that a juvenile will engage in sexually abusive behavior. It is equally unlikely that insecure attachment serves as anything more than a significant element along a developmental pathway, in which insecure attachment serves as a risk factor and secure attachment as a protective factor.

Armsden and Greenberg (1987) write "that the central concern of attachment theory is the implication of optimal and nonoptimal social attachments for psychological fitness" (p. 428). Nothing, of course, could be more fitting or better suited for the population of sexually troubled and abusive children and adolescents with whom we work. However, in recognizing attachment difficulties as a significant pathway and even a risk factor in the development of sexually abusive behavior, we are making a substantial shift in how we envision sex offender specific treatment. This means that, as we adopt an approach informed by attachment theory, our understanding and treatment of both juvenile and adult sexual offenders will move away from cognitive-behavioral, psychoeducational, and relapse prevention models that have until recently dominated the field and our thinking, towards a psychodynamic model of relationships and connection. Of course, this does not for one moment mean that we will abandon those treatment models, but that they and new ideas, including ideas about attachment, will become incorporated into a more inclusive and integrated assessment and treatment model that recognizes both cognitive and psychodynamic theory and application.

This model will explicitly recognize the role of the treater and the treatment environment as central and critical to the treatment, and move the therapeutic relationship and the therapeutic alliance into the spotlight, as we, after all, address issues of attachment, attunement, social connection, and relationship.

CHAPTER 7

The Assessment and Classification of Attachment

In observing behavior in large numbers of people, we seek commonalities that allow us to make inferences about typical human experiences, such as attachment. By sorting those behaviors into groups of similar behaviors we not only condense and organize information, but are able to infer meaning about the behavior of populations rather than just individuals. In effect, we create schemes that are themselves models of the internalized schemes and models that we believe drive and organize individual behavior. This level of organization often results in classificatory schemes, which is certainly the case with attachment theory.

However, classificatory schemes create their own difficulties, and must be used in an informed manner. For instance, organizational schemes often create typologies, and these can be problematic. With respect to the evaluation and treatment of sexual offenders, for instance, it has been difficult to come up with typologies that allow different sexual offenders to be classified into different "types" of sexual offense categories. The same is true of any type of categorization scheme, including the classification of attachment, in which it is difficult to produce typological categories that are mutually exclusive. That is, we cannot easily create exhaustive typologies in which people can be seen to fit into only *one* category without also fitting into another category. The result, although useful, is often a limited typology in which individuals may be "force fit" into the closest available category, thus neglecting other important information about the person. This leads to models that simplify data without capturing the complexity of the phenomenon, although they may give the appearance of completeness.

Classification systems of all kinds are simply too limited to capture the complexity of human life. We must keep this in mind as we examine the assessment and classification of attachment. Of particular note, however, are the models of Patricia Crittenden, who recognizes a dynamic-maturational model of attachment; Kim Bartholomew, who conceptualizes attachment categories as the byproduct of a dynamic interrelationship between mentalized representations of self and representations of others; and Chris Fraley and Phillip Shaver, who describe attachment from the point of avoidance-approach behaviors and experienced anxiety. Each of these models goes beyond the simple assignment of attachment into discrete categories, and recognizes dynamic and changing interactions.

These are dimensional models that recognize the continuous, or gradated, quality of attachment and, in Crittenden's case, the explicit role played by developmental changes over time. Nevertheless, some variant of Ainsworth/Bowlby's original conceptualization of secure and insecure attachment remains at the center of virtually every attachment scheme.

THE CLASSIFICATION OF ATTACHMENT

In the original strange situation process, Ainsworth and her colleagues observed children under controlled experimental conditions, grouping toddlers based on similarities in behaviors that they believed were related to patterns of attachment. Rather than providing descriptive names or assigning value to any particular group, Ainsworth simply labeled the groups A, B, and C. It was only later that descriptive labels were applied to each group, identifying attachment behavior as either *secure* (group B), *insecure avoidant* (group A), or *insecure ambivalent* (group C). Main and Solomon (1986) later reclassified a number of the children in earlier studies into group D, devising a fourth category of attachment behaviors that they named *disorganized-disoriented*.

Although these group labels are intended to be descriptive only, the labels used (secure or insecure) nevertheless imply that a positive or negative value is attached to one group or another. However, in attachment theory each form of behavior is considered as an adaptive variant of attachment, neither positive nor negative, designed to gain and maintain proximity to an attachment figure. The premise is that children *will* attach to a perceived caregiver, and are hard wired to do so, regardless of the quality or the reciprocity of the relationship. Attachment labels are intended only to identify the type of attachment behavior displayed by the child, rather than pass judgment on one variant or another.

Secure Attachment

The secure pattern reflects in the child an internalized sense that the caregiver, and eventually others in the environment, are responsive, reliable, and can be depended upon. Through processes described in earlier chapters, this translates into a internalized positive sense of others and a positive sense of self.

The insecurely attached child, on the other hand, is described as "more likely to become caught up in a cycle of selective perception of the world as unpredictable or threatening, and thus shows less exploration, less competence, and greater helplessness. This, in turn, could lead to a greater likelihood of behaving in such a way as to increase the probability that experiences will be adverse" (Armsden, McCauley, Greenberg, Burke, & Mitchell, 1990, p. 684). Whether secure or insecure, we recognize that children eventually engage in the world in such a way as to affect it as much as it affects them, in a dynamic interplay. The product thus becomes the producer, in which the child becomes "an active participant in shaping and creating experience . . . (bringing) to each new developmental challenge all of his or her prior experiences, and the child and the context become mutually transforming" (Egeland & Carlson, 2004, p. 28).

Insecure Attachment: Anxious/Ambivalent

Although both patterns of insecure attachment are considered to contain elements of anxiety, it is this type that is usually most closely associated with anxiously driven thoughts, feelings, and behaviors. Insecure anxious/ambivalent (or resistant) attachment reflects an internalized uncertainty about the primary caregiver's availability or responsiveness, at the same time that the infant experiences a need for the caregiver's attention. Not only unsure of the caregiver, the child is also uncertain about his or her own capacity to attract or be worthy of the required attention. This leads to behavioral patterns that are anxious, dependent, and needy, and sometimes also rejecting or angry as frustrations and doubts about the parent are expressed through externalizing behaviors. Ambivalence about and resistance to the relationship are shown by the child, who simultaneously needs and rejects, cares for and is angry at, and wants and doubts the parent (and eventually others).

Bowlby (1979) describes this child living in constant fear of separation from the attachment figure, triggering attachment behaviors that Johnson (2003) describes as hyperactivated. Anxious, clinging, and aggressive behaviors escalate, becoming heightened and intense in order to draw and maintain attention from the parent, described by Bowlby (1980) as the "over-ready elicitation of attachment behavior" (p. 39). Resistant children, then, experience the attachment figure as unreliable and perhaps unpredictable, learning that attention can only be assured with a great deal of effort on their part. In the strange situation, these (group C) infants are extremely distressed by separations and often refuse to be comforted upon reunion. Hence, exploratory and independent behaviors are consequently foreshortened and limited due to separation fears and preoccupation with the caregiver.

This attachment pattern is characterized and driven by affective (emotional) strategies to both maintain attachment relationships and for self-regulation and equilibrium, rather than cognitive strategies that are not driven by feelings and require the ability to detach from anxiety.

Insecure Attachment: Avoidant

Although also considered anxious in origin (and sometimes referred to as anxious avoidant), this attachment pattern reflects a more distant or detached attitude towards both relationships and emotions. Consequently, anxiety is more clearly associated with ambivalent attachment, and avoidant attachment is linked to a detached form of insecure attachment. Also built upon a lack of confidence in the caregiver's capacity, the avoidantly attached child has internalized the expectation that the caregiver, and, later, others, will not only be unavailable but may actively reject or ignore the child. Bowlby (1980) describes this as the partial *deactivation* of attachment behavior, and "overtly the opposite of anxious attachment (or) . . . that of compulsive self-reliance" (1979, p. 138).

In the strange situation, avoidant infants (group A) appear to intentionally ignore the mother upon reunion, often showing no more interest in the parent than in the stranger. Accordingly, over time the child appears detached and distant from attachment (and other) relationships. However, within a non-optimal child-rearing environment, it is believed that detached behavior represents an organized strategy that allows the child to maintain proximity and connection to a parent it has come to experience as unreliable.

Unlike the affectively driven strategies of the anxiously (ambivalently) attached child, avoidant attachment is closely associated with cognitive strategies. Crittenden (1997, 2001) describes these as tactics employed by children who have not learned how to elicit the desired level of caregiving, but have learned not to make demands that might cause the parent to further retreat from the relationship, and thus avoid negative consequences by seemingly disengaging and remaining distant from the relationship.

Disorganized Attachment

The disorganized attachment pattern (also referred to as disorganized/disoriented) reflects a pattern of behavior that is considered disconnected and sometimes bizarre, lacking an obvious or coherent system or arrangement behind the behavior, and at times even dissociated. Described by Solomon and George (1999b), in young children observed during the strange situation, behaviors upon reunion lack organization or obvious rationale and reflect little capacity to handle stress. These infants behaved unpredictably and engaged in behaviors that were sequentially and sometimes simultaneously contradictory, such as approach and avoidance behaviors, and showed incomplete and sometimes slowed or frozen movements and facial expressions, as well as other behaviors and behavioral expressions that appeared confused and disconnected. Prior to Main and Solomon's (1986) conceptualization of disorganized attachment (type D attachment), in Ainsworth's original strange situation experiments children with these behaviors had been assigned to an unclassifiable category.

The infant's experience of the parent as frightening or frightened is considered a primary and likely cause of disorganization (Schuengal, Bakermans-Kranenburg, van Ijzendoorn, & Blom, 1999a; Schuengel, Bakermans-Kranenburg, & van Ijzendoorn, 1999b; Solomon and George, 1999a, 1999b). In the first case, the parent is experienced as both the protector and, at the same time, the cause of the danger. An obvious and sad example of this, of course, is the parent who actively abuses the child and is thus the source of fear and the source of protection.[1] Remaining close to the parent or avoiding contact both cause distress. The second hypothesized primary cause for disorganized attachment, lies at the other end of this same dimension.

The frightened (rather than frightening) parent is experienced by the child as somehow inept, incapable, or her/himself frightened and anxious. Under conditions that activate the attachment behavioral system, Solomon and George (1999b) cite as a primary cause of disorganized attachment the inability or failure of the caregiver to adequately respond to, and thus deactivate, the child's attachment behaviors (which only occur when attachment

---

[1] It is this situation that is also hypothesized to form the basis of traumatic attachment, or an attachment bond formed as the direct result of the attachment figure serving as the controller and cause of the abusive relationship. Although the concept is not particularly well defined, it implies that attachment is inevitable in almost every case, even under adverse conditions. The term suggests that attachment develops even within and against a backdrop of trauma, and in which attachment is intimately shaped by developmentally traumatic events which are imprinted into the attachment experience, and therefore the central nervous system.

needs, and hence needs for security, are met). In this scenario, the parent is considered on the frightened side of the frightening/frightened equation, due to the parent's inability or lack of desire to resolve the child's anxiety. In either case, frightening or frightened, imprinted into the internal working model, the disorganized child experiences the attachment figure as incapable of providing protection, and even as the source of danger, and experiences itself as vulnerable and helpless. This presents an untenable and unresolvable situation, resulting in a psychic organization that is disorganized, fragmented, and incoherent, because the child simultaneously seeks physical closeness and mental distance from the caregiver (Fonagy, 2001b).

This model is similar to that proposed by Kernberg (1976), who describes the roots of borderline personality lying in the young child's experience of the parent as either the source of frustration and therefore potentially threatening, or unable to resolve frustration, and therefore incapable. In his view, the origins of pathology lie in deficient object relations embedded into the child's mental map. This idea is reiterated by Schore (1994), who describes the experience of being raised by a dysregulating parent who initiates but is unable to repair misattunement and breaks in attachment. Disorganized attachment is believed to be often linked to the experience of having either a frightening or frightened parent—the parent who is either the source of the threat or unable to resolve the danger and soothe the child.

Although the disorganized pattern can be linked to a secure or insecure attachment style (perhaps itself reflecting disorganization), it is most often linked to anxious ambivalent attachment, typically associated with affectively-driven experiences and behavior rather than underlying cognitive strategies. In fact, it is *only* disorganized attachment that is considered to be linked to the later development of functional psychopathology and mental illness, and West, Rose, Spreng, and Adam (2000) write of accumulating evidence that more closely implicates disorganized attachment with psychopathology than with organized forms (secure or insecure) of attachment. Indeed, some have written that disorganized attachment *itself* is pathological. Zeanah (1996), for instance, considers disorganized attachment to be a severe attachment disorder that indicates that the child is *already* disordered.

DISORGANIZED ATTACHMENT IN ADOLESCENTS

What happens to disorganized attachment in children as they grow up? Holmes (2004) describes adolescents and young adults with disorganized attachment as controlling, aggressive, unable to self-soothe, unable to disengage from painful relationships, and prone to dissociation, and he links disorganized attachment to the development of borderline personality disorder. Fonagy (2001b) similarly relates disorganized attachment to the development of controlling and violent behaviors in adults, writing that, by midchildhood, patterns of early disorganized attachment have evolved into rigid behavioral strategies for controlling situations and people, including aggression. In adults, he considers disorganized attachment to be reflected in fragmented self-representations and a need for control over others. Indeed, we have already seen (Chapter 6) that both insecure and disorganized attachment is more prevalent than secure attachment among clinical populations of children and adolescents.

However, as we shall see, it is not entirely clear how to recognize or measure attachment in older children and adolescents, including disorganized attachment. In fact, descriptions of disorganized attachment in adolescents and adults usually do not even slightly resemble the behaviors demonstrated by disorganized young children, and rarely show the active symptoms of dissociation that Holmes suggests is linked to adolescent disorganization. Indeed, for the most, Holmes and Fonagy's descriptions suggest that the odd behaviors evident in disorganized infants disappear in most adolescents and adults, instead somehow resolving into rigid, controlling, aggressive, and/or other antisocial character structures. Descriptions of these behaviors in adolescents and adults as evidence of disorganized attachment not only seem to more reflect the development of insecure avoidant and/or antisocial personality structures, but do not meet the conditions of "frank disorganization" described by Hilburn-Cobb (2004) in adolescents and adults who demonstrate a complete failure of organization. In fact, it is due to the lack of resources demonstrated by this latter population that disorganized attachment is most linked to psychopathology, in which we are witnessing, not aggressive or controlling behaviors, but psychopathological ideation and behavior. Even in this population, dissociation itself is a relatively rare condition, and still a subject of some uncertainty in terms of both diagnosis and prevalence (American Psychiatric Association, 2000).

As a result, in adults, we are more likely to see *unresolved* attachments, rather than behaviors that suggest disorganized attachment, at least as it is manifested by young children. Adults and adolescents who exhibit a level of behavior and confusion similar to those young children are likely to be considered psychiatrically disturbed, and are relatively rare in the general population, as predicted by attachment theory. Adult attachment schemes thus tend to use the descriptor *unresolved/disorganized* in assessing adult attachment, rather than *disorganized/disoriented*. We should, thus, be careful in describing disorganized attachment in adolescents, and ascribing the cause of controlling and distant, and even frankly antisocial, behavior as disorganized attachment. If we follow the evidence shown by disorganized infants and toddlers, we recognize that disorganized attachment is manifested in deeply disturbed ideation and behaviors that reach a psychiatric level, rather than behaviors that more reflect disturbed but insecure attachment.

ATTACHMENT STRATEGY

Regardless of descriptive labels or variants on those labels, the three primary patterns of observed attachment behaviors (secure, insecure avoidant and insecure anxious) are considered to have organized strategic value, designed to ensure that the child has access to an attachment figure. As attachment is conceived as a hard-wired tool for evolutionary survival, every child is biologically compelled to seek attachment to someone, even if the attachment figure is insensitive and not attuned to the needs of the child, unavailable, neglectful, rejecting, malicious, or abusive.

Crittenden (1997, 2000a, 2000c, 2001; Crittenden & Claussen, 2000) describes the capacity of the securely attached child to balance affective and cognitive strategies for forming relationships with and maintaining proximity to attachment figures, integrating these into a flexible and effective whole. However, the insecure forms of organized attachment are considered to be more closely related to either affective *or* cognitive strategies. Crittenden asserts that the anxiously attached child does not use, or necessarily trust, cognitive strategies, instead engaging in and relying upon affectively driven behavior to maintain caregiver proximity, attention, and engagement. Avoidant attachment, on the other hand, is typically associated with cognitive strategies. Crittenden characterizes this attachment pattern by a cognitive style of attachment behavior in which affect and emotion are not to be trusted and the child instead learns to use cognitive strategies to maintain proximity.

Patterns of attachment, then, reflect organized behavioral *strategies* for developing and maintaining attachment. Each pattern, or attachment type, results from the child's adaptation to caregiver and environmental circumstances, reflecting the capacity for goal-corrected behavior in children as they eventually come to recognize and respond in the most adaptive manner to the social environment in which they are reared. The disorganized category is the exception, representing an inability or significant lack of capacity to form a coherent and cohesive set of behavioral strategies. It represents a pattern of attachment behavior that is not organized, or does not seem to be, and appears disoriented, erratic, and irrational. This attachment pattern, most associated with the development of psychopathology, perhaps reflects a disjointed and disoriented, and even dissociated approach to forming and maintaining attachment. Indeed, despite links between insecure attachment and later difficulty, disorganized attachment, as noted, is the only attachment type significantly linked to later pathology. However, it is not clear whether disorganized attachment contributes to or leads to later pathology, whether disorganization results from or is evidence of a prior pathology, or whether a common factor leads to the coexistence of psychopathology and disorganization and is thus responsible for both.

Relatively few individuals are categorized as disorganized in attachment, but when they are the classification denotes a lack of coherence in thinking and behavior, at least as it pertains to maintaining attachment, and consequently reflects a lack of organized attachment strategy. Although rare in the general population, among clinical populations there is a far greater incidence of disorganized attachment. Hilburn-Cobb (2004) describes behaviors characteristic of disorganized attachment as inexplicable, anxious, and labile, often with inappropriate or bizarre affect mismatched with the situation, with "frank disorganization" demonstrated by the failure of organization. She describes disorganized children and adolescents struggling to maintain attachment relations, and more extreme "frankly" disorganized adolescents lacking any control system whatsoever.

Crittenden (1997) does not specifically recognize this classification, and in most cases considers disorganization to be a temporary, destabilizing condition. Children who might be classified as disorganized in other systems are classified by Crittenden as A$^+$/C$^+$, considered to be emotionally vulnerable much of the time, prone to dysfunction under low stress conditions, and blending and vacillating between unintegrated affective and cognitive strategies, neither of which may be effective.[2] These children display both avoidant and ambivalent behaviors, and may at times appear disorganized, but Crittenden essen-

---

[2] Crittenden has recently added the "+" modifier to her A/C and AC categories, to distinguish well-adapted cognitive (A) and affective (C) strategies from those that are overlaid with compulsive or coercive strategies and may be maladaptive or dangerous (P. M. Crittenden, personal communication, October 2004).

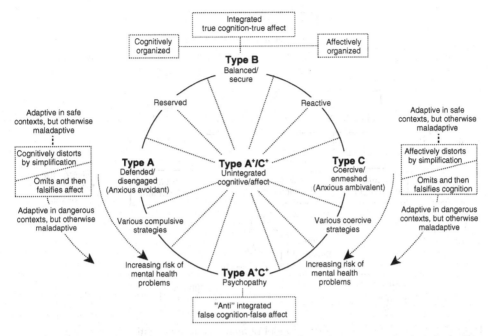

Figure 7.1 Crittenden's dynamic-maturational model of attachment organization, including "standard" attachment labels: secure, avoidant, and ambivalent. The dashed lines represent gradated attachment categories among major types B, A, & C and A+/C+. (Synthesized, and with kind help, from Crittenden [1997, 2000a, 2001] and personal communication, 2004)

tially considers *all* attachment behaviors to be adaptive to particular relationships and circumstances.

A variant of Crittenden's model is shown in Figure 7.1, synthesized (and much simplified) from her work over several years, including more commonly used attachment designations, although these are not terms typically used by Crittenden. As a dimensional model, attachment classifications can fall at graduated points, as sub-types, between the major types (A, B, C, and A+/C+), shown by the intersecting dashed lines within the circle. In Crittenden's model, as children age and mature their models and strategies of attachment may change (hence dynamic-maturational).

Figure 7.2 outlines attachment strategies organized into a hierarchical attachment schema, in which attachment types are discrete, representing a *categorical* and dichotomous model of attachment classification.

THE CLASSIFICATION OF ADULT ATTACHMENT

Attachment in adults is most typically classified into types that closely approximate those of childhood (secure, insecure avoidant, insecure anxious, and a disorganized variant). Although a number of assessment measures have been designed to measure and classify

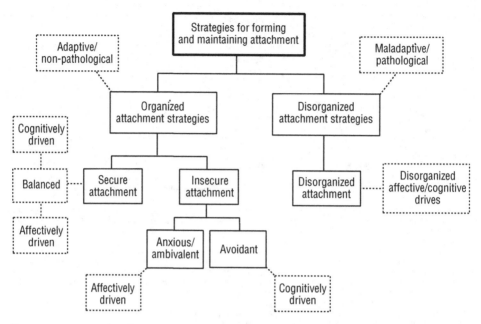

Figure 7.2 Hierarchical-categorical model of attachment organization and security

adult attachment, the "gold standard" is the Adult Attachment Interview (AAI) against which other adult tools have anchored their designs and measured their validity. Thus, the categorical system of the AAI is both the adult correlate to the attachment classification system derived from the childhood strange situation and the attachment system that serves as the basis of most other adult classification systems, most of which use romantic relationships to assess attachment.

However, it is important to recognize that the AAI does *not* measure a pattern of attachment in adults, but instead measures the experience of childhood attachment as reported by adults during structured interviews. In asking "What is being assessed?," Hesse (1999) writes that rather than assessing secure or insecure attachment, the AAI assesses adults "as being in a secure versus insecure *state of mind with respect to attachment*" (p. 421). Using the AAI, four corresponding patterns of adult attachment experiences have been devised, which largely reflect the experience of adults in their relationships with their own parents. These four categories in adults, often used or from which variants are drawn, are *secure/autonomous*, *dismissing* (matching the insecure avoidant category in children), *preoccupied* or *enmeshed* (insecure anxious), and *unresolved/disorganized* or *disoriented/disorganized* (disorganized).

Bartholomew and colleagues (Bartholomew & Horowitz, 1991; Bartholomew & Shaver, 1998; Griffin & Bartholomew, 1994) also define four prototypical adult attachment patterns. Drawn from the interaction between two dimensions, self-representation and representations of others, this model does not identify a disorganized category at all. Instead it identifies three insecure attachment patterns, rather than the two identified in most childhood and adult models. *Secure* attachment results from a positive sense of self and others and is, of course, the equivalent of secure/autonomous attachment. The *preoccupied* attachment classification is characterized by a negative self model and a positive model of others, and is the counterpart of insecure anxious ambivalence in which the individual is highly dependent on others for acceptance and affirmation. Bartholomew breaks insecure avoidant attachment into two prototypes that she identifies as either *dismissing*, which is the result of a positive sense of self and a negative model of others, or *fearful* attachment derived from a negative self-image and a negative sense of others.

Bartholomew's model is dimensional, recognizing that attachment is more like a continuous attribute that lies along gradated continua rather than a concrete quality that exists in discrete categories. That is, one can be more-or-less anxious rather than anxious or not anxious, or more-or-less avoidant. Nevertheless, as shown in Figure 7.3, her model does define four prototypical attachment categories that result from the interaction between two dimensions—self-representation and representations of others. The model also incorporates the alternative anxiety and avoidance dimensions identified by Griffin and Bartholomew (1994), and defined as the key dimensions by Fraley and Shaver (2000),

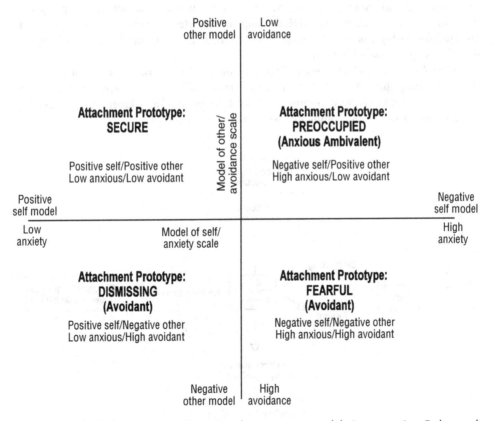

Figure 7.3 Bartholomew's two-dimension four-category model, incorporating Fraley and Shaver's anxiety and avoidance scales, and including approximate childhood equivalent labels. (Adapted from Bartholomew & Horowitz, 1991; Griffin & Bartholomew, 1994; and Fraley & Shaver, 2000)

who regard these as more basic and applicable to the attachment process, than the dimensions of self/other representations identified by Bartholomew.

Fraley and Shaver consider that Bartholomew's dimensions force a perspective that may not fit actual psychological processes, as well as being psychologically too sophisticated. In the first case, for instance, they write that the idea that anxious-preoccupied individuals hold a positive view of others, as shown on Bartholomew's "other" continuum, is unlikely to fit the actual psychological profile of many ambivalently attached individuals. The same is true in the case of dismissing-avoidant individuals who, along the "self" dimension, must be considered to hold a positive view of themselves, also quite unlikely in many actual cases. In the second case, as other species, in addition to precognitive infants, show attachment behaviors and yet do not have the capacity to hold reflective and representational ideas such as those implied by the self/other dimensions, it must *not* be necessary to have the capacity to form internalized views of self and others. Fraley and Shaver, instead, consider the avoidance/anxiety dimensions to be more basic and universal. Still, it must be said that their dimensions also fail to hold up in the real world for some of the same reasons they apply to the Bartholomew dimensions. It is quite unlikely that dismissing individuals, for example, are necessarily low in anxiety. It is equally true that individuals preoccupied with relationships nevertheless sometimes show high avoidance to relationships, or to put it another way, some individuals fearful of relationship are nonetheless preoccupied with them.

Figure 7.4 shows the relationship between adult and childhood attachment classifications, including the AAI and Bartholomew categories. This is followed by Figure 7.5, which provides an overview, comparison, and description of attachment types, including those characteristics most commonly associated with each type.

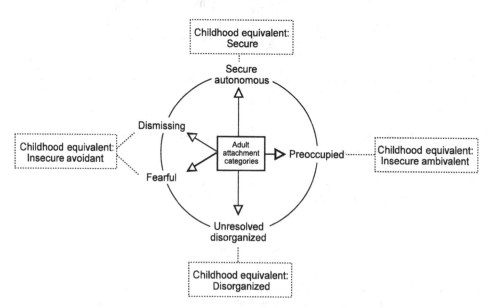

Figure 7.4 Adult attachment categories (including Bartholomew), with childhood equivalents

Attachment type	Sense of security	Alternative descriptions	Affect/ cognitively driven	Self- representation	Representation of others	Behavior
Secure	Secure	• Balanced • Stable • Autonomous	Both (balanced)	• Independent • Interdependent • Confident	• Available • Responsive	• Well adjusted • Adaptive
Insecure ambivalent	Anxious	• Resistant • Preoccupied • Enmeshed • Coercive • Dependent	Affect driven	• Incapable • Dependent • Self doubting	• Rejecting • Not available • More capable	• Needy • Clingy • Angry • Resistant
Insecure avoidant	Anxious	• Dismissing • Detached • Defended • Fearful • Neutral • Limiting	Cognitively driven	• Independent • Self-reliant	• Unreliable • Untrustworthy • Not capable	• Distant • Hostile • Antisocial • Controlled
Disorganized	Anxious	• Disoriented • Unresolved	Scattered	• Poorly formed	• Confused • Uncertain • Unresolved	• Disorganized • Labile • Contradictory • Irrational

Figure 7.5 Overview of attachment types, with examples of typical characteristics

CLASSIFICATION: CATEGORICAL OR DIMENSIONAL?

Crittenden and Bartholomew note that it is not necessarily appropriate or accurate to describe attachment falling into distinct and discrete categories, and instead assert that attachment behaviors are dimensional, with shades and blends of attachment behaviors rather than discrete extremes. Holding that there is no evidence for a true attachment typology, Brennan, Clark, and Shaver (1998) also favor a dimensional approach to classifying attachment styles, writing that categorical models can only be justified on the basis of convenience. Fraley and Waller (1998) describe attachment "types" (or distinct categories) as inadequate to "capture the natural structure of attachment security" (p. 108), describing adult attachment as a variable on which people differ in degree rather than by type of attachment. Fraley and Spieker (2003) assert that the primary difference between the categorical and dimensional models is that attachment in people varies continuously rather than categorically.

Nevertheless, the most popular and common models of attachment classification are eventually categorical, rather than dimensional. This includes the non-typological models of Bartholomew (Bartholomew & Horowitz, 1991) and Fraley and Shaver (2000), which, although conceptualizing attachment along two dimensions, nevertheless describe adult attachment as falling into one of four attachment prototypes despite an underlying dimensional structure. Although they hypothetically allow for shades of attachment, these models do not actually allow for graded differences in attachment categories. This is not true of Crittenden's dynamic-maturational model, which, although having several anchor points and labels (type A, B, and C, or defended, secure, and coercive), identifies multiple gradations and combinations of attachment strategies that form a continuous circle of finely distinguished attachment behavior that covers many real-life circumstances, also recognizing change over time and by social context. Unfortunately, Crittenden's model is complex, and ironically the lack of clear categorical language makes the model complicated to use and fully comprehend. We see, then, the trade off between complexity and utility: the loss of nuance in Bartholomew's model is compensated by its usefulness and simplicity, whereas the subtlety and sophistication of Crittenden's model is weakened by its complexity and changing language when applied in different settings and in different circumstances.

However, dimensional models recognize (i) that people change over time and in different contexts, (ii) that attachment must be measured as a point along a continuum of possible points, rather than assigned as a particular fixed type (hence, people are more-or-less secure, rather than "secure" or "insecure"), and (iii) that attachment categories are the result of multidimensional interactions, described by Fraley and Spieker (2003, p. 425): "In fact, without at least two dimensions, the key distinctions that have been highlighted by attachment theory and research cannot be represented. It is for this reason that we have emphasized a two-dimensional system over a single dimension of security." They also argue that although attachment *behaviors* are likely to developmentally change over time, the underlying *dimensions* that shape these behaviors are not likely to vary across development.

Despite their support for dimensional over typological models, Fraley and Spieker acknowledge that data do not support one classification scheme over the other. On this point, Waters and Beauchaine (2003) conclude that "attachment theory is indifferent" to the structure of attachment classification, whether categorical (taxonomic) or dimensional. In other words, regardless of how they are assessed, categorized, and reflected back, the basic ideas and principles of attachment theory are believed to be sound and do not depend on classification models to prove their validity as descriptions of social functioning and psychological development.

CHAPTER 8

Measuring Attachment

It is difficult to measure attachment, and obviously requires a clear working model of what attachment means and what attachment behaviors look like in the real world and under defined conditions. For the most part, attachment studies have been directed towards very young children, up to and including pre-school, and these largely involve observations and interpretations of observed behaviors. Next to young children, attachment patterns have most been studied in adults, both with respect to their memories and descriptions of their relationships with their own parents and in romantic adult relationships. Although a number of self-report paper-and-pencil questionnaires have been developed to measure adult attachment, mostly aimed at romantic relationships,[1] for the most part the *Adult Attachment Interview* (AAI) is the preferred form of attachment study in adults.

The AAI attempts to measure *coherence* in the capacity of adult subjects to narratively describe and reflect upon their early and ongoing relationship with their own parents and lessons learned, as well as their desires for their own children. Through providing an autobiographical description of their own experience, the AAI measures the current level of coherent, cohesive, and rational thought in the individual. This measure of coherence is considered to be de facto evidence of a well-integrated sense of self, which both reflects and is a product of a balanced and secure childhood attachment experience, thus giving rise to the secure attachment designation in the adult. For Siegel (1999), such coherence is evidence of the individual's capacity for integrative bilateral brain functioning, using and blending left and right brain processes, a reflection of the early attachment experience in which the attuned caregiver develops and enhances in the child the capacity for such integration and self-regulation.

Nevertheless, administering the AAI is a costly and time-consuming process, and, as with studies of young children, requires observation or direct interaction and later interpretation following a code book that classifies, defines, and recognizes previously coded behaviors. Although the AAI is sometimes used with adolescents, it is designed specifically for adults and for this reason, as well as its impracticality, is rarely used in studies of adolescent attachment. For that matter, it is seldom used in assessing attachment in adults, in which case assessment is instead measured by self-report questionnaires.[2] Even

---

[1] For instance, the Experiences in Close Relationships Inventory, Relationship Questionnaire, Relationship Scales Questionnaire, Peer Attachment Interview, Family Attachment Interview, and History of Attachments Interview, all of which have been developed by Shaver, Fraley, Bartholomew and their colleagues.

[2] Baldwin and Fehr (1995) concluded that attachment self-reports are invalid because they measure the relational schema of the moment, rather than an enduring internalized attachment experience.

when the AAI is used, it is not measuring attachment *behaviors*. Instead, through a semi-structured interview, it is designed to access the experiences of attachment embedded in the internal working model, through the spoken narratives of adults, largely about their own parents.

In fact, it is not entirely clear how to assess attachment in either adults, older children, or adolescents. This is especially true when one considers that the nature of attachment as a physical survival mechanism in children is no longer a necessity for adults, nor, usually, for adolescents. In fact, as stated repeatedly, it is not clear what attachment means in adults and adolescents. Although there is a great deal of emphasis on adult attachment, it is still not an area that is well defined or understood, and requires a great deal more investigation (Crowell & Treboux, 1995). As a result, many of the self-report adult attachment instruments in use measure romantic and other intimate relationships, on the assumption that such relationships may adequately be considered attached relationships.[3]

In addition to instruments that specifically aim at recognizing and assessing attachment in adults, however, there are many other measurement tools available that measure aspects of social relatedness and connection in adults and adolescents, including measures of empathy, emotional loneliness, and personal security. Unlike adult attachment measures, these do not purport to assess attachment per se, and are not based on attachment theory. In studying adult attachment, the use of other instruments requires the researcher to find ways to weave these into a model of adult attachment that may or may not match the ideas of attachment theory. The same is, of course, true in research on adolescent attachment.

ASSESSING ATTACHMENT IN ADOLESCENTS

Although the AAI is sometimes used to assess attachment in adolescents, it is a stretch. This is primarily because the interview asks about the subject's experience as an adult, as well as asking several questions about the subject's own children. This first presumes, of course, that the subject has children, and in the case of adolescents stretches the point further, having to substitute an "imagined" child in place of a real child. The interview is, in fact, designed for adults who are also parents, but has been stretched and "tweaked" to allow its use with both adults who are non-parents and adolescents who have not necessarily even yet reached late adolescence, late alone adulthood.

However, other adolescent assessment measures are also limited, if only because they depend entirely on self-report rather than observations (as in infants) or interviews (as in the AAI), both of which allow interpretations to be derived from clinical experience rather than self-reported answers. Self-reports not only depend on the comprehension and honesty of the subject, but also upon the construction of the self-report instrument itself. Such instruments must be based on variables that accurately reflect the underlying constructs, thus having construct validity. That is, questions must actually tap into variables that directly address "attachment," rather than, for example, anger at parents or self-

---

[3] Fraley and Shaver (2000) describe romantic relationships as a legitimate target for assessing attachment in adults, although this practice is criticized by Rutter (1997) on the grounds that concepts of attachment in children should not be extended to sexual relationships.

esteem, or even, as Baldwin and Fehr (1995) note, relationships as they are experienced at that moment (rather than underlying and enduring aspects of attachment).

Of course, this means that we must fully understand the construct being assessed, and hence have the ability to operationalize it in the form of a questionnaire. This is not true of the state of our knowledge about attachment in adolescents. Accordingly, although it is easy to describe aspects of relationships or social connection that we wish to explore through self-report, these may not be valid indicators of attachment. For instance, the Inventory of Parent and Peer Attachment (IPPA), described below, includes a measure of peer relationships, but such relationships are clearly not considered by attachment theory to represent attachment. This variable, then, cannot be said to be a valid measure of attachment (according to attachment theory). Because the IPPA does assess peer relationships, however, as an aspect of *attachment* rather than *affiliative* relationships, and the IPPA is accepted as a valid measure for the assessment of attachment, it de facto rewrites or modifies attachment theory without the empirical evidence to do so. To use a term common to attachment theory, the definition and inclusion by the IPPA of peer affiliations as attached relationships is not lawful. Until we clear up what truly represents attachment in adolescence, despite being a useful measure and yielding some good information, it is quite possible that, at least in this regard, the instrument is not measuring attachment at all. Indeed, this reflects a flaw in the construction of attachment theory itself, because it is not at all clear what attachment looks like at different ages, including adolescence. Other than observing attachment behaviors in young children, for whom attachment is most clearly defined, this makes it exceedingly difficult to recognize and assess attachment, then, in older children, adolescents, and adults.

RECOGNIZING ATTACHMENT IN ADOLESCENTS

Lopez and Glover (1993) describe the belief that the parent–adolescent relationship promotes or inhibits adolescent separation and individuation, and facilitates the development of a stable sense of self in the adolescent. For the most part, then, attachment theorists have begun to associate the present experience of attachment in adolescents with past and current parental relationships. Adolescent attachment is therefore most typically assessed by exploring and measuring thoughts, feelings, and behaviors evoked in adolescents by or directed towards their parents. This includes use of parents as a base of support, nature of the relationship, quality of communication, reliability and capability of parents, and so on. The outcome of such assessment is assignment to a classification type believed to be related to attachment status. Attachment across the life span is believed to be connected to attributes of self-esteem, self-regulation, independence, and social competence. Accordingly, the relevance and accuracy of adolescent attachment measures is studied by comparing the resulting attachment-related classification to independent measures of such attributes, in which "characteristics of secure attachment will be associated with social competence" (Kenny, 1994, p. 400).

June Sroufe (1991), for instance, connects parental control and affect, as well as family characteristics and structure, to the resiliency and level of personal control found in adolescents. Her study of 41 adolescents and their families linked adolescent ego resiliency with positive family functioning, and both adolescent under- and overcontrol were considered the results of emotionally unsafe families. With respect to undercontrol, in which children are easily stimulated and lack the ability or willingness to regain control (suggesting the affectively driven anxious attachment mode), families were characterized as highly stimulating, unrestrained, and lacking limits, and either threatening or with blurred boundaries around adult–child roles and relationships. In the case of the overcontrolled child, described by Sroufe as rigid, suppressing emotions, and maintaining tight personal control based on fears of vulnerability (resembling descriptions of cognitively driven avoidant attachment), the family is described as emotionally unsafe and threatening. In their study of 121 young Scottish criminal offenders, aged 15–22, Chambers, Power, Loucks, and Swanson (2000) note a high level of parental overcontrol, and link high levels of anxiety and depression in adolescents with low levels of perceived parental care, thus implicating both quality of care and parental control and protection with adolescent functioning. As they use the Parental Bonding Instrument, an attachment-based instrument described below, they are clearly linking adolescent–parent attachment to adolescent functioning.

In their study of 131 adolescents, aged 14–18, defined by the researchers as moderately at-risk (based largely on family socioeconomic status), Allen, Moore, Kuperminc and Bell (1998) also linked attachment status to psychosocial functioning in the adolescents. Using a range of measures of attachment and social functioning, they concluded that adolescents assessed with secure attachment to parents showed greater social competence and less emotional distress and/or delinquent behaviors than adolescents assessed as insecurely attached in their parental relationships. They suggest that security derived from attached parental relationships generalizes to the capacity for effective functioning in a range of social situations and interactions. In a later study of 117 moderately at-risk adolescents, aged 16–18, Allen et al. (2002) found support for the idea that attached relationships to parents predict increased social skills development over time. On the basis of their study of 213 non-clinical adolescents, aged 12–19, using an attachment tool that was the forerunner to the IPPA, Greenberg, Siegel, and Leitch (1983) also provide support for the belief that the quality of parental relationships is linked to self-esteem and satisfaction with life. They report that high-stress life events were moderated by positive parent–child relationships and also report that the quality of parental, more than peer, relationships is influential in predicting a sense of well-being, supporting the idea that family relations bear a causal influence on well-being.

INSTRUMENTS AND THEIR IDEAS ABOUT ADOLESCENT ATTACHMENT

Each of the instruments described below contains ideas about what it means to be attached as an adolescent or young adult, stated or inferred in their defined scales. They clearly capture important and useful information about the relatedness of adolescents and young adults to their parents and, in some cases, to peers. However, it is not entirely clear that the information captured actually measures attachment in adolescents (particularly as we don't quite know what that means). This is partly true because these instruments are limited to assessments of attached relationships to parents, rather than the more global model of attachment that we assume develops during adolescence and into adulthood, that is far broader in scope and certainly free of the dependence upon parents experienced by young children.

That is, even if we assume that measuring the feelings of the adolescent towards or about the parent(s) accurately reflects adolescent–parent attachment, it is not entirely clear that *adolescent–parent* attachment is the same as that larger and more *global* model of attachment. Such a global model is described by Overall, Fletcher, and Friesen (2003). They theorize that internal working models of relationships that are limited to specific types of relationship, such as relationships with family members, friends, and romantic partners, are nested under and governed by a larger internalized model of relationships. As a specific class of relationship, nested within Overall and colleagues' global relationship model, it is not clear whether a measurement of adolescent–parental attachment accurately represents the perhaps more complex and more complete experience of attachment in adolescence.

Finally, as we consider the assessment of adolescent attachment through self-report, we must further ask, following Baldwin and Fehr (1995), if it is possible that self-reports of adolescent–parent relationships are transitory, based on passing feelings or experiences of that moment rather than the enduring qualities considered intrinsic to attachment. However, as noted by Lyddon, Bradford, and Nelson (1993) in their review of adult and adolescent self-report measures, we must also evaluate the utility of these tools in helping to illuminate the therapeutic process and thus help clients to recognize, address, and overcome relational problems and make changes in internal working models. They write that "perhaps the most important contribution of attachment measures lies in their ability to provide reliable and valid means for assessing changes in clients' working models over the course of therapy" (p. 394).

Each of the instruments described below has been subjected to tests of validity and reliability, and each is built on some variant of attachment theory, although none directly results in or attempts to classify an attachment status. There is, instead, an assumption that relationship security, satisfaction with parental relationships, and feelings about parents are attributes that are tied to and accurately reflect an adolescent's attachment status. Consequently, each largely proposes the importance of the parent as an enduring attachment figure, and hence a figure who enhances internal security, provides confidence, and can be counted on as a source of safety and support from which exploration can occur. As primary attachment figures and caregivers, parents are considered to have helped to instill in the adolescent child the ability for self-regulation, the capacity to cope with stress, a sense of independence, a confidence in the parent, and a desire for an ongoing relationship with the parent. Accordingly, we expect to see these attributes of attachment reflected in self-reports, as well as being able to match reported experiences with and feelings about parents (positive or negative) against observable real-life behaviors that demonstrate such attributes in the child.

Although none of the available adolescent measures assigns adolescents to any specific or direct attachment type (such as secure or insecure), such attachment classifications are often made when using adult attachment tools, such as the AAI, the Relationship Questionnaire (RQ), or Relationship Scales Questionnaire (RSQ). However, Bartholomew (2004) warns that neither the RQ nor RSQ is intended to be used as a categorical measure of attachment, and outcomes should be described with respect to the subject's general orientation to close relationships or orientation to a specific adult, peer relationship.

Inventory of Parent and Peer Attachment

The IPPA, authored by Armsden and Greenberg (1987), descended from the earlier Inventory of Adolescent Attachments (Greenberg, Siegel, & Leitch, 1983), is probably the most commonly used of the adolescent attachment self-report instruments, and is based on the conceptual framework of attachment theory. Like the AAI, the IPPA attempts to tap into the internal working model, in this case by assessing bilateral aspects of the affective/cognitive dimension of attachment, tapping into positive experiences of trust in attachment figures and negative experiences of anger or hopelessness that result from unresponsive or inconsistent attachment figures. The IPPA was originally based on a sample of 179 college students, aged 16–20, although it has since been used with adolescents as young as age 12. The most current version of the IPPA comprises three sets of 25 questions, each in a mother, father, and peer category, regarding how well each of these figures serves as a source of psychological security. For each figure, attachment subscale scores are yielded in the areas of *Trust* (degree of mutual trust), *Communication* (quality of communication), and *Alienation* (extent of anger and alienation), which coalesce to yield attachment scores in either a high or low *security* classification (but not security of attachment, although it is implied that security equals attachment). Following their original study, Armsden and Greenberg concluded that self-esteem and satisfaction with life are highly related to the quality of parent and peer relationships, and adolescents classified as high security appear well adjusted.

Adolescent Attachment Questionnaire

The AAQ, developed by West et al. (1998) is based directly on the three-category classification system of the AAI. It is based on two sample populations, one of which comprised a clinical population of 133 adolescents aged 12–19. The second was a non-clinical group of 691 adolescents in the same age range. The AAQ is also a self-report, consisting of three scales consisting of three questions each. The *Availability* scale measures the adolescent's confidence in the parent, the *Goal-corrected Partnership* scale assesses the adolescent's sense of empathy with the parent, and the *Angry Distress* scale assesses the amount of anger towards the parent. High scores on the availability scale correspond to secure attachment, low scores on the goal-corrected partnership scale correspond to dismissing (avoidant) attachment, and high angry distress scores correspond to preoccupation (ambivalent) attachment. The authors do note that although designed to correspond to the AAI, the scales cannot be said to directly measure security or insecurity in the relationship.

Adolescent Unresolved Attachment Questionnaire

The AUAQ, also developed by West et al. (2000), was normed on the same two samples used in the development of the AAQ, and is intended to assess the nature of disorganized, or unresolved, attachment in adolescents, measured along three scales. Based on a total of 10 questions, the *aloneness/failed protection* scale assesses perceptions of parental care and responsiveness, the *fear* scale measures fear about loss of the parental relationship, and the *anger/dysregulation* scale evaluates emotional responses to perceived lack of care. Adolescents in the clinical sample also completed the AAI, and this resulted in a rather unwieldy classification in which these adolescents were classified either in some variant of the AAI unresolved/disorganized classification or a second classification that incorporated all of the other non-disorganized AAI categories. The authors report that, although the AUAQ scales correlate well with the AAI unresolved classification, these scales cannot be used to classify individuals as disorganized, and this can only be done through the use of the Adult Attachment Interview. Based on *a priori* assessment as unresolved/disorganized, the authors conclude that the AUAQ scales can be "regarded as assessing unresolved adolescents' perceptions of self and their attachment figures only" (p. 502), admonishing that the scales should not be regarded as a direct measurement of unresolved attachment.

Parental Bonding Instrument

Authored by Parker, Tupling, and Brown (1979), the PBI is designed to measure the quality of the attachment bond between parent and child, as perceived by the child, although it was designed for and normed upon *adult* children (fifth-year medical students) and their experience of their parents as remembered prior to age 17. The PBI comprises 25 self-report questions scored in two dimensions, as experienced by the child; in their review of self-report measures of parent–adolescent attachment, Lopez and Glover (1993) describe the PBI as reflecting actual, rather than imagined, parental behaviors. *Care* measures affection and empathy at one end and indifference and emotional coldness at the other, while *Control/Overprotection* ranges between intrusion and prevention of independence to independence and autonomy. Based on the way they rate their parents, subjects are grouped into one of four types of attachment bonds with classifications resulting from the interaction between the care and control continua: optimal bonding (high care, low protection), affectionate constrained bonding (high care, high protection), affectionless controlled bonding (low care, high protection), and absent or weak bonding (low care, low protection). Chambers et al. (2000) report that the PBI may be used to recognize levels of parental contribution to psychological and behavioral difficulties, with respect to levels of parental care and control as perceived by the subject.

Parental Attachment Questionnaire

The PAQ, developed by Kenny (1987), is based upon Ainsworth's ideas about attachment and intended for use with late adolescents and young adults ages 18–21, and considers that parents continue to serve as a secure base even into late adolescence. Normed on 173 first-year college students, the PAQ is now a 55-item questionnaire that measures the perceived quality of parental relationships, interest in interaction with parents, emotional behavior directed towards parents, and help seeking behavior and satisfaction with help received from parents. The PAQ attempts to provide an adult analog to the variables observed in the strange situation, resulting in three subscales: *Affective Quality of*

Relationships, *Parents as Facilitators of Independence*, and *Parents as Source of Support*.

Despite these few tools, however, the assessment of attachment in adolescents falls into somewhat of a limbo, between the assessment of attachment in adults and the assessment of young children up to about age 7 for whom there are a series of useful measures.[4] In the case of both adolescents and latency age children between approximately ages 7 and 12 (for whom there are virtually no attachment measures), this is largely due to our lack of clear understanding about attachment in this age range, falling between the clearly *dependent* form of attachment found in infants and young children and the *romantic* and *child-rearing* forms of attachment found in adults.

MEASURING ELEMENTS OF ATTACHMENT

We can only consider measuring attachment when we define it in a way that allows us to recognize elements that comprise the construct, each of which is amenable to description and observation. In addition, by doing this we can recognize transformations in attachment throughout the life span. In fact, as a construct standing alone from its constituent parts (i.e., its subscales), "attachment" has little meaning.

However, we can deconstruct attachment by recognizing that it comprises several distinct components, including attachment strength, attachment security, and attachment behaviors, as well as the individual's subjective experience of attachment and desire to have social relationships. Each of these can be understood and measured separately from any other, and put back together to define attachment status, or attachment type, as a composite scale that reflects the accumulation of observations or measurements on each subscale. Furthermore, we can also recognize a pathological extension to each of these subscales, with extremes outside of each end of what we can consider the normal range of variation in a non-clinical population, as shown in Figure 8.1.

1. *Attachment strength* stresses the strength of the social connection, along a continuum running from strong to weak. Weakly attached individuals do not feel strongly connected to others, and may even feel isolated. The pathological extremes are disconnection and enmeshment.
2. *Attachment security* reflects the level of trust and confidence that *relationships* (and not individuals) will meet emotional needs, from insecure and uncertain to secure and confident. The pathological extremes are paranoid and grandiose.
3. *Attachment experience* involves the individual's subjective experience of relationships as either satisfying or not satisfying emotional needs. The pathological extremes are alienation or unrestrained fulfillment.
4. *Attachment behaviors* demonstrate the manner in which an individual engages in relationships, from distant and self-oriented to fully engaged and mutually oriented.

---

[4] These include the strange situation, of course, as well as Crittenden's Preschool Assessment of Attachment (8 months to age 5), the Cassidy–Marvin System (ages 3 and 4), the Main–Cassidy system (ages 5–7), and the Attachment Q-Sort (infancy through age 5).

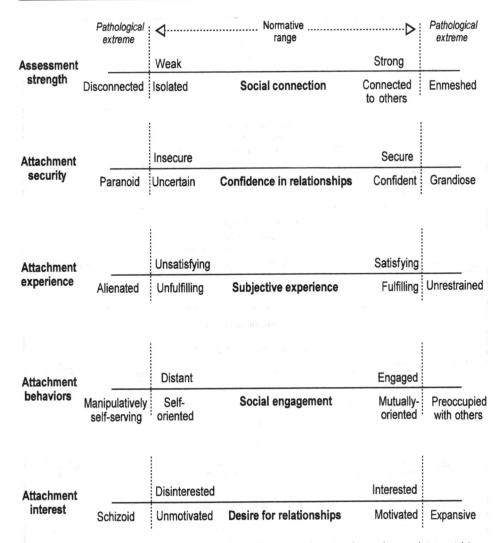

Figure 8.1 Attachment construct subscales indicating suboptimal attachment lying within a range of normative functioning, and pathological outliers

The pathological extremes are manipulative self-serving and preoccupied with others.

5. *Attachment interest* gauges the individual's desire to form relationships from unmotivated to highly motivated. The pathological extremes are schizoid and expansive.

These scales are easily turned into a clinical assessment instrument ("clinical" here means assessment based on the judgment of the evaluator, rather than through self-report or derived through psychometric measurement), such as the *Dimensions of Attachment Assessment scale* shown in Figure 8.2, which includes the construct scales with ordinal scores.

1. Attachment strength
Social connection
(weak to strong, with pathological extremes)

Pathological Disconnected	Very isolated	Somewhat isolated	Cannot assess	Somewhat connected	Very connected	Pathological Enmeshed
1	2	3	0	4	5	1

2. Attachment security
Confidence in relationships
(insecure to secure, with pathological extremes)

Pathological Paranoid	Very uncertain	Somewhat uncertain	Cannot assess	Somewhat confident	Very confident	Pathological Grandiose
1	2	3	0	4	5	1

3. Attachment experience
Subjective experience in relationships
(unsatisfying to satisfying, with pathological extremes)

Pathological Alienated	Very unfulfilling	Somewhat unfulfilling	Cannot assess	Somewhat fulfilling	Very fulfilling	Pathological Unrestrained
1	2	3	0	4	5	1

4. Attachment behaviors
Social engagement
(distant to engaged, with pathological extremes)

Pathological Self-serving	Very self-oriented	Somewhat self-oriented	Cannot assess	Somewhat mutually-oriented	Very mutually-oriented	Pathological Preoccupied
1	2	3	0	4	5	1

5. Attachment interest
Desire for relationships
(disinterested to interested)

Pathological Schizoid	Very unmotivated	Somewhat unmotivated	Cannot assess	Somewhat motivated	Very motivated	Pathological Expansive
1	2	3	0	4	5	1

Attachment subscale score	Overall attachment status	Consistency across attachment subscales
__ Strength	__ Strong	__ Consistent
__ Security	__ Moderate	__ Variable
__ Experience	__ Weak	__ Highly variable
__ Behaviors	__ Pathological/disturbed	
__ Interest	__ Cannot assess	

Figure 8.2 The Dimensions of Attachment Assessment Scale. The lower the score the greater the level of concern for attachment-related problems along any particular dimension, with the exception of zero scores which represent an inability to assess. Scores can be compared and assessed below the dashed line

Attachment status is a term synonymous with attachment classification, category, type, and pattern; there seems to be very little difference in the meaning and use of any of these terms, all of which appear to reflect the same idea, namely that of providing a composite "handle" by which we can easily describe the manner in which an individual is attached to other people. When we ask how someone is attached we are usually interested in global representations of attachment to people in general, rather than one individual. In the case of the DAAS, attachment status or attachment type is a composite measure derived from the accumulation of observations or measurements along each subscale, which together reflect an overall pattern of attachment.

With a simple model, it is possible to describe the individual as an attached person both in general and, if one chooses, with respect to a particular relationship. For the most part, though, as we hold that "attachment" is an experience that shapes and colors *all* relationship experiences for the individual, it makes sense to apply this model to the individual and his or her overarching experiences in all relationships. This most closely approximates "attachment" as we generally mean it when we describe an individual as strongly or weakly attached, and mirrors the global internal working model of relationships described by Overall et al. (2003), that includes perceptions of all social connection and personal security. It is also simple to conceive of scales that assess the position of the individual along each dimension, by either self-report or observation, and a means to synthesize these into a global assessment of attachment.

The intention here, however, is not to develop or further define a model for assessing or measuring attachment. The only present goal is to describe attachment as an overarching construct made up of individual dimensional components, and define and outline the nature of these dimensions so that: (i) "attachment" can be demystified and deconstructed, (ii) such dimensions can be more easily understood and observed as separate constituents, and (iii) attachment can be reconstructed and described in a meaningful manner, and in a manner that recognizes that it is not a unidimensional trait that resides in the individual, or in any particular relationship.

Further at the extreme/pathological ends of each subscale, we see behaviors that reflect a disturbance in psychological functioning. These allow us to recognize that attachment pathology is quite unusual, and may in fact be the result of a pre- or coexisting psychiatric condition, and also recognize the range of attachment experiences, both secure and insecure, that are considered to fall within the normative range. Nevertheless, if we consider measurements at the low end of the scales to be both suboptimal and attachment deficits, we can also see how the accumulation of multiple deficits contributes to what we might consider attachment disturbances or disorders. Beyond this, it is presumably attachment patterns that fall at the extreme, pathological ends that result in disorganized attachments.

CONCLUSION: OBSTACLES TO THE ASSESSMENT OF ADOLESCENT ATTACHMENT

Part of the problem with assessing attachment in adolescents and adults is that attachment theory bases its ideas on attachment in early childhood, despite recognizing in principle that, of course, attachment changes as it nears and then enters adolescence. However, because it is asserted that attachment does not change in its structure after the phase of goal-corrected partnership, completed by age 4, we are stuck with the idea that adolescent and adult attachment is driven by the same structural elements that motivate attachment in very young children. As childhood attachment is directly connected to adults who provide physical and psychological safety and guide growth, this forces us to think of all attachment figures throughout life as parents, or bases of emotional, if not physical, security. This requires that we conceptualize attachment figures as *only* those who meet these childish (literally) emotional needs for survival and anxiety reduction.

However, as it has moved into human development over the life span, rather than early development, attachment theory has been forced to tweak and modify its ideas, now asserting, for instance, that, actually, attachment *can* involve non-attachment figures, such as peers. Moreover, romantic relationships also count, even if we cannot count on such figures being more than transitory, and especially in late adolescence and early adulthood when one may have many romantic partners. If romantic partners *can* be counted as attachment figures, in the limited sense intended by attachment theory, given the failure of so many romantic relationships, including marriages, one wonders why most adolescents and adults do not eventually become insecure as they learn that they cannot depend on their adult attachment figures. However, what is constant and enduring, is *not* the adult relationship but our internal representation of relationships and what we can expect from them. This is what holds our relationships together in adulthood, most notably beginning in late childhood and developing throughout adolescence. In some people, it is the fragility of this internal model that explains the fragmentation and incoherence in cognitive images of self and others, and is reflected in disorganized or unresolved relationship-related behaviors.

Consequently, as long as attachment theory is unable to reconceive its ideas and continues to define "attachment" as a relatively rare occurrence limited to only one type of relationship, it will be unable to fully recognize or meaningfully explore attachment beyond childhood. Indeed, this shows in the operational inconsistencies and contradictions that exist within attachment theory itself, as well as adolescent and adult assessment attachment measures that allow peers and romantic partners to be counted as attachment figures when they are not the caregivers that attachment theory insists they must be in order to "qualify." In reality, of course, as children become adolescents they require less and less "caregiving" and more and more partnership until, as they enter adulthood, they require only partnership, often reaching the point where they themselves become the caregivers.

CHAPTER 9

Disordered Attachment or Attachment Disorder?

I have several times used the term "attachment deficit" as roughly describing what we are trying to get at when we discuss problems in attachment and the development of relationship bonds. These deficits clearly imply that the ability of an individual to engage in relationships or feel attached to other people is, in some way, impaired and does not function optimally. The point is clear, and probably doesn't need more of an explanation, although what may not be clear is the psychological depths that an attachment deficit implies. In any model involving internal representations of the external world, relational skills are located in the mental schemata that stimulate, recognize, and respond to external situations in which relationships are available and can be developed.

In turn, the ability to engage in social relationships and become attached to other people, thus experiencing an emotional bond, implies a sense of social relatedness—that is, the feeling of being connected to others and part of and able to influence a larger world that lies outside of oneself. In an attachment model, such a sense of social relatedness is embedded within the internal working model. Hence, the internal working model, once again, is seen as the container, assimilator, and synthesizer of experience and the source of thought, reflection, and action. Consequently, it is also the target for treatment. Beyond the ability to engage in satisfying social relationships, however, the presumption is that attachment deficits also lead or contribute to troubled emotions and dysfunctional behaviors, and in some cases the development of more serious maladaptations and psychopathology.

This seems like a perfectly reasonable way to describe difficulties in attachment experiences that lead to or significantly contribute to psychosocial impairments. Whether we call these attachment deficits, disturbed or disrupted attachments, attachment disorders, or disorders of attachment, each label appears to serve the same purpose of describing disturbances in the formation of attachment as a root cause behind another disturbance, such as impaired relationships or an affective or behavioral problem. However, "disorders of attachment" (rather than attachment disorders) implies a constellation of related attachment difficulties, which in turn suggests that we know enough about disturbed attachments to be able to form a spectrum of attachment-related disorders—and we don't. This is one of the great weaknesses, if not the great weakness, in using a term like "attachment disorder" in the first place. It is just too global, lacking in much specificity.

DO ATTACHMENT DISORDERS EXIST?

Although attachment theorists consistently point to the development of troubled behaviors, poor self-image, and unsatisfying relationships in those who have developed insecure patterns of attachment, they are not willing, in most cases, to define the attachment pattern as an attachment disorder, or even as a deficit. As well described by now, attachment patterns, secure or otherwise, are considered adaptations to the environment in which the child was raised. Similarly, theorists do not describe the *cause* of the insecurity as a disorder of attachment; instead, the origin of the insecurity is considered to lie in early developmental experiences with primary caregivers. Describing an attachment disorder as the *cause* of attachment difficulties suggests that the problem lies in the individual child, and not the environment. Hence, in neither case do we describe attachment patterns as attachment disorders. Attachment theory also does not recognize a *lack* of attachment as a disorder because, for the most part, it is held that attachments virtually always form, even if insecure or disorganized.

To this end, Greenberg (1999) writes that few children with insecure attachment are considered to have an attachment "disorder." Consequently, when social relationships and related social functioning are so impaired as to be considered a mental health disorder, it is usually assumed that there is some other cause of the disorder, although it may well combine with or be potentiated by disrupted and insecure attachments. Richters and Volkmar (1994), for example, suggest that reactive attachment disorder of infancy or early childhood (RAD), described as relatively uncommon (American Psychiatric Association, 2000), may be better explained as a facet of atypical development rather than a disorder of attachment, in part because the sometimes extreme behaviors seen in RAD resemble behaviors seen in autistic spectrum (pervasive developmental) disorders. However, in recognizing that children diagnosed with RAD do appear to have primary differences in social relatedness, quite possibly reflecting social-emotional development rather than neurobiology (as in pervasive developmental disorder), they note also that the condition may be caused by pathogenic maltreatment rather than early suboptimal attachment experiences. That is, RAD may actually be a disorder resulting from *maltreatment*, rather than the failure to attach or a reaction to the attachment process.

Similarly, Hanson and Spratt (2000) write that behavioral and emotional problems in children with histories of early maltreatment are presumed to stem from their attachments to caregivers, but there are frequently comorbid behavioral and psychiatric problems in these children that extend far beyond insecure or disorganized attachment, reflecting the multiple deficits described by Richters and Volkmar. From this perspective, the very distinct problems in social behavior and relatedness at the heart of the RAD diagnosis may have their origin in pathogenic factors other than attachment, in which case the disordered attachment diagnosis becomes *descriptive* rather than *causal*. In fact, it is clear that although many disturbed children and adolescents have histories of insecure attachment, many children who are insecurely attached do not exhibit major psychiatric disorders in childhood or in later life.

Still, Zeanah (1996) asserts that attachment disorders *do* exist, both as a product of insecure attachment and the cause of further psychiatric disturbance. He writes that not only does insecure attachment place some children at risk for later problems, but due to the severity of the insecure attachment, the child is *already* disordered in some cases. Such disorders of attachment represent a deeper and more pervasive disturbance in safety and security than that typically reflected by insecure attachment, "thus, disordered attachments are all insecure attachments but most insecure attachments are not disordered" (p. 42). Recognizing the possibility that insecure attachments may not represent disorders at all, Zeanah nonetheless proposes that extremes that fall outside the normative range of insecure attachment represent attachment disorders (see, for instance Figure 8.1, Chapter 8).

THE DIAGNOSIS OF ATTACHMENT DISORDER

Diagnoses of disorders are made on the basis of presented symptoms. However, the resulting diagnosis is not considered the *outcome* of the symptoms, but the *cause*. To consider a diagnosis the sum of the symptoms is merely using a short label to describe, rather than explain, pathology. Accordingly, the use of a term like "attachment disorder" presumes that *it* is the cause of the symptoms, and not the outcome. In addition, mental health diagnoses follow a medical model, in which the problem resides within the individual, regardless of how it got there. Consequently, as we believe the cause of disordered attachment to be the social environment, and not the child, we are unlikely to diagnose an attachment disorder, thus ascribing the problem to the individual.

As stated, this does not preclude us from describing attachment as disordered, which is neither the same thing as a diagnosis of attachment disorder nor an explanation of the cause of attachment difficulties. It is simply a description of attachment difficulty, or the nature of the problem rather than the cause. Similarly, we may refer to the inability to form secure relationships as an attachment deficit, clearly implying that the strength of attachment skills is suboptimal or in some way impaired. Attachment-related weaknesses that lead to mood or conduct disturbances may also be described as attachment deficits. Finally, we may refer to patterns of attachment that contribute or lead to significant psychosocial difficulties as disordered. Attachment theory also recognizes that beyond secure and insecure forms of attachment, the *disorganized* form contributes to the most severe forms of later functional difficulty, and in some cases is considered to be linked to the development of psychopathology, the only form of attachment to be linked directly to significant mental health problems. Still, the concept of "attachment deficit" is not part of the nomenclature of mainstream attachment theory, and few attachment theorists use the term "attachment disorder".

With this in mind, the diagnostic use of "attachment disorder," rather than being used to explain the cause of attachment difficulties (clearly, we hypothesize this to be suboptimal attachment experiences), is instead used to describe the nature of the problem and provide an explanation for *other* symptoms, such as depression, anxiety, conduct disorder, and even dissociation and psychosis, that we believe result from attachment-related problems. Indeed, when used at all, the diagnosis ascribes disordered attachment as the cause of some other emotional or behavioral disturbance. Even so, there are no widely accepted diagnostic systems in place to diagnose attachment disorders in older children, adolescents, or adults.

DIFFERENTIAL DIAGNOSIS

For infants and young children aged 4 or younger, the Diagnostic and Statistical Manual (American Psychiatric Association, 2000) includes a diagnosis of *reactive attachment disorder of infancy or early childhood* (RAD). This is typically defined by disorganized and sometimes seemingly irrational, contradictory, and otherwise significantly disturbed social behaviors. To meet the diagnosis, these must be coupled with either disinhibited and indiscriminate social relatedness to others, or inhibited attachment behaviors in which the child shows a failure to respond in an age appropriate manner in most social situations. When linked to a history of pathogenic care, these behaviors are considered disorders of attachment. As noted, Richters and Volkmar note the possibility that the condition described in RAD may actually have less to do with attachment, and more to do with other features of atypical development.

The International Statistical Classification of Diseases and Related Health Problems (ICD-10, World Health Organization, 1992) provides a similar diagnosis, also with onset prior to age 5, although broken into *reactive attachment disorder of childhood* and *disinhibited attachment disorder of childhood* (essentially, the DSM RAD diagnosis broken into two separate diagnoses), also with onset prior to age 5. For children aged 3 and younger, a slightly different take on childhood attachment problems is presented in *The Classification of Mental Health and Developmental Disorders of Infancy and Early Childhood* (DC: 0–3), produced by the Zero to Three organization (National Center for Infants, Toddlers, and Families, 1994). The diagnosis of *Reactive Attachment Deprivation/Maltreatment Disorder of Infancy* is included as an affective disorder among a larger group of disorders of infancy and early childhood. The diagnostic label speaks for itself, asserting that this is a disturbance in affect produced by the deprivation of appropriate attachment experience or active maltreatment.

Although other diagnostic labels and systems have been proposed for infants and young children, none have taken any particular hold. Nevertheless, two systems in particular are far more detailed than the single RAD type diagnosis, offering more specificity within the diagnostic category of disturbed attachment. These do postulate the existence of an "attachment disorder." Zeanah (1996) proposes three types of attachment disorders, including *non-attached* attachment disorder, in which the infant shows no preferred attachment to anyone; *disordered* attachment that represents disturbances in the child's relationship to the parent, in which the child engages in either excessively clingy or recklessly risky behaviors; and *disrupted* attachments that follow the child's experience or perceptions of loss of a primary attachment figure, or grief as described by Bowlby (1980) that results in distressed and detached behaviors. Incorporating this differential classification, Zeanah et al. (1993) presented five specific subtypes of attachment disorders, aimed at specifically exhibited attachment behaviors rather than a more general set of behavioral or relational symptoms: *Type I*, non-attached attachment disorder; *Type II*, indiscriminate attachment disorder; *Type III*, inhibited attachment disorder; *Type IV*, aggressive attachment disorder; and *Type V*, role-reversed attachment disorder, in which the young child appears to be excessively worrying about the parent's well-being. Like RAD, but unlike the diagnostic scheme proposed by Brisch, described below, these diagnoses apply only to young children (aged 1–5). Also, unlike Brisch's diagnostic model, in this model symptoms need be present in only a single attachment relationship. The age range for the diagnosis, however, limits its use to young children. Its value and use is even further weakened by the fact that symptoms need be displayed in only *one* attachment relationship, rather than across a range of social situations, as well as the lack of specificity in defining the length of time that symptoms must be displayed before the diagnosis can be made.

Also aimed at specific attachment behaviors, Brisch (1999) writes that an attachment disorder diagnosis cannot be made on the basis of insecure attachment per se, as insecure attachment falls within the normative range of functioning. Instead, Brisch requires disturbed behaviors in interactions with a variety of attachment figures to be manifested as stable patterns both across situations and longitudinally, and for at least six months. Although asserting this typology of attachment disorder can be applied in defined circumstances to both children and adolescents, Brisch is not clear about the age at which symptoms of attachment disorders must first appear. Presumably, although stating that his typology can be applied to adolescent attachment disorders, there presumably is a continuity between attachment-disordered behaviors that first appear in early childhood and those evident, in Brisch's model, during mid-childhood and adolescence. He describes seven diagnoses of attachment disorders in children: (1) no signs of attachment behavior, (2) undifferentiated attachment behavior, (3) exaggerated attachment behavior, (4) inhibited attachment behavior, (5) aggressive attachment behavior, (6) attachment behavior with role reversal, and (7) attachment disorder resulting in psychosomatic symptoms. Although offering a little more specificity and focus than the model of Zeanah and colleagues, it is not clear that these same symptoms cannot be more adequately explained by or subsumed under other, existing diagnostic (non-attachment) categories. Like other attachment diagnostic schemes, Brisch's model is more theoretically driven than empirically supported. In addition, of course, it has no relevance in diagnosing attachment difficulties in adults, but probably should as attachment difficulties are presumed to continue into and throughout adulthood, which is the idea behind connecting attachment deficits to adult attachment.

Elizabeth Randolph (2000) also describes "attachment disorder," although she distinguishes it from reactive attachment disorder, and provides a typology of four subtypes. In the absence of an autistic spectrum disorder or developmental disability, Randolph considers an attachment disorder (AD) marked by: (i) a history of disrupted attachment prior to age 2, such as history of maltreatment, serious illness in the infant or parent, maternal psychiatric illness, multiple changes in primary caregivers, or being raised institutionally, (ii) onset before age 6 of significant emotional or behavioral problems, (iii) inappropriate or disturbed social relationships, such as indiscriminate attachment to others or lack of apparent attachment, and (iv) signs of conduct disordered or oppositional behaviors. She considers ADs to be found in the four subtypes of anxious, ambivalent, avoidant, and disorganized, although stresses that these have no relationship to the standard model of secure/insecure and organized/disorganized attachment. Despite her disclaimer, these can each be largely understood through descriptions of insecure and disorganized attachment already provided in prior chapters. Most recently, Randolph has changed the subtype names to isolated (avoidant), evasive (anxious), defiant (ambivalent), and bizarre (disorganized).

Clearly, Randolph conceptualizes attachment deficits as the explanation for behavioral problems in children when they also display relationship problems prior to age 5 or 6, and at that or a later time develop symptoms consistent with a diagnosis of conduct or oppositional defiant disorder. The value of such a diagnosis is that it legitimately recognizes that, in the absence of other explanations (such as childhood illness, autistic spectrum conditions, variants of mental retardation), developmentally early troubled social behaviors may represent problems in the child-rearing environment. However, as we have seen, it may be maltreatment, rather than attachment, ranging from neglect to abuse, that is the root of these problems. This is of special importance as there is no empirical proof that attachment experiences cause early childhood problem behaviors. Although it may be that children with such problems also have deficit attachment experiences, we must also remember that correlation does not imply causation.

Nevertheless, Randolph and others suggest that correlation in the case of attachment *does* imply causation. Further, they assert that what they refer to as attachment disorders are the underlying cause of, or heavily implicated in many, if not most, child and adolescent disorders. These authors legitimately recognize that the presence of very early behavioral problems (prior to age 5) is quite likely associated with and heightened by early bonding, relational, and caregiver experiences, but go on to infer that these early experiences are not simply developmental vulnerabilities, but are the *cause* of later behavioral and psychiatric difficulties. Indeed, one of the great problems with the use of the attachment disorder diagnosis, if we can consider it a legitimate diagnostic label, is that it is usually applied so globally and, often, so indiscriminately, that it is rendered incapable of informing differential diagnosis. It becomes a "shotgun" diagnosis, hitting all symptoms in its path.

For instance, based on their study of 19 boys aged 5–10, Clarke, Ungerer, Chahoud, Johnson, and Stiefel (2002) assert that attachment insecurity is associated with attention deficit/hyperactivity disorder. Although they acknowledge that not all of the ADHD children in their small study were assessed with insecure attachment, they nonetheless write that the "prominence of social deficits in ADHD provides further evidence of striking similarities between the developmental outcomes of insecure attachments and the difficulties seen in children with ADHD" (p. 181). However, even assuming a correlation, they also describe the difficulty in ascertaining directionality—that is, does the quality of caregiving contribute to the development of ADHD symptoms, or do the challenging behaviors of ADHD lead to disturbed interactions in child–parent relationships?

UNDIFFERENTIATED DIAGNOSIS

Although attachment theory has not been broadly applied to clinical populations, there is recently a greater focus on the application of attachment theory in understanding and treating psychopathology. However, Kelly (in press) has written that the lack of consensus about the validity and value of attachment disorder makes the usefulness of such a diagnosis questionable. Nevertheless, the term "attachment deficit" or "attachment disorder" is used with increasing frequency, implied as a diagnosis of causation rather than a description of symptoms, although used in this manner the term remains unsupported by the literature of attachment theory.

In fact, other than the diagnostic classifications of attachment disorder described above, other diagnostic descriptions are so broad that they virtually recognize and diagnose all troubled behavior in children and adolescents as attachment disorders. They are thus of very limited utility, and lack any ability to discriminate between troubled behaviors in children and adolescents or provide the means for differential diagnosis. This includes Randolph's model in which she expansively describes attachment disorder as a severe disorder of childhood that subsumes (but is not limited to) attention deficit/hyperactivity disorder, conduct disorder, oppositional defiant disorder, bipolar II disorder, psychotic disorder not otherwise specified, schizoaffective disorder, major depressive disorder, dysthymic disorder, intermittent explosive disorder, and posttraumatic stress disorder (2000, pp. 2–3).

Although Levy (2000) does not provide a set of related diagnostic categories or typology of attachment disorders, in a similar mode he groups the causes of attachment disorder into three categories: (1) parental/caregiver contributions (e.g., abuse and neglect, depression, psychological disorders); (2) child contributions (e.g., difficult temperament, prematurity, fetal alcohol syndrome); and (3) environmental contributions (e.g., poverty, stressful and violent home and/or community). He writes that the most common causes of attachment disorder are abuse, neglect, multiple out-of-home placements, and other prolonged separations from the primary attachment figure. Following or linked to these circumstances, it appears that Levy considers virtually all childhood and adolescent problems to be caused by attachment malformation, which is the result of almost any damaging condition within the parent, child, or environment. Levy (2000, p. 9) describes the outcomes of attachment disorder in children as low self-esteem; needy, clingy, or pseudo-independent behavior; extreme oppositionality; lack of conscience and empathy; inability to give and receive genuine affection and love; anger, aggression, and violence; incapacity for genuine trust, intimacy, or affection; negative, hopeless, and pessimistic view of self, family, and society; lack of empathy, compassion, and remorse; behavioral and academic problems at school; the perpetuation of the cycle of maltreatment and attachment disorder in their own children when they reach adulthood; and/or "identification with the evil and the dark side of life" (2000, p. 10). This, obviously, defines a very wide range of troubled behavior in children as "attachment disordered," virtually eliminating other alternative diagnoses.

In fact, the range is so broad that, attachment disorder diagnosis or not, it suggests that the cause of almost all emotional and behavioral problems in children is impaired attachment. Remember, in its use as a diagnosis, the term "attachment disorder" is considered the *cause* of these problems, not merely a description of the role that attachment difficulties or deficits play in the formation of such problems or as a factor contributing to developmental vulnerabilities. In general, it is this line of global and expansive thinking about attachment disorder that renders it weak and incapable of discrimination.

Many clinicians are informed by attachment theory, but are not otherwise affiliated with any particular school of thought about attachment theory. In such cases, the term "attachment disorder" is most typically used descriptively and diagnostically (rather than as a diagnosis) to describe implicated or suspected causes of problems. But as an actual diagnosis, "attachment disorder" is often associated with an attachment-informed therapeutic mode that is referred to by many of its practitioners as "attachment therapy," or AT. Although this loose school of therapy, derived from ideas about attachment, has many supporters who practice an applied version of attachment theory, it also has many detractors[1]

---

[1] Mercer (2002), for instance, writes that despite the assertions of AT writers and their use of attachment-informed vocabulary, there is no significant connection between AT and attachment theory.

and represents only a small percentage of those whose work is informed by attachment theory. However, for AT practitioners, most troubling childhood behaviors appear to be the result of attachment difficulties and, hence, attachment disorders.

Some treatment centers for AT therefore endorse and embrace attachment disorders in the same global and extreme terms described above. As an illustration, on their websites the Attachment and Treatment Training Institute (Evergreen Center, 2004) and the Institute for Attachment and Child Development (2004) post descriptions of the behavioral, cognitive, affective, relational, and developmental symptoms that embrace the symptomatology of virtually every troubled child, including "identification with evil and the dark side of life" (Evergreen Center, 2004). This is not true in all cases, of course, and the website of ATTACh (Association for Treatment & Training in the Attachment of Children, 2004) offers a far more reserved, limited, balanced, and less hyperbolic description of attachment disorders and problems in children, more in keeping with the tenets of attachment theory.

In fact, it is not that the models and perspectives of Randolph, Levy, and others aligned with "attachment therapy" are poorly informed. On the contrary, they are well versed in the literature of attachment theory; indeed, Levy's descriptions fit well with the ideas of Bowlby and the attachment theorists in that compromised attachment sets the basis (through the internal working model) for many life difficulties. The major difficulty with models like those of Randolph and Levy is that, although they accurately count deficits and disturbances in attachment as significant contributors to dysfunctional behavior and possibly many childhood and adolescent psychiatric diagnoses, they are so broad as to have no useful diagnostic value. They use the term "attachment disorder" so broadly as to render it purely descriptive or so all-inclusive that it subsumes virtually all other disorders.

ATTACHMENT DISORDERS IN OLDER CHILDREN AND ADOLESCENTS

Randolph (2000) quite clearly distinguishes between attachment disorder and reactive attachment disorder, primarily it seems because she considers RAD to be a symptom *of* attachment disorder. In general, however, when "attachment disorder" is used as a diagnosis to explain troubled emotional, behavioral and relational disturbance in children, it is often used synonymously with RAD. This is an inaccurate description, however, as RAD is a diagnosis used in the case of infancy and very early childhood, whereas attachment disorder, whether used as a diagnosis or as a more general term used to describe disturbed attachments or attachment deficits, is typically applied across the life span, from childhood to adulthood.

The RAD diagnosis is often used carelessly and casually, without further explanation and, as noted, as a synonym for "attachment disorder," therefore applying the RAD diagnosis to an age range far above that for which it is intended. Kathy Seifert is doing much work in trying to understand the relationship between disturbances in attachment and troubled behavior in adolescents and adults, including violence. In her work (2003a, 2003b), she frequently refers to attachment disorder as though it was a clearly defined and fully operational construct, and, in fact, appears to be referring to reactive attachment disorder of infancy or early childhood (it is important to remember the qualifier on the RAD diagnosis—that is, "of infancy or early childhood"). Equally clear, she applies the disorder to adolescents and adults. However, although it is sometimes diagnosed in older children, and even adolescents, it is clear that the RAD diagnosis is intended for *young* children. It is of little use in diagnosing attachment difficulties or deficits in older children, adolescents, or adults, although we may conceive of attachment problems as central to their functioning and the development and enactment of behavioral or psychological pathology. I was recently surprised to see the RAD diagnosis applied to a 50-year-old patient described on a website specializing in treatment through neurofeedback, although they applied a non-DSM diagnosis of "Reactive Attachment Disorder of Adulthood." Inventing diagnoses in this way may help to make the case for the treatment being sold, but has no empirical basis and simply weakens the legitimacy of diagnoses of attachment disorders.

Further, it seems improper to diagnose a reactive attachment disorder in a child older than perhaps age 7 or 8, given the intent of the diagnosis. If the diagnosis has not previously been made (and each of the diagnostic systems described above require diagnosis prior to age 5), it is incorrect to diagnose RAD past age 5, unless the symptoms were clearly present but simply undiagnosed. However, in the event that the diagnosis has been present (and, therefore, the symptoms) since early childhood (prior to age 5), then by age 8 or 9, it can hardly be called reactive. In such circumstances, despite the origins of later behavior in earlier reactive attachment, by latency age the disorder has evolved into something that likely resembles a conduct or affective disorder, and should be diagnosed as such, noting the attachment origins of later behavioral, affective, interactional, and diagnostic developments.

In fact, RAD aside, and it is my clear contention that it is a diagnosis not appropriate for children past 8, we have no model of attachment disorder to apply to adolescents or adults. No widely accepted diagnostic labels have yet arisen for this age range to identify psychiatric or behavioral difficulties that result from an attachment impairment. Accordingly, without the benefit of an age-matched operational model of attachment in adolescents and adults, it is difficult to apply the idea of "attachment disorder" as a comprehensive explanation for or link to current behavior. Thus, in our work with adolescent and adult sexual offenders, it is difficult to say what "disordered attachment" looks like, and we must therefore substitute other constructs that we can more easily operationalize, such as emotional loneliness, trust in others, security in relationships, or empathy,[2] assuming that these are either the same thing as attachment, elements or sequelae of attachment, or reasonable facsimiles. Work with adult sexual offenders also asserts that early attachment experience and classification does predict, or at least contributes to, later attachment difficulties and the development and enactment of sexually abusive behavior. There is little evidence for this, however, in part because we lack an adequate understanding of what we mean, what to look for, and how to diagnose such attachment difficulties.

---

[2] Although these are also difficult constructs to define, and particularly empathy for which there is no clear definition. Nevertheless, these are typically the sort of things we assess in adolescents and adults when looking for evidence of "attachment."

ATTACHMENT-INFORMED DIAGNOSTIC FORMULATION

It seems that a majority of troubled and criminal populations of adolescents and adults have experienced difficult and disrupted childhoods. As the expansive model of attachment disorder conceives of virtually every disorder of affect and behavior as a reflection of attachment difficulties, if preceded or accompanied by difficult childhood experiences, then virtually every delinquent or emotionally troubled child, adolescent, and adult meets the criteria for attachment disorder. There is, then, little point in having an attachment disorder diagnosis as everyone in this population has the diagnosis. As Rutter and O'Connor (1999) have written, if so many behavioral and psychiatric disorders are linked to attachment insecurity, then a diagnosis of attachment disorder loses its ability to explain much.

Diagnoses of attachment disorders, then, are contraindicated. In the first place, this is because it is not clear that the emotional/behavioral disturbance is the direct result of disrupted attachment, and this is certainly not a conclusion postulated or supported by attachment theory. On the contrary, attachment theory tells us that suboptimal attachment and attachment deficits are neither pathological, nor, in most cases, linked to psychopathology. In the second place, a diagnosis of attachment disorder has little relevance because it is so broad and global as to lack all utility. This is not to suggest that attachment difficulties (or deficits) are not significant in the development of later psychosocial difficulties, and even mental health diagnoses, or that attachment problems are not present in current behaviors and relationships. In fact, as attachment theory insists that patterns of attachment are relatively stable through the childhood years and beyond, attachment deficits are quite likely to remain active throughout adolescence and into adulthood.

It is when "disordered attachment" is used *descriptively*, rather than as a diagnosis, that it serves an important and instrumental role in pointing to the function of earlier attachment and related social experiences in the development of current cognitions, affects, and behaviors. Consequently, it is absolutely clear that attachment should neither be disregarded nor go unassessed. On the contrary, any comprehensive psychosocial or mental health assessment must include an attachment perspective, thus viewing the individual through an attachment lens. Nevertheless, this doesn't mean that we should provide a diagnosis of attachment disorder, rather than a diagnosis formed by and more relevant to presenting symptoms.

In fact, while recognizing and accepting that deficits in attachment, including RAD, may well be a significant factor in the development of later behavioral and mental health disorders, it is not necessary to have an attachment disorder diagnosis because other diagnostic labels can quite sufficiently explain the presence of current symptoms. It is nonetheless important to recognize the role of attachment in the etiology of mental health and behavioral disorders that result in standard (non-attachment) diagnoses, and include this in the formulation of diagnoses. An attachment-informed framework can achieve this goal, just as an attachment-informed model of treatment can provide for the development of suitable treatment interventions.

CONCLUSION: THE HOLY GRAIL?

As we have seen, there is no essential model of attachment disorders for adolescents. By mid–late childhood, earlier disordered attachment experiences have been incorporated into character, absorbed into and displayed through aspects of psychosocial functioning, including social relationships, emotional stability, mental coherence, and behavioral control. In a clinical population aged 9 or older, earlier attachment difficulties are no longer "reactive" but are instead reflected through other diagnoses, including disruptive behavioral, anxiety, and affective disorders. In fact, reflecting the perspective embraced by attachment theory, Greenberg (1999) writes that it is quite clear that insecure attachment does not reflect and is not a measure of psychopathology. Instead, he warns that the enthusiastic use of attachment theory to inform assessment and treatment may lead to over-interpretation in our search for the "Holy Grail of psychopathology" (p. 472).

In any circumstances, Rutter and O'Connor (1999)—who are critical of the attachment disorder diagnosis, which they consider to be only loosely informed by attachment research—write that even when an attachment problem is evident, "it is by no means self-evident what form treatment should take" (p. 833). In noting, then, that we lack a method of reliably assessing the construct of attachment disorder, Kelly (in press) suggests that attachment self-report measures are best suited as a means to guide and inform clinical judgment, rather than as proof of diagnosis. Consequently, before we move on to address clinical issues among juvenile and adult sexual offenders, I remind the reader that, despite its great utility in understanding both human development and behavior, the attachment concept is not likely the next white horse that will carry us to the treatment horizon from which all answers are laid out before us.

Prepared with a basic framework and knowledge of the developmental dynamics of attachment, we now break from theory. However, it is important that we recognize that there are many pathways to and explanations for particular behaviors. Although an attachment-informed perspective offers a useful way to conceptualize and interpret human development and behavior, it seems likely that human beings are richer and far more complex than our theories about human functioning. Accordingly, although we can endlessly create models, it is important to keep in mind the factors that combine to shape the ways in which consciousness, character, and behavior unfold, many of which we are simply unaware of and remain invisible to us.

Nevertheless, I hope the reader finds an attachment-informed framework to be of use as we move on to the next chapter where, through a single case study, we specifically look at the hypothesized relationship of attachment to the development and perpetration of sexually abusive behavior. Regardless of any direct relationship or the lack thereof, it is obviously true that juvenile and adult sexual offenders are first and foremost social beings with the same needs for security as anyone else, and as susceptible to the effects of early childhood development and ongoing socialization experiences. Even if attachment theory does not allow us to see a clear pathway between attachment and the onset of sexually inappropriate and abusive behaviors, minimally it does provide us with a means of recognizing the effects of attachment experiences on sexually aggressive children and adolescents.

CHAPTER 10

Applying the Attachment Framework: An Attachment-driven Case Study

This chapter uses a single case study to illustrate the application of attachment ideas to a case of juvenile sexual offending, and the development of an attachment-informed case formulation. However, no brief study (even if does take up an entire chapter) can possibly be presented in all its complexity. Furthermore, in synthesizing or blending cases, it is difficult to highlight attachment issues as clearly as in *actual* cases. In fact, when one begins to assume and use an attachment-informed perspective, given the complexity, great difficulties, and developmental challenges often experienced by the children and adolescents with whom we work, it is difficult to fabricate or synthesize case studies that are as pointed or as focused as actual cases. Accordingly, although significant changes have been made in order to ensure anonymity and protect confidentiality, many of the elements presented in this study reflect actual case details.

In reading this case the reader is encouraged to think in terms of the principles and ideas of attachment theory, and the rearing environment and its possible effects on the adolescent described. Beyond this, consider also the impact of the family rearing environment on the *parents* of the offender as *they* grew up. Think about the *intergenerational* transmission of attachment patterns, bearing in mind the belief among attachment theorists that the adult attachment pattern of the parent (as assessed by the Adult Attachment Interview), and especially the mother, is believed to predict the attachment pattern evident in the child by 1 year of age. Fonagy et al. (2000), for instance, describe the parents' internal working models *prefiguring* the child's security of attachment, and their assumption, largely typical of attachment theory, that the quality of the infant's attachment to the parent is intrinsically linked to the parent's internal working model: "the child is likely to be securely attached if . . . the parent's internal model of relationships is benign, dominated by favorable experiences" (p. 269).

Following the details of the case we apply an attachment framework to focus on, not simply the effects of early experience on early development, but also the impact of early attachment experiences on the internal working model (including the sense of self and others, metacognition, schemata and automatic thinking, and felt security), and its implications for recent and current behavior, and trajectory for the future. In terms of forensic risk assessment,[1] in the context of attachment theory a *secure* pattern of attachment is a protective factor, and *insecure* and/or *disorganized* attachment a risk factor.

THE CHILD BEHIND THE SEXUALLY ABUSIVE BEHAVIOR

This case has been chosen from among hundreds, all of which are both tragic and complex, and any of which demonstrates that juvenile sexual offending is far from a mundane behavior that just happens, or behavior that is simply overlaid on a child or adolescent who is otherwise a pretty regular kid or just another delinquent. Perry's case and his history is not at all unusual for those children and adolescents who engage in sexually inappropriate and sexually abusive behavior to the point where they are admitted into the system for treatment. These are typically troubled children with problems far greater than sexually coercive behavior alone, and with histories that point to the developmental and emotional disturbances and milestones that contribute to their eventual engagement in sexually inappropriate and damaging behavior.

In fact, the sexually abusive behavior that these juveniles manifest often pales by comparison to the events in their own histories, which frequently involve serious disruptions and difficulties. These include neglect, domestic violence, and family dysfunction, and, as many readers will be aware, histories of overt physical and sexual abuse are quite common in juvenile sexual offenders. Effective treatment for these children and adolescents will involve at least an equal, and usually a far greater, emphasis on their histories, the current level of emotional or psychiatric acuity, and/or characterological aspects of their behavior, rather than simply their sexually aggressive behavior. That is, good treatment focuses on the *whole* child, and resists seeing the juvenile as a simply a "sexual offender." Treatment is, accordingly, applied to far more than the sexually aggressive behavior that brought the juvenile into treatment. Thus, although the *target* of the treatment is sexually abusive behavior, the *focus* of the treatment is on the *source* of the problems *behind* the behaviors. Treatment is often and typically about understanding and overcoming the obstacles of *prior* development that present themselves in *today's* affect, behavior, and personality, and creating a treatment environment and set of relationships that can rehabilitate developing dysfunctional characterological attributes of psychic organization.

Furthermore, the shifts and changes we seek in treatment, and particularly those related to experiences and patterns of attachment, can only occur over time. They cannot happen through workbooks, revelations and epiphanies (so called "ah ha" moments), or short-term treatment, and they certainly cannot be rushed or hastened. A six month intensive treatment program, no matter how well designed or how well delivered, can simply not provide the experiences of life that bring about such change. The internal working model shifts and changes, and in Piaget's terms, accommodates and adapts, only over time.

Remember, also, that although some of the children with whom we work may become adult sexual offenders, many will not, despite difficult histories. Think here about those

---

[1] Forensic work is not addressed in this book, but is central to our work and abundantly addressed in the general juvenile and adult sexual offender literature (see, for instance, Calder, 2000; Doren, 2002; Rich, 2003; Ryan & Lane, 1997).

201 high-risk children in Werner and Smith's (1992) study, and recall also that by age 18 one-third were doing okay, and by mid-adulthood almost all "had staged a recovery of sorts" (p. 193).

ATTACHMENT-DRIVEN CASE STUDY

An attachment-driven approach to case study contributes to developing treatment interventions by providing an understanding of *past* shaping events, many of which remain *current* and *active* in the internal working model. This allows a deeper understanding of past and current behaviors, likely future behaviors and experiences if things remain unchanged, and the development of targeted treatment interventions that are individualized and can bring about change. Of course, in the case of an attachment model, in developing treatment interventions there will be a particular focus on the internal working model, or the set of dispositional representations, into which is embedded images of self and others, and relationships (the self-in-society).

In any case, presenting case studies represents more than simply describing cases, but selecting the right level of detail and getting to the heart of the case, formulating an explanation for behavior and a resulting direction for treatment. In developing case study skills, one has not only to look at cases but to learn *how* to look and what to look *for*. In the cases of an attachment-informed study, not only is an attachment perspective revealed in understanding juvenile sexual offenders, but we learn *how* to apply an attachment-informed perspective.

However, in order to make attachment theory useful, and particularly in clinical settings, it must be synthesized into a format or framework that makes it capable of being applied. Accordingly, by recognizing the elements of attachment disturbance in personality, behavior, interactions, and relationships we can imagine and devise simple measures that can assist and inform us. The attachment-informed formulation for the study presented here is based upon, but not rigidly directed by, the 20-item *Inventory for Attachment-informed Analysis of Behaviors (IAAB)* and 12-item *Attached Relationship Inventory (ARI)*, each of which serves as a lens through which to examine behaviors and a guide for analysis. These provide a framework and structure by which to ask exploratory questions and formulate and frame answers that can help us to understand behavior from an attachment perspective.

The *Inventory for Attachment-informed Analysis of Behaviors*, shown in Figure 10.1, was designed solely for this case study. It is neither intended, nor purported, to be an exhaustive, definitive measure of attachment elements, nor does it have any psychometric properties. It is simply a guide for thinking about important elements of attachment, with particular reference to the internal working model and the formation and maintenance of ongoing social relationships. It is age sensitive, meaning it must be applied in an age-appropriate manner. For instance, some elements are more or less useful or meaningful at different chronological ages or points in cognitive development, and some, such as items 18 and 19, are not at all relevant for young children.

Using these 20 questions to consider attachment to parents, other individuals, and social values, one can conduct an analysis of behavior leading to an interpretation of attachment-related attitudes, experiences, and behaviors. Such an analysis is based on an observational

1.	Representation of Self	*Sense of self, self-image, self-esteem, personal identity, etc.*
2.	Self-agency	*Sense of self as capable of acting upon the world and others.*
3.	Self-efficacy	*Sense of self as capable of satisfactorily accomplishing goals.*
4.	Self-regulation	*Capacity to contain and stabilize thoughts, emotions, and behaviors.*
5.	Experienced security	*Sense of security and trust in self and environment.*
6.	Representation of others	*Sense of others as reliable, trustworthy, caring, etc.*
7.	Social connectedness	*Sense of belonging to social group larger than self.*
8.	Parental connectedness	*Sense of connection to and relationship with parents.*
9.	Parental security/model	*Sense of parents as reliable, trustworthy, competent, caring, etc.*
10.	Proximity behaviors	*Organization of behaviors intended to maintain proximity to others.*
11.	Signaling behaviors	*Methods for expressing and communicating needs to others.*
12.	Exploratory behaviors	*Level/type of risk-taking behaviors when away from security figures.*
13.	Capacity for intimacy	*Ability to feel comfortable and engaged in intimate relationships.*
14.	Empathic connection	*Vicarious understanding, concern, and support for others.*
15.	Perspective taking	*Ability to assume point of view of another person.*
16.	Metacognition	*Capacity to recognize and reflect upon thoughts & feelings of self/others*
17.	Goals of behavior	*Purpose and drives behind sequences or patterns of behavior.*
18.	Congruency of social norms	*Approval of/desire to conform with common social norms.*
19.	Response to social norms	*Capacity to meet social norms through legitimate means.*
20.	Moral decision making	*Understanding and use of moral means to acquire goals.*

Figure 10.1   The Inventory for Attachment-informed Analysis of Behaviors (IAAB)

and/or interview process, rather than answers to dichotomous or multiple choice questions that yield categorical assessments of attachment. In principle, this is the same sort of process that lies beneath the assignment of attachment category through the use of the Adult Attachment Interview and the strange situation, in which assessments of attachment are *interpreted* rather than derived from self-reports on questionnaires. Far from measuring or classifying attachment, an inventory like the IAAB provides a concrete structure for viewing and analyzing behavior from an attachment perspective, and thus contributes to the development of an attachment-informed framework.

Shown in Figure 10.2, a second inventory of attachment-related relationships, the *Attached Relationship Inventory*, provides an additional way to analyze and make sense of behaviors, again bearing in mind an attachment framework.

In the case of both measures, an "inventory" implies taking stock of and assigning meaning and value to a series of items. However, unlike an inventory of physical items, an inventory of human experience cannot be easily defined in terms of quantity or the existence or non-existence of a particular item (although, in some cases, it is reasonable to assess a human quality in this manner—for instance, it is possible to not have any perspective taking skill at all, as in the case of a very young child or a severely autistic adult). Rather, an inventory of human experience is assessed through an interpretation of behavior, in terms of its quality and form, rather than its existence. It is also, in some cases, possible to measure human qualities as a gradated process assessed between two points on a scale, or dimensionally (more of or less of, for instance), rather than dichotomously (for

1. Desire for relationship .... *Does the individual want or seek relationships with others?*

2. Importance of relationships .... *Does the individual see social relationships as important?*

3. Security in relationships .... *Do relationships enhance satisfaction and confidence rather than increase or produce anxiety or doubt?*

4. Security through relationships .... *Do relationships increase or enhance the individual's sense of self-image and social connection?*

5. Confidence in relationships .... *Does the individual believe that other parties in relationships can be trusted to and will care about and make his/her needs important?*

6. Confidence in relationship-building skills ...... *Does the individual believe in his/her ability to form and maintain personal relationships?*

7. Perspective taking .... *Does the individual have the capacity to recognize the needs, emotional states, attitudes, and thoughts of the other person in the relationship?*

8. Caring and giving .... *How giving is the individual with respect to recognizing and meeting the needs of other parties in the relationship?*

9. Reciprocal mutuality .... *Does the individual display mutuality and reciprocity in relationships (give and take), or just seek personal gratification (take and take)?*

10. Derived satisfaction .... *Does the individual have insatiable relationship demands?*

11. Intimacy and boundaries .... *Is the individual capable of close and interdependent relationships without becoming possessive and incapable of separation?*

12. Relationship independence .... *Is the individual capable of close and interdependent relationships without over-dependence or enmeshment?*

Figure 10.2   The Attached Relationship Inventory (ARI)

example, yes/no). Both the IAAB and ARI are tools designed to be used this way, part of an attachment-oriented framework against which to view, analyze, and interpret social relationship behaviors.

CASE STUDY: PERRY, 16-YEAR-OLD JUVENILE SEXUAL OFFENDER

Perry is a 16-year-old adolescent in a long-term residential treatment center for juvenile sexual offenders. At age 15 he was discovered sexually abusing his 6-year-old step-sister, Marcy, by engaging over a two-year period in french kissing, fondling her vagina, and having her masturbate him but not to ejaculation, and fellatio and cunnilingus. He initiated these behaviors when he was 13 and Marcy was 4. There were frequent attempts at both digital and penile penetration, but Perry did not continue past his sister's resistance. He used no aggression, force, or threat, instead depending on his relationship with her and promises of playing and spending time together. Perry was living with his father, step-mother, and Marcy at the time, and he was caught when Marcy's mother entered the room.

Marcy later reported that she did not tell Perry to stop because she felt scared, and later reported "feeling relieved and safe" after the behaviour was discovered and stopped.

Perry told the evaluator, "I wanted to get caught so I could get help." He also reported that although he never used force against Marcy, he hated her and called her a "little bitch" because he did not like the way she treated her younger brother (Perry's half brother). Perry has also referred to Marcy's mother (Perry's step-mother) as "a selfish and manipulative bitch who only does things for her own kids." Perry said that he tried to stop his sexually abusive behavior but could not, describing an addictive and obsessive quality, but also said at one point that "maybe it was to get back at my father, step-mother, and victim for being jerks." Of special note, Perry wrote in his journal that he is angry with himself because he became "another loser sexual offender like the rest of my father's family." This is because Perry's paternal grandfather was jailed for sexually abusing a female neighbor, and his adult daughter (Perry's paternal aunt) recently alleged that Perry's grandfather had raped her in her teens. Two of Perry's paternal uncles have served prison sentences for sexual offenses and one is currently incarcerated, and one is suspected of sexually abusing Perry's father, Jordan, who is their younger brother, when Jordan was in his mid-teens. Jordan himself has been accused of rape by his former wife, Sally, Perry's mother. She alleged that Jordan raped her on numerous occasions during their marriage and that he had an "insatiable" sexual appetite, and she alleged that he attempted to rape her younger teenage sister three times when she and Jordan were themselves teenagers. It has recently been revealed that Perry's younger brother, age 15, has also been sexually abusing Marcy, Perry's victim.

Perry is not a violent or physically aggressive individual. He is dysthymic and experiences episodes of mild–moderate clinical depression, is very anxious and engages in obsessive thinking, engages in scabiomania (skin picking) and trichotillomania (hair pulling), ruminates over minute details, is somatic and worries excessively, has a low tolerance level for frustration, is passive-aggressive, and uses his relatively high intellect (full score IQ of 122)[2] to badger and harangue others until he gets his needs met. By his often irritated and anxious alienation, affect, attitudes, and social interactions, clinicians wonder if Perry is a candidate to be a school shooter. He has a history of social isolation, with few to no friends and no close acquaintances, a few very brief romantic relationships, and he reported in his initial evaluation that he would like to be a government assassin: "No-one listens to me. If I was a sniper I could be independent and take charge." Perry said that he didn't fit in with his few friends at school and had no sense of belonging. He described being able to blend in, but felt that no-one really noticed or talked to him in particular. Perry was frequently enuretic until age 12, and periodically continues to have nighttime enuretic episodes at almost 17. Perry is odd and moody, and even within a residential treatment program for juvenile sexual offenders he sets himself apart from his peers, who themselves are juvenile sexual offenders, reporting after almost one year in residential treatment that he does not trust any of his peers, or most of the staff. He tends to blame others for his problems, and easily falls into a victim stance. Perry generates strong countertransference feelings in his clinicians.

---

[2] Average IQ is represented by scores falling between 85 and 115, with 100 as the mean average. A full score IQ of 122 falls into the above average to superior range (116–130).

Perry tends to blame others for his problems, easily falling into a victim stance. With trichotillomania, Perry pulls hair out of his arms and his head, leaving small bald patches, and has pulled his eyelashes out in the past. He worries about the size of his testicles, and expresses concerns about being teased because of this. Perry reports often worrying about aches and pains, checking his fecal stools, and periodically worrying that people will try to hurt or kill him. He reported past hallucinations of wild animals passing near him, and stated that when younger he could levitate himself, but later acknowledged this could have been a dream. He reports being into the Wicca religion, and believes that "all my life I felt a strong power inside of me, like a magical, powerful force." Perry does not have a history of any substance abuse, although there was significant substance use in his immediate family.

Perry has had several very brief romantic relationships with three same-age girls, none of which lasted more than 3–4 days before the relationships were ended by the girls, usually for another boy, with the exception of his current relationship with a 14-year-old girl. None of these relationships got past the kissing and hand-holding stage, although Perry had already developed sexual experience with his victim and was interested in sexual relationships. He reports he didn't want to risk being sexual with them as "I was afraid of losing them and I'm phobic about being alone." Perry trusts his current 14-year-old girlfriend because "she loves me."

FAMILY HISTORY

Jordan and Sally, Perry's biological parents, divorced when Perry was age 8, and prior to that Jordan was rarely around. There is a history of multiple and frequent moves, and a reported history of periodic local social service intervention during Perry's early years due to reports of neglect and poor supervision at home. Perry has three other younger full siblings from this marriage, and several other younger half siblings and step-siblings from his parents' later marriages. His father has had additional children but his mother, married to a recovering substance abuser, has not. She feels unable to handle additional mothering responsibilities. Jordan won custody of Perry and his younger siblings after the divorce, due to maternal neglect, and Perry lived with his father until age 16, until his sexually abusive behavior was discovered. After moving in with his father at age 8, Perry reports excessive and unnecessary physical punishment by his father, emotional cruelty and abuse, and being treated differently from the rest of the children, all of whom were younger. Perry was home schooled while living with his mother, and past age 8 was enrolled in a number of public and private schools, never remaining in the same school for more than two years. At age 9, Perry went to the school nurse's office in tears, stating that he feels his father doesn't love him. He reports that his father has never been proud of him. Perry's father immediately cut off all contact with Perry after learning of his sexual abuse of Marcy.

Perry reports strained relationships with almost every family member. Interestingly, Perry is entranced by his youngest half brother, whom Perry alleges is mistreated by his older sister, Marcy (Perry's victim). He says that Marcy has been trying to harm her younger brother, age 4, "since he was born," and this is why he doesn't like Marcy. Perry reports feeling fond and protective of his younger half brother, but also sees him as "babied and whiney."

PARENT DESCRIPTION

Perry's mother is an excessive worrier and was over-protective of her children when they were younger. She becomes easily frustrated and overwhelmed, and is dominated by others. She made a decision to not have more children, and reports having little patience with other people's children, which is of particular interest as she runs a small day care service in her home. She was sexually abused by her paternal uncle while growing up, is currently married to a former substance abuser whom she describes as domineering and controlling, and lives with him and his three children from a former marriage. She is not in contact with any member of her own family, despite having many siblings. Her closest ally and confidante is her former mother-in-law, Jordan's mother from whom he is estranged.

Perry's father was himself reportedly sexually abused by one of his older brothers, and it has been reported by Sally, his former wife, that he engaged in sexual offenses himself when younger. Sally also has reported that when they were married she was afraid he may turn his sexual attentions to their children as a result of his "sexual appetite." As noted, Jordan's own father (Perry's grandfather) has served a prison sentence for sexual abuse although he is now deceased, and both of Jordan's older brothers have served prison sentences for sexual offenses. Jordan himself may have been sexually abused by one of his brothers. Jordan appears to be an angry and rigidly controlled man in general, estranged from his own family, including his mother whom he reports has never taken care of him nor supported him and who is now closely allied with Perry's former wife.

Perry's strongest relationship is with his mother. However, he feels she smothered him as a child, and sees her as anxious and incapable, and ultimately unable to take care of him. He nevertheless feels he was deprived of the opportunity to live with her and be taken care of by her past age 8, and still wishes to live with her, feeling loved by her but resentful of her incapacity to take care of him earlier in life, instead allowing him to live with his father through his childhood and early teens. Perry longs for his father's approval, but reports being "angry" with his father for as long as he can remember, with early memories of abandonment by his father. He has life-long experiences of his father as angry and rejecting of him, even after moving with his father, at age 8, and has for many years both sought his father's love and reported feeling that his father doesn't love him. Being around his father is difficult and Perry considers his father to be explosive and dominating, and feels that his father treats everyone else better than he treats Perry. Despite wanting his father's love and attention, and wanting to be recognized by his father, Perry feels that due to the massive conflicts between his parents and the mutual "bad mouthing" that has always characterized their relationship, he has grown up not knowing what to believe, and attributes this, in part, as the source of his uncertainty about almost everything in life.

Attachment Patterns in the Parents

The contrast and similarities between the parents are striking: polar opposites, representing two opposite attachment patterns. Mother is anxious, needy, and loving, incapable and fearful, as an adult latching onto anyone who can lead the way; father is domineering, harsh, rigid and demanding, capable of getting his way, and distant and unforgiving in relationships. Both have had awful family and personal experiences, and continue to have estranged or heavily conflicted relationships with their own parents. Both, also, are heavily controlled by others, Sally because of her anxiety and dependence on others and Jordan because he is still significantly affected by a dominating mother and accusations by his ex-wife, and because he is financially dependent upon his current wife and her family who fund his small and struggling business.

Generally speaking, attachment theory presumes that ambivalently attached individuals form romantic relationships driven by neediness, goals of anxiety reduction and increased self-esteem, and assurance, and tend to be clingy and dependent in the relationship. Conversely, avoidantly attached individuals form relationships for social control, maintenance of self-image, and purpose-driven goals, and tend to be distant and unresponsive to demands placed upon them. When individuals with these attachment styles form a union, it is unlikely that either party will feel satisfied by the relationship which is more likely to be self-defeating for both, and particularly for the ambivalent or emotionally preoccupied partner.

THERAPEUTIC IMPRESSION

Perry seems very much personality disordered, with strongly interlocking personality characteristics that influence and shape his entire way of dealing with the world, compounded by cognitive distortions that impede emotional connection and perspective taking. Despite his IQ, in many ways Perry is alexithymic—that is, has no words by which to recognize, label, and discuss his feelings. The pressure and expectations of therapy sessions, including the structure of sessions, is difficult and anxiety provoking for Perry who seems to feel he is under a microscope.

Therapy is slow moving, and sessions, in which it is difficult for the clinician to connect with Perry, move at a snail's pace. The therapist finds it difficult to move as slowly and as laboriously as Perry who talks in a quiet monotone throughout, rarely making any direct eye or facial contact, usually playing with cards, or some other distraction, throughout the session. Perry depends on "meta" communication instead, such as vacant stares at the table or out the window, silences, and eye rolling to communicate feelings, recognizing that the therapist will understand the meaning of these behaviors. Perry seems uncomfortable or not able to engage in a relationship with the therapist. He shows little capacity for intimacy or tolerance for anything that irritates him, and an inability to assume the perspective of another, and creates treatment conundrums by wanting to do what "he needs to do" in therapy as defined by his therapist, including workbook assignments, but does not want to follow that direction when it makes him feel emotionally uncomfortable or challenges his very rigid sense of self. He thus seeks concrete and simplistic answers and direction, hampered by limited ability to tolerate feelings or conceptualize or reflect on the ideas of others.

Perry is emotionally and intellectually impoverished. He very much wants to be seen and experienced by others as the person he feels he *really* is, but is frustrated by the fact that this is not what people see. He was genuinely hurt when his therapist failed to see or experience him as empathic, and wanted her view of him to be rectified because he felt she and others were not really understanding or seeing the "real" him, as he experiences himself. His attempts to change her mind about him were aimed at being recognized and understood by a person (i.e., his therapist) who is *supposed* to recognize and understand him. This smacks of the sort of expectations a young child reasonably has of its parents, and may well be a significant clue to Perry's early and ongoing emotional and connection experiences with his parents, as well as the power and importance of the therapeutic relationship.

ATTACHMENT-INFORMED FORMULATION

We can use the *Inventory for Attachment-informed Analysis of Behaviors* (Figure 10.1) by which to consider and interpret Perry's thoughts, feelings, attitudes, and behaviors from an attachment perspective, or Perry as the product of his attachment experiences. Perry's sense of self is poor, characterized by ambivalence and confusion. He feels that he can only trust himself and needs to "just make sure," driving ruminative and obsessive thinking and compulsive behaviors, yet also experiences himself as incapable and lacking the capacity to be recognized, seen, or heard by others, or get others to follow his lead. He feels that he blends in and disappears. However, as his greatest fear is being alone, he has thus learned to use his disappearance as a way to stay in the proximity of family and friends, although he has strained or distant relationships with almost everybody, and feels either treated poorly and differently from others, or ignored and unseen.

Fear of Being Unlovable

Perry counts his girlfriend as his most trusted friend. Although she is several years younger than he is and he has never been alone with her, and has barely had an actual relationship with her, this relationship represents Perry being seen by, and important to, someone/ anyone, as well as representing the idea that he is someone who *can* be loved. He trusts her because "she loves me." This relationship is a symbol of both being connected *and* being loved. However, although he wants to be loved, given the choice between feeling loved or being alone Perry will first choose not to be alone, as he feels he cannot be loved by anyone who is of true importance to him; his 14-year-old girlfriend is a surrogate only for other, unavailable objects who might love him and be loved in return. Torn by and in denial of this idea, Perry nevertheless fears that he *cannot* be loved. From the attachment perspective this stems from his relationship with a father whom he believes has never loved him and, Perry fears, disdains him, and a mother who, despite loving him, Perry disdains on some level because she is incompetent, was unable to take care of him, and is anxiety-ridden, an attribute that Perry feels she has passed directly onto him, rendering him afraid of and isolated from the world.

Restricted Imagination and Suppression

Perry is insecure about everything. His affect is almost completely flat and his movements sparse. His feelings are communicated through his obsessively driven behavior, somatic complaints, trichotillomania, and other visible representations of his internal state. Perry depends on these metacommunications[3] to engage with others, almost like sign language. Despite a relatively high IQ, he has little insight into his own thoughts and feelings, is a concrete thinker, and demonstrates little exploration or risk taking in his ideas. However, Perry does engage in imaginative flights that involve isolated fantasy play, such as dungeon and dragon type and other electronic games which require little engagement and interaction with others and to a large degree depend on intellect, and also is interested in mystical spiritual practices such as Wicca and witchcraft. These interests not only require no active engagement with others and can accommodate solitary activity, but they also involve the acquisition and release of power, and the possibility or reality of power over others. Recall that Perry has always experienced and continues to believe that he has an inner strong power, waiting to be released. In this formulation, this is a suppressed sense of humanity and connection, an attachment-longing-to-be-formed, unrecognized by others but vaguely recognized by Perry who mistakes it for a mystical force waiting his whole life for release. The question is will it, like a powerful spring, be uncoiled at some point and, if so, in what manner and form?

Impoverished Metacognition

Perry shows little ability to reflect upon or think about what other people may be thinking or how they are feeling, or chooses not to think about others in this way, and seems virtually unable to assume another perspective. Not surprisingly, he demonstrates little in the way of empathy, although he describes himself as caring about other people and empathic. Nevertheless, although he reports having "empathy for what he did" to his step-sister, Perry reports having no other compassion or feelings for her, and seems to consider her to be a "deserving" victim.

Attachment and Sexually Abusive Behavior

Perry's sexually abusive relationship with his young step-sister possibly met a complex combination of personal needs. It may be seen as a troubled effort to become connected to someone, combined with being seen, commanding respect, and being in charge (if only in the form of fear and domination—much like his father), while also meeting Perry's needs to feel that he was experiencing what he imagined other young men of his age were experiencing—sex! Here, we see elements of social connection, presence and recognition, sexual exploration and satisfaction, the sexual adult rite of passage, and control and social mastery—a pathological equivalent of idealized adolescent identity. We may also see elements of Schachner and Shaver's (2004) hypothesis that in adults, at least, anxiety is associated with the use of sex in order to help to reduce insecurity, and the conclusions of Davis, Shaver, and Vernon (2004) that adult sexual behavior serves attachment functions

---

[3] Metacommunication is communication without, outside of or beyond words, which nevertheless conveys information about some event or experience.

of emotional closeness, reassurance, enhanced self-esteem, and stress reduction, and particularly so for individuals high in attachment anxiety.

Perry's sexual abuse of Marcy also contained elements of revenge against his father and step-mother, as well as punishment of his step-sister because of the way that Perry perceived she treated their younger brother. Perhaps in some poorly realized manner Perry sees himself in his young brother, troubled and alone, the victim of someone who should care for and about him but doesn't. However, in addition to feeling protective of his younger brother, Perry also sees him as babied and whiney, reflecting ambivalence about the need to be protected, intolerance of weakness, and ideas embedded in Perry's experience that, on some level, we own and are responsible for our problems and get what we deserve. Perry is also unable or unwilling to see his step-sister, even at age 6 (4 when the abuse began) as anything more than a spoiled, nasty, and demanding "little bitch," despite her life circumstances and his own life circumstances at that age. No perspective taking, metacognition, or empathy is shown here.

Ambivalence and Social Needs

Perry experiences a strong need for intimacy but fears rejection, thus describing the ambivalent attachment pattern—preoccupation with but ambivalence toward and resistance to the desired object (the relationship, in this case). This pattern sets up a scenario for relationship disappointment and the confirmation of already existing internalized negative schemata and internal scripts that predict failure. These thinking errors (to use sex offender treatment language) confirm lack of worth, lower or maintain already low self-esteem, prohibit further risk-taking behavior, and further depress a sense of self-agency and self-efficacy. It is a self-perpetuating model of social failure that is built upon, maintains, and strengthens already existing templates embedded in the internal working model. With respect to anomic and strain theory, the only way for such an individual to acquire legitimate social goals is through deviant means, demonstrating not so much deviant *ideation* as deviant *means* to accomplish legitimate social goals—in Perry's case, true for many adolescents, he considers sexual relationships to be a legitimate social goal.

Pathological as it may be in the case of all sexually abusive behavior, having sexual contact nevertheless serves to *partially* meet *many* needs: (i) restoring some sense of social connection (especially for the alienated), particularly pertinent as there is almost always some pre-existing relationship with the victim, (ii) creating a sense of adherence to a social norm, in this case sex as normative teenage behavior, (iii) promoting a sense of social competence, (iv) taking and demonstrating social control and self-agency, (v) illusory preparation for later romantic and sexual relationships, (vi) sexual gratification and relief, (vii) reducing anxiety about powerlessness, (viii) fulfilling curiosity about the much desired but mysterious sexual world, and (ix) stress relief and escape from an otherwise troubling and frustrating world. Every instance of sexual offending, of course, is going to meet, or partially fulfill, a different set of needs for different offenders, and in addition to the needs identified here there may be many others. For instance, see Rich (2003, chap. 5) for a more detailed overview of factors that motivate and/or maintain sexually abusive behavior.

Romance, Sex, and Loneliness

With no experience of the mutuality and union that characterize intimate relationships, having experienced only the anxious protection of his mother or the rigid rejection of his father, Perry has developed a lifetime fear of being alone. Driven by messages prevalent in his social environment, Perry assumes that sex relates to social competency and feeling good, embodied by the relentless media propagation of the message that sexual prowess is a means for pleasure and satisfaction and a measure of social normality. He is fearful that if he seeks sex in his few fragile romantic relationships he will fail and be left alone (and his limited romantic experiences have generally lasted only a few days anyway, with girls leaving for other guys). In the case of his current girlfriend, whom he has not known for long and with whom he has never been alone as she is a minor, he is content to simply let the relationship stand, a fragile tribute to the idea that he *can* have relationships, and someone cares for him. In many ways, Perry counts this as all he has, and names his girl-friend as the person he most trusts. Of note, the person he counts as his second most trusted friend is a young woman he met through an internet chat room, although he has never met or seen her, has had contact only several times, and has had no contact for over 14 months.

To be Seen or Not to be Seen: The Desire to be Recognized

For Perry, behaviors are driven by a convoluted need to be seen but not becoming *too* visible (as this may evoke discomfort), the risk of rejection, and demands on already limited emotional energy (remember, he is depressed and flat, as well as anxious), and highlight limited metacognitive skills in which he is challenged to engage with and demon-strate understanding of others. Operational all of the time, this is especially apparent in therapy sessions where he is expected to demonstrate both motivation and insight into self and others, engage in an active relationship, and be present. Perry cannot even look at the therapist. Perry feels, and perhaps is correct, that his parents *were* not and *are* not able to recognize and meet his needs and, as important, see and understand him for who he actu-ally is. He transfers these feelings onto others about him, and particularly his therapist, whom he feels should both recognize and lead him, removing all responsibility for his own actions, much as an infant should be able to depend on its caregiver(s) and in those very early days be recognized and loved, but not held responsible for self.

Trapped Inside

Another goal, related closely to the need to be visible to others, is the need to be recog-nized, understood, and, as a result, loved and able to love back. Perry feels tortured by his experience of being unrecognized for whom he feels he really is, and "trapped" inside of himself. His goal is to feel emotionally comfortable and socially accepted, establishing security in himself and trust in others through feeling attached, recognized, and safe. For Perry, loss of identity, value and meaning, and his inability to know who or what to trust, stem *directly* from insecurity and failure in his parental relationships, mirroring the poor attachment and family relationship experiences of both parents. Perry's sexual behavior, as well as all other social behavior, and even his depression, anxiety, and ruminative thinking, must be understood in this light if one is to understand who Perry is, how he came to be that person, and how one might help him.

An Attached Relationship Perspective

Turning to the 12-item *Attached Relationship Inventory* (Figure 10.2), it is clear that Perry desires and experiences relationships as important, so we can bypass any idea that Perry is schizoid[4] or a sociopath. In fact, Perry is relationship oriented, but derives little security or satisfaction through his relationships, and has little confidence or trust in relationship partners, although he seems to long to have relationships that *will* provide a sense of safety, protection, and well-being.

Perry's capacity to engage in supportive and satisfying relationships is further impaired by his lack of perspective taking and general metacognition, as well as his inability to give and take in relationships, needing more than he can give. It is not clear whether Perry's relationship needs can ever be met as he has never had a relationship that meets even basic psychological needs. It seems unlikely that, unless things change drastically, Perry will be capable of a close relationship without being overly demanding, needy, or enmeshed, or whether he can feel secure in a relationship.

UNDERSTANDING PERRY

Hilburn-Cobb (2004) proposes that: (i) attachment behaviors are designed to ensure stable/regulated internal states, (ii) secure parent–child relationships provide a measure of self-regulation, (iii) secure or not, individuals will struggle to maintain internal homeostasis/regulated stability, and (iv) insecure individuals will engage in anxious behavioral strategies that are suppressed or distorted, but in either case are aimed at proximity, protection, and self-regulation. She describes Perry well when she describes insecure individuals experiencing the ordinary ups-and-downs of daily life as survival issues in which self-regulation is *always* driving emotional reactions to daily events.

We recognize also that both secure and insecure attachments are considered adaptations to the rearing environment, and recall Goldberg's (1997) notion that secure *and* insecure attachment patterns serve protective functions (even if maladaptive or dysfunctional). Consider, then, the protective role that remaining anxious, cutoff, and partially invisible plays for Perry as he deals with others in his daily life, trying hard to remain emotionally regulated in the face of things that, for him, represent great adversity and challenge his sense of security. We also note that Bowlby (1979) described some of the very factors at play in Perry's upbringing when he described the development of suboptimal, or "common deviant patterns of attachment behavior" (p. 136) based on the parent–child relationship. These include one or both parents being persistently unresponsive to the child's

---

[4] A social withdrawal and inability to form relationships, marked by disinterest in relationships and often associated with or considered a rudimentary form of or precursor to schizophrenia.

care-eliciting behavior and/or actively disparaging and rejecting, discontinuities of parenting, persistent threats by parents not to love a child, and threats by parents to abandon the family. He writes that any of these experiences, if repeated often enough, can lead a child, adolescent, or adult to live in constant anxiety about loss of attachment figures, describing this pattern as anxious attachment.

When it comes to defining Perry's attachment pattern or, if we can, an attachment category, he is the person described by both Holmes (2001) and Slade (1999) who write that we cannot simply overlay defined categories of attachment styles onto actual people or think of individuals in terms of single, exclusive, and stable categories of attachment. On the one hand, it is easy to report that Perry is an extremely insecure individual, in a constant state of anxiety about himself and his relationship to everyone else, both anxious *and* avoidant. For Hilburn-Cobb (2004) avoidance *is* a form of anxious attachment, so there is no conflict there, but in most attachment models, anxious attachment and avoidant attachment are separately defined.

In terms of defining an attachment pattern, it is difficult to be any more specific than describing Perry as anxiously and avoidantly insecure. However, although Perry is relationship avoidant and distant in most cases, we also see that he has grasped tightly to several unrealistic relationships that are virtually non-existent, such as with his girlfriend and internet chat room friend. Perry is both avoidant of *and* dependent upon relationships, creating mythological relationships to take the place of real ones.

Actually, Perry is a poster child for both preoccupation and anxiety when it comes to relationships, not because he is ambivalent about them (he wants relationships) but because he fears rejection and being misunderstood. One might argue that his fears are well grounded as he does not appear to be able to understand or care about how others think and feel, and thus relationships are alien to him. Lacking metacognition, the very thing Perry wants is frightening to him: to be loved means loving others; to be understood means understanding others—difficult tasks for Perry. Accordingly, at one and the same time, although he wishes to have relationships he is distant in the few relationships he has and avoids forming new ones. This is because they frighten him, not because he doesn't want relationships. His avoidance of relationships is really played out in his ambivalence about and resistance to relationships, and vice versa (his resistance leads to avoidance), making ambivalence and avoidance flip sides of the same coin for Perry. If one *had* to categorize him, using the Bartholomew model (Figure 7.3, Chapter 7), it would be as fearful-avoidant, in which he essentially has a poor view of himself and of others, and is high in anxiety and avoidance.

One can argue that Perry's behaviors, having reached a pretty pathological state (he is diagnosed with an anxiety disorder, a depressive disorder, trichotillomania, enuresis, and traits of obsessive compulsive personality disorder), are in fact driven by disorganized attachment strategies that combine elements of both avoidance and anxiety. Although, from Crittenden's perspective (Figure 7.1, Chapter 7), she doesn't recognize a disorganized category, Perry perhaps is most closely associated with the A^+/C^+ classification, which combines affect and cognition but fails to integrate them, suggesting a variant of disorganized attachment.

It becomes clear that even in a case in which elements of both anxious and avoidant insecure attachment are obvious, classification is a difficult and artificial task, forcing the clinician to categorize individuals into the nearest best fit, rather than recognizing, not just dimensionality, but *multi*-dimensionality. Perry can best be classified as anxiously and avoidantly insecure with an operational style that is disorganized and contributes to significant mental health problems, albeit never reaching the psychopathological level of "frank disorganization" described by Hilburn-Cobb (2004).

SUMMARY: ATTACHMENT THEORY APPLIED TO REAL LIFE

I hope that this single case study has provided a useful way to apply attachment theory and bring a case to life from the viewpoint of attachment and the internal working model. From this analysis, we can reasonably assert a relationship-disturbed pattern that dominates Perry's ideas and behavior, related to the development of attachment insecurity. Also demonstrated, I hope, is the importance of considering the attachment experiences of the parents, with respect to the intergenerational transmission of attachment experiences and the patterns of family interactions and dynamics that, in Minuchin's (1974) words, "imprints its members with selfhood" (p. 47). In fact, central to any attachment-informed analysis, the content and shape of family history and family dynamic lies at the heart of attachment formation and the development of selfhood and self-in-society. Indeed, West et al. (1998) have noted the role and quality of family relationships in the development of emotional disorders in adolescents, writing that adverse family experiences pose "a relentless threat" to the adolescent's sense of secure attachment (p. 662).

Does this attachment-informed analysis case study produce a more coherent view of Perry's history and his recent and current behaviors? I hope the reader will find it to have been a useful means by which to view Perry in a different light than we might otherwise, and thus understand both motivation and treatment direction, at least in part. We can conclude that Perry's sexually abusive behavior, rather than being the product of deviant sexual arousal—wanting to hurt another individual, wildly out-of-control sexual drive, or genetic heredity (in light of the history of sexually abusive behavior in his paternal family)—is more directly related to attachment difficulties and his view of himself, others, relationships and their availability to him, and his capacity to have a satisfactory impact on the world. Thus, rather than addressing deviant sexual arousal or cognitive distortions per se, treatment is more likely to be productive if it targets self-efficacy and self-agency, works to resolve security and efficacy in relationships, helps self-regulation of anxiety, and increases perspective taking and the realization of empathic states.

Does this mean that we shouldn't provide treatment that addresses boundaries, thinking errors, dysfunctional behavioral cycles, relapse prevention plans, and so forth, much described in the literature that addresses comprehensive treatment for juvenile sexual offending? Not at all. In fact, working hand in hand with what has become "conventional" assessment and treatment for juvenile sexual offenders, an attachment-informed *evaluation* goes beyond risk assessment and moves towards depth in formulation, and attachment-informed *treatment* includes and moves beyond the cognitive-behavioral and psychoeducational language of sexual offender treatment. It becomes integrated with that treatment, rather than replacing, sidestepping, or paying short shrift to it, adding an understanding of developmental dynamics, internal working models, and psychodynamic relationships.

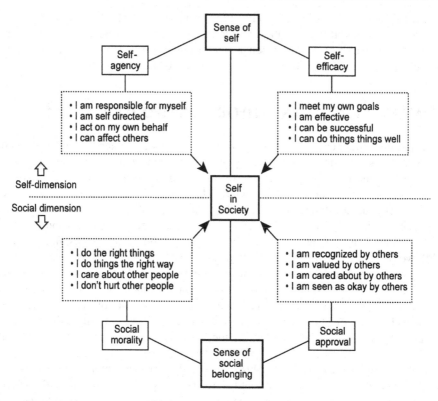

Figure 10.3   Self-in-society: Self-image and personal identity

However, with respect to any analysis, it's a mistake to see treatment and clinical for-mulation through only a single lens. This is equally true whether the lens is that of attach-ment theory or that of any other theory. This would be akin to thinking that the way we see the universe, through visible light, is the only way to see it. Using this analogy, we know that we can see the universe and anything in it through radio waves, x-rays, ultra-violet, gamma rays, light, and even sound. Each is no more than a limited and narrowly defined bandwidth along a far broader band. It's important to narrow our bandwidth and tune in for clarity and pinpoint accuracy, but it is also important to know that there's a much broader band out there and the bandwidth we are using represents one thin slice and not the whole thing. We need to consider this in our analyses, and not limit ourselves by trying to understand everything through one narrow bandwidth. In particular, we must not come to believe that the single bandwidth is "it"—the one lens that will reveal all.

Because people are multidimensional, it is important to apply multidimensional theo-ries and multidimensional approaches to our understanding of people. In examining a diamond, each facet in itself offers much information. However, it would be a mistake to believe that each facet offers the only view or perspective. As the diamond is turned another facet is revealed, and then another. All of these facets add up to a deeper, richer, more complete view and the possibility of a more complete explanation.

CONCLUSION: SELF-IN-SOCIETY

Figure 10.3 provides an overview of the forces that shape the formation and experience of self-in-society, from both the internal/self and the external/social domain. In this simple model, selfhood is defined by, or the product of, self-agency and self-efficacy, or a sense of personal capacity and competence. From the social domain, connection and belongingness are shaped and fostered by the twin forces of social morality and social approval. Where self-efficacy means doing things right, social morality means doing the right things. Parallel to this is our experience of being recognized by others for both what we do and who we are. As we conclude this chapter, I invite the reader to reconsider the experiences of Perry from the perspective of these four forces, in which internal and external conditions come together in our sense of self as we exist in society.

CHAPTER 11

Presumed Links: An Attachment-driven Pathway to Sexual Abuse

For the past few years, dating back to around 1990, it has become increasingly common to see not only attachment deficits linked to the development of sexually abusive behavior, but also social skills and social competence. For the most part, in this context, social competence is, more-or-less, heavily defined by the capacity to understand and appropriately act upon moral social imperatives, experience empathy for others, and develop intimate social relationships. Linked to these underlying elements, social competence is evidenced by twin behavioral and emotional strands. That is, social competence is mirrored in behavior that is socially appropriate and results in the achievement of socially appropriate goals (appropriate and effective social behavior) *and* emotional satisfaction derived from interactions, relationships, and behaviors in the social setting, including a sense of accomplishment in the social environment (social satisfaction). These ideas are, of course, linked to the agentive self and self-efficacy, both central elements in the formation of self-in-society, or the social self and its impact on selfhood and personal identity.

SOCIAL INCOMPETENCE AND CLOSE RELATIONSHIPS

Rather than serving as a categorical measure of one's capacity to behave effectively and derive satisfaction from social behaviors, prosocial behaviors and social satisfaction are dimensional, each lying along a continuum. That is, some people are more socially competent than others, social competence changes over time, and social competence may vary under different circumstances. Nevertheless, social competence embraces the idea that one can be and feel successful in the social environment, whereas social inadequacy suggests that the behavior of the individual neither achieves social goals nor results in a sense of social satisfaction. That is, the individual is socially incompetent.

Central to the idea of social competence are the constructs of empathy and intimacy which, of course, are related. Empathy is considered a prerequisite to adult intimacy (or close relationships, and not necessarily sexual intimacy). And intimacy, which may, but often does not, result from empathy, is nonetheless unlikely without empathy. Although neither empathy nor intimacy is required to live safely in society, for sexual intercourse, or for sexual reproduction, they are nevertheless considered central to a sense of social relatedness and social satisfaction, and serve to drive prosocial behavior. In addition to serving as social satisfiers within the individual, empathy and intimacy are also protective factors against antisocial behavior. Conversely, one can easily argue that an absence of either results in social alienation (lack of social connection) and increases the possibility of antisocial behavior.

Figure 11.1 illustrates a simple model (although, at first glance, it may not look simple) that breaks social competence into its behavioral and emotional constituents, linking competence to empathy and intimacy, sense of selfhood (self-in-society), and ultimately social behaviors. Because, in any linear model, outcomes always lead to feedback and reinforcement, the illustration shows how the outcome of social competence serves to further reinforce social competence or social inadequacy.

As we have tried to understand not only forces that drive *towards* sexually abusive behavior, we also have looked for factors that fail to prevent or restrain the behavior. Such a notion is central to control theories of criminology that ask *not* why some people are criminal, but why more people do *not* engage in antisocial behavior. The notion of social competence addresses both sides of the equation. On the one hand, as in strain theory

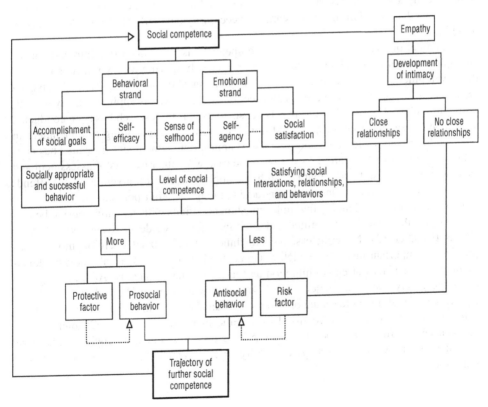

Figure 11.1   A model of social competence, selfhood, and social behaviors

(Chapter 4), a lack of social competence drives people towards delinquent or socially deviant behavior in order to meet goals that are not otherwise achievable, and on the other fails to restrain socially incompetent individuals from victimizing others in pursuit of those goals. Like attachment theory itself, then, social competence by its presence or absence somewhere along a continuum, serves as both a risk *and* protective factor. In fact, social competence is a central component of attachment theory in which it is believed that the level of social competence is an outcome of the attachment experience. The ability to tolerate difficulty and adversity, a form of social competence in and of itself, builds towards increased social competence in a self-fulfilling and positive cycle.

Indeed, Hudson and Ward (2000) note that in many conceptualizations of adult sexual offending, social competence is heavily implicated in the causal pathway to sexual offending. Given the hypothesized relationship between social competence and attachment, several groups of researchers have formulated ideas regarding the development of sexually abusive behavior driven by attachment difficulties. Described in this and the following chapter, these ideas reflect the current thinking that links social relatedness and attachment to adult sexual offending. Social deficits that result from attachment deficits are conceptualized as the links between attachment theory and theories of sexual offending, and the causative factor that results in sexual abuse. This model, now prevalent and increasingly so in the sex offender specific literature, hypothesizes, in part at least, that adult sexually abusive behavior, often with children, "may be in the service of underlying social needs that in and of themselves are not necessarily deviant" (Hudson & Ward, 2000, p. 497).

This model of social deficits, or social competence, is very much tied into and part of an applied model of attachment theory that is presently driving a new understanding of the developmental pathways that, in some people, contribute or lead to sexually abusive behavior. Of special note, however, with exceptions, this model is applied entirely to adult sexual offenders. The primary reason is because, to date, little research has been conducted with juvenile sexual offenders; beyond this, our limited understanding of attachment in older children and adolescents and the lack of appropriate attachment measures has contributed to the lack of research. As has been the case with other aspects of assessment and treatment, it may also be true that research and applied work with juvenile sexual offenders always lags behind similar work conducted among the adult population.

In addition, the broad model that links attachment deficits with sexually abusive behavior is largely theoretical, with limited and often inconsistent evidence to support its propositions (Chapter 12). Nevertheless, the attachment deficit/sexual coercion model does provide an important means by which to conceptualize and follow a link between developmental experiences of early childhood and later criminal behaviors. And, although we can largely only apply the model to adult sexual offenders, given the lack of any significant research with juvenile sexual offenders, we can also recognize that for many, sexual-offending behavior can be recognized as a crime of relationships (see Chapter 13). As Hudson and Ward (2000) note, these are crimes driven as much by social needs as by sexual interests, which is perhaps especially true of sexually abusive adolescents and children.

OPERATIONAL DIFFICULTIES

Hudson and Ward (2000, p. 497) write that hypothesized social deficits

> paint a picture of the typical offender as being socially inept, sexually preoccupied, socially isolated or at least having limited skills with respect to close relationships, and having a hostile, unempathic style of relating to others . . . deficits in social competency, specifically those aspects relevant to close relationships, are clearly viewed as being central to sexual offending.

This is, of course, in most cases, a caricature of the adult sexual offender. In part, however, these deficits in social skills lie in the realm of relationship building and the formation of close relationships that lead to a sense of social connection and belonging, as well as the development of interpersonal relationships that are satisfying and constitute attached relationships. But social skills deficits extend beyond relationship-building skills. From an attachment perspective, social skills also include the essential skills of metacognition, or the ability to reflect on the minds of self and others, contributing directly to the development of empathy for others, and the capacity for self-regulation and distress tolerance. Both metacognition and self-regulation skills contribute to the experience of self-agency and the capacity for self-efficacy, and are thus central components in the process of building and maintaining social relationships. The capacity for relationship building, or the interactional component of social behavior, is itself partly contingent upon the primary social skills of metacognition and self-regulation, as depicted in Figure 11.2.

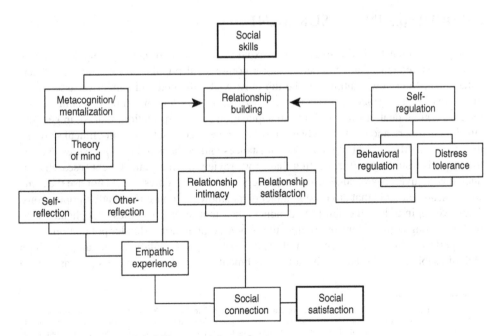

Figure 11.2 From social skills to social satisfaction

However, although we commonly talk about social deficits in juvenile and adult sexual offenders, by which we mean a lack of social competence (or social efficacy), Mulloy and Marshall (1999) have noted that, "we need a clearer identification of just what it is we expect when we claim that sexual offenders have social deficits so that we can more definitively examine the hypothesis that they are deficient in these skills" (pp. 95–96). Nevertheless, despite this lack of clarity, magnified by little actual evidence to support an attachment-driven hypothesis for the development of sexually abusive behavior, our ideas continue to be driven by theory rather than empiricism. Indeed, disregarding their own criticism of definitional weakness, Mulloy and Marshall write that "despite the problems . . . there appears to be no doubt that attachment styles are an important area of dysfunction in sexual offenders" (1999, p. 106). Although an attractive idea, with important treatment implications, there is no clear empirical evidence for this perspective. However, although we have little evidence that social skills in sexual offenders are any more relevant than social skills deficits in non-sexual criminals, or indeed, among groups of non-forensic clinical subjects, we continue to emphasize our belief that social skills *are* significant in understanding sexual offenders.

Although, the idea of social skills and attachment deficits has obvious appeal at face value, and is apparent in some sexual offenders, we nonetheless have little evidence that social skills deficits are essential to the development of sexually abusive behavior rather than criminal or antisocial behaviors in general. And, of course, in discussing social skills we are only *indirectly* discussing attachment, using the idea of social skills deficits as a proxy for attachment deficits, often measuring concepts such as empathy, intimacy, and security in relationships, taking these as indirect evidence of attachment difficulties.

DIFFICULTIES IN MEASUREMENT

As opposed to our limited research with sexual offenders, there is far greater consistency in the measurement of attachment among a non-clinical population, in which the Adult Attachment Interview continues to be the most well-validated and supported assessment tool. This is an impractical instrument, however, as it is lengthy, time consuming, and requires a great deal of training for both application and interpretation. Indeed, in general, attachment theory and related study has most often been conducted in non-clinical settings, thus facing a different set of testing circumstances and perhaps reduced pressures. Nevertheless, it is troubling and frustrating that as we review the little attachment research conducted with juvenile and adult sexual offenders, we review studies that do not use the same well-researched tools that are used in attachment studies of non-clinical adult populations. Thus, we begin to lose the ability to conduct consistent research studies or replicate them, or draw strong comparisons or contrast to the non-clinical, non-offender population.

In part, attachment research with clinical and forensic populations[1] is hampered by a lack of usable tools. In fact, of the adult attachment instruments we have, many are aimed

---

[1] In attachment and social deficit studies, forensic populations most typically include adult sexual offenders, non-sexual violent criminal offenders, and non-sexual and non-violent criminal offenders. Sometimes sexual offender groups are broken into rapists and child molesters, and sometimes include prison and community populations of sexual offenders, and in some cases, a non-criminal offender group is also included as a comparison group.

at adult romantic relationships, and themselves may be measuring a different construct than the one we really want to reach. As a result, tools that measure intimacy, emotional loneliness, attitudes towards others, empathy, and self-esteem are included with, and sometimes substituted for, attachment measures. Although the use of measures that can be cross-referenced against (and add validity to) other measures may strengthen and make more robust research design, they can also confuse the design as multiple constructs are being assessed, rather than just "attachment." The inclusion of measures designed to assess constructs, such as empathy, intimacy, or loneliness, and using these also to measure or in some way reflect attachment (for which they were not designed), may actually weaken the ability to adequately or accurately interpret outcome data. Here, we risk confusing one construct for another, and blurring the boundaries between them, such as assuming that empathy or security in relationships also implies attachment.

Further, we recognize that the best way to assess attachment is through indirect measures, such as observation or interview. Recall that in both the AAI and the strange situation—the gold standards for measuring attachment—attachment is assessed, not by self-report, but by the careful analysis of heavily trained observers. Accordingly, regardless of the construct they are designed to assess, as almost all of the measures typically used in studies with sexual offenders involve self-report, data are further weakened. Finally, putting to one side the reality that we have limited tools to measure attachment, and even allowing for the practice of using measures that assess related, but non-attachment, measures, an additional and serious limitation on our assessment of attachment is that different instrumentation is used in different studies of attachment within the sexual offender field.

Partly reflecting the limited quality and capacity of attachment assessment instruments available to researchers, there is a wide disparity in the choice of instruments used to assess attachment in forensic research, as well as research design. This make it difficult, of course, to compare results across different studies, and makes it impossible to replicate studies. It's no wonder we come up with so many mixed, confusing, and contradictory results in studies – and we do. As noted, the evidence supporting or pointing to a link between attachment and the development of sexually abusive behavior is both weak and inconsistent, and continues to be largely theory driven and, hence, hypothetical.

EVIDENCE OF ATTACHMENT DIFFERENCES

Despite well-conjectured ideas linking attachment to sexually abusive behavior, efforts to prove or find evidence for this connection – not just correlation – have failed to produce anything we can consider significant. Central to most of these ideas, attachment is considered *causal*, and not just correlated, although any well-constructed model of attachment and sexually abusive behavior recognizes attachment as one element in a *multicausal* pathway that leads to sexual offenses. Attempts to find a link, then, seek not just coexistence of attachment difficulties, but intend to demonstrate that attachment deficits among sexual offenders prefigure and are a cause of, or at least significantly contribute to, the development *and* the maintenance of sexually abusive behavior. Here, disordered attachment is not considered just a comorbid condition found among sexual offenders, but a causative factor. That is, the very existence of a pattern of attachment deficits among sexual offenders, distinguishing this population from other forensic and non-forensic populations, would be considered prima facie evidence of a causal connection. Further refining the attachment-sexual offending link, there is an expectation that distinct patterns of insecure attachment will distinguish among types of sexual offenders, and most notably between adult child molesters and adult rapists.

However, a note of caution is due, not only because we have not, thus far, found a distinguishing pattern that separates sexual offenders from other forensic populations, but even if we did, this would not necessarily support the idea that attachment deficits are the cause of, or maintain, sexually coercive behavior. We must always bear in mind the principle that correlation does not imply causation.

However, if attachment *is* significant in sexually abusive behavior, we would expect to see differences in attachment patterns between groups of sexual offenders and non-sexual criminal offenders, and between sexual offenders and the general population. To begin with, then, as about 67% of the general population is considered secure in attachment and about 33% insecurely attached, we expect to see a significantly higher percentage of sexual offenders with some variant of insecure attachment, and we also expect to find differences in attachment security between sexual offenders and non-sexual criminal offenders. And, in the event that insecure attachment is high in both sexual and non-sexual offenders, we expect to see different types of insecure attachment among the two forensic groups, again teasing out differences based on attachment status rather than behaviors. However, in the relatively few studies so far, such differences have been inconsistently supported, and sometimes not supported at all, most often finding no significant difference between sexual offenders and other non-sexual groups of criminal offenders. For the most part, when a pattern of attachment difficulties is assessed as present, it appears more as a general risk factor for the development of socially deviant behavior, including criminal behavior in general, rather than sexually abusive behavior.

The pathway to healthy attachment is a promising and exciting road to search as we strive to understand the development of sexually abusive behavior. Indeed, it is likely that attachment *is* a significant variable in the development of dysfunctionality, and sometimes antisocial behavior, as well as opening avenues by which to further understand and treat sexual offenders. It seems equally unlikely, however, that attachment will turn out to be any more than an important contributing factor in a convoluted multidetermined pathway that sometimes leads to sexually abusive behavior, rather than a, or *the*, causative factor in the etiology of sexual abuse.

However, it is possible that the failure to support a theory of attachment differences is due to a lack of adequately designed or well enough controlled studies, or our present inability to design instruments sufficiently capable of sensitive measurement. In this case, the issue is one of design, measurement, and/or instrumentation rather than theoretical construct. It is also possible that we do not see attachment differences between groups of sexual offenders and non-sexual criminal offenders, and sometimes between offenders and the general public, because there is no global difference between groups, in which case the theory of attachment differences is inadequate or incorrect.

LINKING ATTACHMENT DEFICITS TO JUVENILE SEXUAL ABUSE

Even if not *the* central component, if attachment deficits are central in adult sexual offenders, we would obviously expect to see such deficits in juvenile sexual offenders as well.

This is especially pertinent, as, unlike other aspects of disordered adult behavior—such as personality disorders, which may not emerge until early adulthood—attachment patterns are typically considered to be established by 12–18 months of age, and stable throughout childhood and adolescence, en route to adult attachment patterns. This makes it all the more important to assess attachment in juvenile sexual offenders, as well as the stability of such patterns into adulthood. If there is a pathway from early attachment deficits to adult sexually abusive behavior, as proposed by Marshall and others, we can expect this pathway to be evident also in juvenile sexual offenders, and in the sexually reactive children who sometimes prefigure adolescent sexual offenders. That is, adolescent insecure attachment and social skills deficits should presage adult deficits, as attachment is a feature of child development, considered to be relatively stable from early childhood onwards.

Of course, if attachment is a significant component, we will also expect to see differences in the attachment classifications of juvenile sexual offenders and those of: (i) non-sexual juvenile delinquents, (ii) emotionally troubled but non-forensic adolescents, and (iii) non-clinical and non-forensic adolescents. Further, because, as far as we know, the majority of juvenile sexual offenders do not recidivate or develop into adult sexual offenders, we can also expect to see differences in attachment patterns between: (i) juvenile sexual offenders who continue into adult sexual offenders and (ii) those who do *not* go on to become adult sexual offenders. This obviously requires not only an adequate and valid definition of attachment in adolescents, but also the application of tools sensitive enough to measure such attachment. Additionally, of course, this requires the implementation of *prospective* (rather than retrospective) or longitudinal attachment research studies that track juvenile sexual offenders over time, including juvenile sexual offenders who do not sexually recidivate as adults and juvenile sexual offenders who do.

This is a large research agenda, then, with respect to juvenile sexual offending. It is perhaps more significant than similar work with adult sexual offenders because, if attachment is central, it is critical to recognize and address the attachment issues that *must* also be present in adolescent sexual offenders (as attachment is developmental, and not emergent). Without such research, of which barely any has yet been conducted, we cannot say much more, other than note expected outcomes in juvenile sexual offenders if attachment is a significant factor. That is, we would expect to see:

- The same sort of attachment deficits in juvenile sexual offenders as in adult sexual offenders.
- Differences in attachment between juvenile sexual offenders and non-sexual juvenile delinquents.
- Differences in attachment between juvenile sexual offenders and non-offending (non-forensic) juveniles.
- Differences in attachment among "types" of juvenile sexual offenders (although we do not yet have an adequate typology of juvenile sexual offenders).
- Differences in attachment between those juvenile sexual offenders who desist from sexually abusive behavior prior to adulthood and those who persist into adult sexual offending.

In fact, although attachment has been increasingly identified as a key variable in adult sexual offending, little has been written about attachment in the development of juvenile sexual offenders. Thus far, almost all of the limited literature that has been produced has been based on male adult sexual offenders, and quite often child molesters rather than rapists, often generated by one of several small research groups. Accordingly, in order to explore and understand the nature of attachment in juvenile sexual offenders it is both relevant and important to also review and understand the literature on attachment and adult sexual offending. Not only is this work informative, but like most of the research interest in our field, work with adult male sexual offenders precedes work with juvenile and other special populations of sexual offenders.

However, attachment research with juvenile sexual offenders is underway. Although they have yet to publish significant data, in progress are several studies exploring attachment in the development and maintenance of juvenile sexual offending, including studies by Michael Miner of the University of Minnesota, David Burton of Smith College, and Barry Burkhart of Auburn University.

Adding to the complication of associating attachment patterns with the onset of sexually abusive behavior is Smallbone's contention (Smallbone, in press-a, in press-b; Smallbone & Wortley, 2004) that, contrary to statistics frequently cited, many adult sexual offenders do not engage in sexually coercive behavior *until* they reach adulthood, after first engaging in other non-sexual criminal activities. Regardless of attachment pattern, if many adults do not engage in sexually coercive behavior until adulthood, then this clearly means that attachment can *not* be the instrumental factor as attachment patterns are already in place by adolescence. In this case, although attachment may play a role in the pathway to sexual offending, factors not apparent until full adulthood are more pertinent than attachment in determining the onset of sexually abusive behavior.

Smallbone's contention that many adult sexual offenders do not engage in sexually abusive behavior until age 30 or later is a further confounding variable. It makes a proposed relationship between attachment difficulties of childhood and later adult sexual offending even more tenuous than it already is, as adult sexual offenders obviously pass through adolescence en route to adulthood. It makes more sense to expect that adult sexual offenders have engaged in, at least, a variant of sexually troubling behavior as adolescents, thus providing a pathway that directly connects attachment difficulties in childhood to the onset of sexually abusive behavior in adults.[2]

FROM ATTACHMENT DEFICIT TO SEXUAL OFFENSE

As attachment is developed during infancy, it is obvious that if it is a factor in adult sexual offending then it must also be a factor of some kind in juvenile sexual offending, or at least in those juvenile sexual offenders who go on to become adult sexual offenders. This suggests concerns immediately, as many/most juvenile sexual offenders do not become adult sexual offenders. This raises the idea that in reviewing similar cases and outcomes retrospectively (seeking commonalities, for instance, by looking backwards to the possible roots of the problems) one comes up with clusters of similar factors. In this case, we

---

[2] It may also be that Smallbone's contention is incorrect, and that the typical belief that a significant percentage of adult sexual offenders did indeed engage in sexually abusive behavior as adolescents is correct (for instance, Abel, Osborn, & Twigg, 1993; Knight & Prentky, 1993; Prentky, Harris, Frizzell, & Righthand, 2000).

see early attachment and bonding difficulties and challenges as one of these factors, as well as histories of troubled and maltreated childhoods. However, if one starts with those factors postulated to be key and works forward, prospectively, one is not likely to see the same outcomes in every, or even most, cases. This is a misleading trap to fall into, and we must be careful to discuss *commonalities* in populations of juvenile and adult sexual offenders rather than *profiles*, recognizing early childhood experiences as *risk* factors rather than pathologies with certain outcomes. This is as true for classifications of attachment, as for any other childhood risk (or protective) factor.

To date, there has been relatively little in-depth material on the subject of attachment in sexual offenders. The field has instead most often relied on generalized descriptions, explanations, and theorizing mostly found in single chapters within larger edited books or a relatively few articles describing research into the area, most often generated by various permutations of relatively few researchers who work closely and collaborate with another, and hence produce similar ideas. As described, much of this work remains theoretical only, and in some cases is clearly contradictory. Descriptions of attachment difficulties theorized to exist among juvenile and adult sexual offenders often do not provide adequate or in-depth exploration of the construct, and rely on poorly defined ideas. Furthermore, they frequently pay little or no attention to the large body of related literature that exists outside of the forensic field, with little reference made to the huge literature of attachment theory itself.

For instance, although some of the better defined and researched literature within the sexual offender field asserts that failures in attachment are significant to an understanding of sexual aggression, there is little in the field of attachment theory itself that suggests that attachment is actually related to the development of pathology. Nevertheless, the premise in the sexual offender literature is that presumed difficulties in attachment are associated with the development of sexually abusive behavior. It is hypothesized that the failure of individuals to form early secure attachments with their parents leads to the development of insecure adult (and presumably, adolescent) attachment styles. This, in turn, compromises their capacity to form and maintain stable and satisfying romantic and other intimate relationships, as well as contributing or leading directly to other related deficits, such as loneliness, powerlessness, low frustration tolerance, anger, and interpersonal conflicts. Somehow, it is proposed, in some individuals a consequence of deficits in intimacy skills is transformed into coercive sexual activities in order to satisfy emotional needs. In this view, sexual offending is a distorted attempt to build interpersonal closeness in the absence of the social and psychological skills required to build emotionally satisfying relationships.

Marshall and his colleagues (for instance, Marshall, Hudson, & Hodkinson, 1993; Marshall & Marshall, 2000; Marshall, Serran, & Cortoni, 2000) argue that an insecure attachment style renders people vulnerable to sexual offending, and particularly sexual offenses against children. He recognizes this as a developmental vulnerability, and hence a risk factor rather than *the* cause (Marshall & Eccles, 1993), but considers that when individuals with this vulnerability are exposed to other predisposing or precipitating factors, they are more likely than securely attached individuals to engage in sexual abuse. One of the key variables in this attachment-linked model is that attachment deficits, or weak attachment experiences, make the child more susceptible to being a victim of childhood sexual abuse, which thus adds a significant factor to the pathway along which sexualized coping, conditioned sexualized behavior, and sexually coercive behavior may later develop. Indeed, Alexander (1992) describes the ongoing sequelae of insecure parent–child relationships as not only creating vulnerabilities and setting the pace for later adjustment difficulties, but also active elements in creating children who are susceptible to being sexually abused within the family.

Alexander writes that insecure relationships within the family are often found in the homes of families characterized by sexual abuse, and asserts that family characteristics are the most significant predictors of increased risk for child sexual abuse. Such risks include absence of a parent, maternal unavailability, marital conflict and violence, the child's poor relationship with the parents, and the presence of a step-father. Alexander considers the insecurely attached child to be more susceptible to sexual abuse because of his or her need for emotional support and recognition, which may come, in a perverse manner, from a family perpetrator. Further, the insecure and poorly attached child may be recognized by the perpetrator as accessible because of the child's reduced ability to otherwise get needs met, understand and recognize emotions and thoughts in self and others, and seek help to stop the abuse. In addition, Alexander reports that the long-term effects of family sexual abuse are mediated, and therefore may be reduced or heightened, by the level of support received from the non-abusive parent.

Marshall's model is shown in Figure 11.3. Once an offense has been perpetrated, through the establishment of cognitive distortions that support the accompanying ideation, attitudes, emotions, and behavior, the behavior is likely to repeat. Attachment style is thus a significant variable in Marshall's framework, and has been identified by others as central in the etiology of sexual offending. Marshall suggests that these problems lead to a primary reliance on sexualized coping, including the early onset of masturbation and sexual acts with others, providing the offender with a way to deal with and avoid difficulties related to a history of family and childhood problems, as well as current difficulties and frustrations. In this model, ongoing sexually active and coercive behavior becomes a *conditioned* response that builds on sexualized coping, such as excessive masturbation, and aims these individuals towards ongoing sexual coercion. In keeping with attachment theory, Marshall suggests that individuals with disturbed attachment experiences do not adequately develop self-regulatory skills, and thus rely on externally based means of self-regulation.

Supporting Marshall's general perspective, Beauregard, Lussier, and Proulx (2004) agree with Knight and Sims-Knight (2004) that abusive and neglectful childhood experiences lend themselves to aggressive, and sometimes sexual, fantasy taking. From their study of 118 sexual offenders, Beauregard et al. assert that deviant sexual arousal results from sexually inappropriate childhood experiences within the family, the use of sexualized coping and behaviors during childhood and adolescence (such as the use of pornography), and impulsive and antisocial childhood and adolescent behavior.

Lyle (2003) explored the link between attachment and sexualized coping in a sample of 110 male college undergraduates. Measures of sexualized coping including what was defined as compulsive masturbation, as well as sexual fantasies. Although a relationship between attachment and sexualized coping was found to be modest, it was nevertheless sufficient to support the hypothesis. Aside from the relationship to attachment status, Lyle notes that over half the men in the sample engaged in compulsive masturbation, which on its own suggests that males may engage in compulsive masturbation for reasons other than coping or dealing with stress (or may not recognize stressful contexts in which the use of

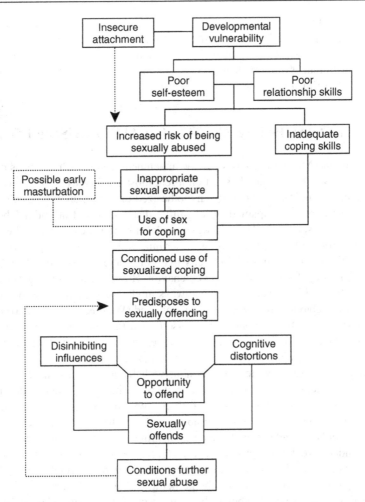

Figure 11.3 Marshall's attachment-linked pathway to sexually abusive behavior. (Modified from Marshall & Marshall, 2000)

masturbation increases). Using the Parental Bonding Instrument, the Inventory of Parent and Peer Attachment, and the Experiences in Close Relationships Inventory, Lyle found the strongest predictors of sexualized coping behavior to be related to parental scales linked to insecure attachment,[3] with particular respect to anxious insecure attachment, but not avoidant insecure attachment.

Although attempts to link specific forms of sexualized coping behavior to childhood sexual abuse were not supported by the study, Lyle nonetheless reports that a relationship between early sexual abuse and later sexualized coping was mediated by parental attachment. That is, in support of Alexander's premise, the quality of attachment with parents

---

[3] The reader should recall that these tools do not yield direct attachment "styles," such as insecure or secure, but are assumed and interpreted to reflect security and insecurity in relationships (see Chapter 8).

has a significant impact on the effects of childhood sexual abuse, in which those subjects with the strongest parental bonds were the least likely to use sexual coping to deal with stressful experiences, including that of being sexually abused. Lyle concludes that the quality of attachment is important in the development of compulsive masturbation and other sexualized forms of coping.

DYSFUNCTIONAL PATHWAYS TO SEXUALLY ABUSIVE BEHAVIOR

Ward, Hudson, and Marshall (1996) describe attachment-driven difficulties as one of five primary pathways to the sexual abuse of children, most notably when the perpetrator has deficits in interpersonal functioning. It is hypothesized that children will be substituted for adult sexual partners, accompanied by cognitive distortions and attitudinal beliefs that allow the sexual misconduct. The pathways model distinguishes between the long-term and short-term roots of sexual offending, describing a developmental process by which early vulnerabilities result in social deficits that contribute to, or, from Marshall's perspective, set the stage for sexually abusive behavior. However, in asserting multiple pathways that *lead* to child molestation, the pathways model does not attempt to explain why sexually abusive behavior *continues* and is maintained (Ward & Sorbello, 2003). For this, we would turn to Marshall's model which asserts that the resulting sexual, and perhaps relational, satisfaction serves as a reinforcer for sexual arousal to children and as a conditioned response that supports further sexually child molestation.

The four primary pathways to sexually abusive behavior are described by Drake and Ward (2003b) as interactive with one another, with one primary pathway predominant over the others in its link to sexual abuse. A fifth pathway occurs as the result of multiple primary deficits. In pathway one, sexual abuse is driven by attachment-related intimacy and social skill deficits, and not by deviant sexual arousal. Along this path, insecure attachment is considered to be the primary causal factor, leading to failures in establishing healthy and satisfying adult relationships (Ward et al., 1996) in which the child, according to Ward (2003), is experienced by the perpetrator as a pseudo-adult.

Along pathway two, sexually abusive behavior is caused by distorted sexual scripts that involve deviant arousal, interacting with dysfunctional relationships that catalyze deviant arousal into sexual behavior. Ward (2003) describes this pathway as attachment-related also, asserting a dysfunction in attachment style in addition to a distorted sexuality, perhaps linked to childhood sexualized experiences or history as a victim of sexual abuse.

The third pathway is characterized by emotional dysregulation. Here, incapacity for self-regulation and an inability to tolerate, cope with, and work through dystonic emotional experiences leads to inappropriate behavioral solutions used to address and remedy emotional distress or needs. Although not stated outright, there is also an assertion of social deficits, with particular regard to difficulty identifying emotion and experiencing empathy with others (Ward, 2003). The fourth primary path involves cognitive distortions and antisocial beliefs that drive and support take-what-you-need, antisocial, and sexualized behaviors. This appears to be the only pathway not conceptualized as directly linked to deficits in attachment or social skills, and is a reflection of pro-criminal attitudes.[4]

---

[4] Although, recall from Chapter 4, Fonagy et al.'s (1997a, 1997b) perspective that criminal thinking and behavior result from an inability to mentalize—itself a consequence of deficits in attachment.

The fifth pathway is driven, not just by interactions between pathways, but by multiple dysfunctional mechanisms that work across multiple pathways. With the possible exception of the fourth pathway, the pathways model is largely a model of sexually abusive behavior driven by attachment and social deficits.

Connolly (2004) tested the pathways model in a study of the family experiences of 13 male child molesters using narrative interviews rather than the usual self-report measures. Upon analysis, she found that 10 of the sample fit into one of the pathways, not only partially supporting the pathways model as a viable means for understanding the etiology of sexually abusive behavior, but also suggesting that "developmental trajectories, or individual pathways, have been influenced by a building block of behavior and experience" (p. 56). In describing the ability of the pathway model to incorporate biology, social factors, early childhood experience, learning history, and social learning, as well as environmental restraints and opportunities, Connolly is describing attachment theory at work. The pathways model, shown in Figure 11.4 overleaf, is then very much in line with a model in which sexually abusive behavior is driven by deficits in attachment and social skills.

DISORGANIZED ATTACHMENT AS A PROPOSED CAUSE

Smallbone and Dadds (1998, 2000) and Smallbone (2005) argue that the link between attachment style and sexual offending occurs because adult sexual offenders experience an overlap between the attachment, caregiving, and sexual systems of their childhood and early adolescence. They conjecture that children who experience child abuse may develop a disorganized attachment style that leads to sexual behavior when they experience high levels of stress. According to this model, sexual abuse of a child occurs when individuals with patterns of disorganized attachment experience stress, have multiple behavioral systems triggered, and have access to a child. Burk and Burkhart (2003) also focus on the role of disorganized attachment in the development of sexually abusive behavior, with controlling sexual strategies used by the sexual offender as a means to re-establish an internally experienced state of emotional and cognitive organization.

Although supporting the overarching premise of Marshall's model, Burk and Burkhart identify gaps in his framework that fail to describe how stressors that may be attachment-related actually lead to the adoption of sexually abusive behavior. They assert that the model is incomplete because it fails to provide an explanation of motivation that is sufficient to initiate the use of sexually coercive behavior in the first place. They argue that disorganized attachment is a disorienting and emotionally and cognitively uncomfortable experience, and that the very same conditions that lead to disorganized attachment in the first place also lead to the delayed onset of attachment in some individuals, and the subsequent development of controlling attachment strategies. Such strategies are designed to regain control over, and make predictable, an otherwise uncomfortable interpersonal environment, and thus serve to stabilize the internal emotional state. Like Marshall, they argue that these individuals begin to use sexual behaviors, including masturbation, as pleasurable coping mechanisms. In addition, they note that exposure to maltreatment, aggression, and sexual behaviors, including personal sexual victimization, during childhood is an experience common in the lives of many sexual offenders. Burk and Burkhart thus contend that in sexual offenders these elements combine and result in the use of sexual coercion

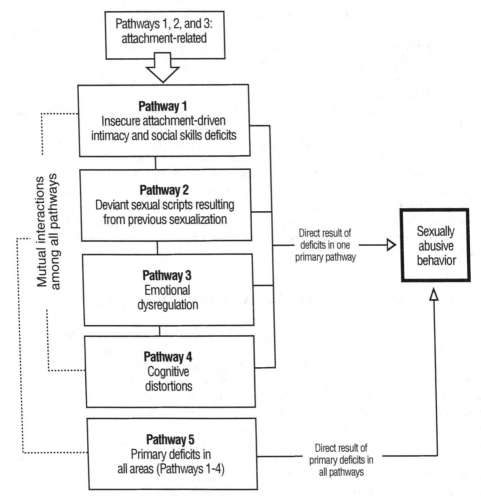

Figure 11.4 Five pathways to sexually abusive behavior (Ward, 2003)

to fill a self-regulatory need that the attachment-disorganized individual is otherwise unable to fill. They add that the physically gratifying properties of the sexual act, as well as the "pseudo-intimacy" provided by the sexual act, reflect a control strategy designed to regain cognitive and emotional equilibrium.

Although more complex than Marshall's work, Burk and Burkhart are attempting to make the Marshall model more complete rather than proposing an alternative. Whereas the Marshall model more generally considers insecure attachment to be a constitutional predisposition to sexually abusive behavior, Burk and Burkhart consider disorganized attachment to be the central predisposer, thus making the Marshall model more complete from their perspective. However, although adding detail, or filling an "explanatory gap" as they describe it (p. 489), their model nonetheless remains highly theoretical. It, too, fails to explain why many individuals encountering very similar early life experiences, including disorganizing and disrupted attachment experiences and early forms of maltreatment and abuse, don't later resort to sexually abusive behaviors. It also raises the question of why and how juvenile sexual offenders, most of whom do not continue on as adult sexual offenders, manage to overcome these very conditions that presumably (in this model) led to their engagement in sexually abusive behavior in the first place.

Smallbone (in press-a) amends Marshall's model, in an "attachment-theoretical revision" that also addresses disorganized attachment as a central feature missing from the Marshall model. He asserts that sexual offenders confuse and blend attachment, parenting, and reproductive behaviors/strategies, catalyzed into sexually abusive behaviors by other forces such as psychosocial environment and situational variables. According to Smallbone (2005), childhood disorganized attachment plays a significant role in this process because it may lead to a confusion and inability to functionally separate the three behavioral systems (attachment, caregiving, and reproductive). Under conditions that should, in the attachment organized individual, trigger the attachment *or* caregiving behavioral system, Smallbone argues that, in the attachment-disorganized individual, the sexual behavior system is instead activated, or all three systems (attachment, caregiving, and sexual) are engaged. This results in the use of sexual behaviors in service of emotional security, in which empathy is overridden by more immediate anxiety-driven emotional needs (Smallbone, in press-a; Smallbone & Dadds, 2000). In particular, Smallbone is critical of the way that "attachment" is described as a stable trait in individuals rather than a changing variable that is in constant interplay with the sometimes competing and sometimes overlapping parenting and sexual behavioral systems, as well as other environmental and personal variables.

Fonagy (2001b) provides some theoretical support for the position that disorganized attachment is related to the development of controlling and violent behaviors in adults, although assumes a different approach. He writes that, by mid-childhood, patterns of early disorganized attachment have evolved into rigid behavioral strategies for controlling situations and people. As a result, early disorganized attachment is associated with the development of aggressive behavior in these children, described also by Lyons-Ruth (1996). Fonagy believes that disorganized attachment in adults, reflected in fragmented self-representations, manifests itself as a need for control over others, and asserts that this, in part, provides the basis for male violence against women. Holmes (2004) also associates control and aggression with attachment-disorganized adolescents and adults, whom he also describes as unable to self-soothe when faced with emotional turmoil, unable to disengage from difficult situations and painful relationships, and liable to dissociation.

PROBLEMS WITH THE DISORGANIZED HYPOTHESIS

Recall that attachment theory holds that *only* disorganized attachment is related to the development of pathology, and insecure attachment itself is neither pathological nor maladaptive, albeit suboptimal. However, although disorganized attachment is implicated in the development of sexually abusive behavior by Burk, Burkhart, and Smallbone, and to a lesser degree by Fonagy (who is describing a broader range of male sexual violence against women, including domestic abuse, as well as rape) and Holmes (who links disorganized attachment to the development of borderline personality), there is no empirical evidence for this position. Of the studies of attachment and sexual offending, only one has so far attempted to directly measure disorganized attachment, and it finds no evidence for the proposition that disorganized attachment is an active link in sexually abusive behavior.

Baker and Beech (2004) explored the idea that adult sexual offenders experience disorganized attachment, and that such disorganization could be explored and revealed through self-reported attachment instruments. In this case, the authors considered disorganized attachment in terms of evidence of dissociation, often considered an outcome of or evidence of disorganized attachment (Chapter 7) and described by Holmes (2004) as common in disorganized attachment, and multiple internal working models and representations of attachment that shift over time. Their study included 20 sexual offenders of adult women, 15 non-sexual violent offenders, and 21 non-criminals, using the Relationship Scales Questionnaire (RSQ), the Young Schema Questionnaire (YSQ), and the Dissociative Experiences Scale II (DES). However, the Adult Attachment Interview is the assessment instrument most typically and most successfully used to assess disorganized and unresolved attachment in adults, rather than the DES or any other measure of dissociation or disorganization. Although the inclusion of the DES offers a measure of dissociative experiences that can be cross-referenced to the attachment measure (RSQ), like the other instruments used, it is quite transparent and easily susceptible to manipulation by the user, thus weakening the study.

The study hypothesized a relationship between dissociation, variability of attachment style over time (and thus a loosening of coherent and consistent internalized experiences of attachment), early maladaptation, and sexual offending, with variability data collected four times, approximately every three weeks. On their first hypothesis, Baker and Beech failed to find that sexual offenders show a variability in their self-reported attachment patterns over time, and thus may not have the multiple and disconnected internal working attachment models proposed by the authors. The second hypothesis was also not supported, in that the sexual offenders did not show more variability over time in early maladaptive schemata than the non-sexual criminal offenders, although both groups showed more variability than the non-offender group, supporting this as a general factor in the development of antisocial behavior. The third hypothesis was mostly unsupported with respect to changes in their interpersonal relationships, measured by staff observers along four checklist scales that measured belligerence, withdrawal, egocentricity, and distress, showing variability only on the distress scale. The fourth, and perhaps most important hypothesis in this case, that sexual offenders would report more dissociative experiences than either non-sexual criminal offenders or non-offenders, was also not supported, although again both sexual offenders and non-sexual criminal offenders reported more frequent dissociative experiences than non-offenders.

Thus, despite conjecture that disorganized attachment is involved in the development of sexually abusive behavior, central to Burk and Burkhart's thesis and, to a lesser degree, Smallbone's, there is no empirical support for this position. Indeed, sex offender theorists, in this case, seem to be blending, and even confusing, insecure and disorganized attachment. In addition to a lack of supporting evidence, the description of disorganized attachment as predispositional for sexually abusive behavior, or indeed any criminal behavior, falls outside of descriptions of disorganized attachment found in mainstream attachment theory, and further does not fit the data with respect to the relatively rare incidence of disorganized attachment. That is, disorganized attachment appears to be a much rarer phenomenon than sexual offending, and, indeed, as described in Chapter 7, descriptions of disorganized attachment in adolescents and adults as aggressive, controlling, and rigid do not resemble the level of frank disorganization and disorientation shown in attachment disorganized young children, and described by Hilburn-Cobb (2004) as evidence of disorganized attachment in adolescents.

Although, sexual offenders may be driven by attachment insecurity, and may indeed experience an overlap between competing behavioral systems, this is not likely to constitute or be driven by disorganized attachment which is more likely to show as troubled and dysfunctional social behavior in every psychosocial domain, including clear psychiatric disturbance. In children and adolescents, disorganized attachment is more likely to be evident in a psychiatric population, predominantly appearing as mental illness and severe psychopathology rather than as antisocial behavior. In adults, we are likely to see a similar presentation of disorganization as psychopathology, rather than criminal behavior, or embedded into clear personality disorders resulting from significant unresolved trauma and other early experiences. Further, Holmes (2004) describes attachment-disorganized adolescents as "liable to dissociation" (p. 183), but this is not a quality typical of juvenile or adult sexual offenders, again suggesting that we see no evidence of disorganized attachment.

ATTACHMENT AND ADOLESCENT SEXUALITY

As we struggle to understand the relationship between juvenile sexual offending and attachment, Tracy, Shaver, Albino, and Cooper's (2003) contention that childhood attachment style is directly related to adolescent sexual behavior may be far more to the point. They assert that childhood attachment styles are directly related to the development of sexual and romantic behavioral patterns in adolescents and young adults, and sexual attitudes and the use of sex as a tool to get emotional needs met are related to earlier patterns of attachment. Insecure attachments lead to the use of sexual relationships as a means for gaining control and meeting personal needs, rather than sexual and romantic relationships that would be considered emotionally healthy and satisfying, bearing a slight similarity to the Burk and Burkhart model regarding emotional and cognitive equilibrium. In fact, Smallbone and Dadds's ideas about the overlap between the sexual, parenting, and attachment behavioral systems appear to be drawn from Shaver's earlier work in which he and his colleagues assert that romantic love is an amalgam of those three behavioral systems (Shaver, Hazan, & Bradshaw, 1988).

Belsky argues still further (Belsky, 1999b; Belsky, Steinberg & Draper, 1991) that early attachment experiences are directly related to the onset of pubertal experiences and sexual behaviors, serving as an evolutionarily prompted strategy. From this perspective, the insecurely attached child grows into late childhood/early adolescence experiencing resources as scarce or unpredictable, other people as untrustworthy, and relationships as transient. This child, he suggests, enters into both puberty and sexual behaviors at an earlier time as a biologically driven imperative in which sexual promiscuity is a means to ensure reproductive certainty. In this conceptualization, emotional satisfaction is not the goal, but sex is a means for reaching out into the world to ensure reproductive survival under uncertain or adverse conditions. Whereas the secure adolescent living in a secure world may biologically/preconsciously feel he has time to reproduce later, the insecurely attached child is biologically pressed into early sexual development and behavior in an otherwise uncertain world. Driven by evolution, sexual behavior in young/pre-adolescents is one result of an attachment pattern (secure vs insecure), presumably in combination with other personal and environmental factors. There is little evidence for Belsky's contention, but it brings us back to the idea that attachment is considered to be a *biological* and not a psychological mandate. Evolutionary-biological early onset puberty also fits with, lends theoretical support for, and provides a process to explain Marshall and Smallbone's suggestion of early onset masturbation in insecurely attached children, which is key to Marshall's idea of early sexualized coping.

CONCLUSION: EVIDENCE OF ATTACHMENT-DRIVEN SEXUAL ABUSE

It may indeed be that attachment is one highly significant component in the development of sexual aggression, combined with the many other elements that are found so frequently in the lives of juvenile and adult sexual offenders. However, the attachment deficit model of sexual offending, in which insecure attachment is an instrumental and causative factor in the development of sexually abusive behavior, fails to overcome the contention of established attachment theory that insecure attachment itself is not a sufficient cause.

Thus, in an attachment-informed model, although the pathway along which sexually abusive behavior may later develop is set in motion by attachment experiences, behavioral pathology (and one must consider sexually abusive behavior pathological, and particularly in adults) is *not* the product of insecure attachment and must therefore be caused by other factors, albeit perhaps potentiated by attachment difficulties. Hence, the model is more complex, and hence less simplistic, than that described by Marshall and others. Nevertheless, Figure 11.5 illustrates and synthesizes the ideas presented in this chapter, in which the attachment system is linked to the caregiving and reproductive behavioral systems as suggested by Smallbone (and Shaver et al., 1988, and Belsky, 1999a), and follows the Marshall model in recognizing attachment deficits as developmental vulnerabilities that are sometimes later potentiated by other risks and crystallized into sexually abusive behavior. It connects attachment to sexually abusive behavior through the biological interplay between the attachment, caregiving, and sexual systems, as well as the interaction between biology and emotional development over time and in the context of early negative learning experiences and social messages regarding sexuality and sexual behavior. In this model, sexually abusive behavior ultimately reflects dynamic maturational and biological changes over time, from childhood to adulthood, and the incorporation of social skills or social deficits into the internal working model, mediated by the development and incorporation of psychosocial restraints (and hence, behavioral and emotional regulation) into a pathway that may ultimately lead to sexual aggression.

Chapter 12 turns our attention to the evidence that supports or fails to support the attachment hypothesis, as well as evidence of empathy, intimacy, and other social skill deficits in sexual offenders. The specific focus, however, is not on the presence of attachment and social deficits in sexual offenders, but the prominence of those deficits as features that dis-

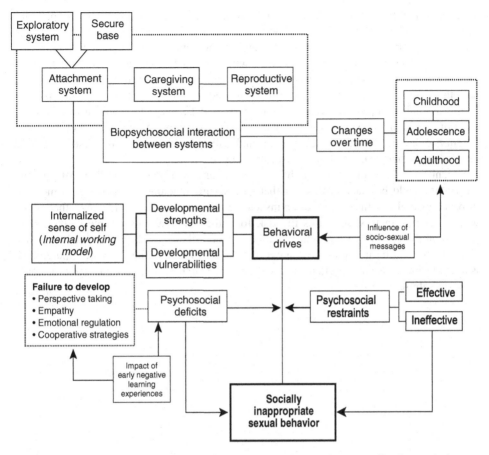

Figure 11.5 Applying an attachment framework to understanding sexually abusive behavior

tinguish sexual offenders from the larger and inclusive population of juvenile and adult criminal offenders.

However, for now we can say that ideas about attachment and social skills deficits as instrumental in the development of sexually coercive behavior have utility. They inform our thinking about the nature of sexual abuse as a crime of relationships, driven by social needs that cannot otherwise be met by individuals unable to easily tolerate stress or impose self-regulation; such individuals are thus motivated to use antisocial means for taking what they want, in a variety of ways specific to individual perpetrators. An attachment perspective is not limited to sexual crimes, however, but appears relevant to all sorts of antisocial and criminal behavior. Nevertheless, although all forms of crime involve victimization, it is the unique nature of sexual abuse as a crime of *relationships* that makes attachment theory an especially intriguing and relevant approach to both understanding and rehabilitating sexual aggression.

The attachment–social deficits pathway, shown in Figure 11.4, illustrates one way in which attachment deficits may be linked to sexually abusive behavior. In the case of attachment theory with non-clinical populations, attachment insecurity sets the pace for life difficulties and dysfunctions, but with a population affected and influenced by many other pathognomic factors, such as family neglect and home, domestic violence, and exposure to sexual victimization, in combination with other factors unknown to us (and, which may always remain unknown), we see a shift towards pathological behavior that would not otherwise occur in the absence of this range and combination of pathognomic factors. In this visualization, we can recognize attachment deficits as elemental in the development of later difficulties, including sexually abusive behavior, but it is the *range* and *combination* of normative, albeit suboptimal, and pathognomic factors that leads to sexual aggression, rather than attachment insecurity per se.

Greenberg (1999), one of the authors of the Inventory of Parent and Peer Attachment, writes "it should be made quite clear that an insecure attachment is not itself a measure of psychopathology. In some cases an insecure attachment may set a trajectory that, along with other risk factors, increases the risk for either externalizing or internalizing psychopathology" (p. 477). He reminds us that, as a contributory risk factor, attachment will show its greatest influence in the context of *other* risk factors. The conclusion here, then, is that attachment is an important, and even critical, *general* risk factor but is not the cause of sexual abuse.

The Evidence for Attachment-driven Sexual Offenses

Currently, one must mostly turn to the adult literature to review research that explores the link between attachment style and sexually abusive behavior, as virtually none has been conducted with juvenile sexual offenders. At this time, mentioned in Chapter 11, of those studies of which I am aware, only three groups of related research projects are in progress that specifically examine attachment in juvenile sexual offenders. Most of this adolescent-oriented research is in relatively early stages, with little yet published. In fact, although far more work has been conducted with adult sexual offenders, in the relatively limited research with both adult and juvenile sexual offenders, despite assertions that are more hopeful than certain, little has been established that points to any significant relationship between adult sexual offending and attachment deficits, other than on a theoretical basis. To this end, it is important to bear in mind Smallbone and Dadds's (2000) note that we lack sufficient empirical support for a relationship between attachment and sexual offending.

This notwithstanding, there is consistent evidence linking attachment deficits to behavioral problems, including the development of sexually abusive behavior. The question, however, is more about exclusivity and specificity than contribution. That is, the central issue is whether attachment deficits serve as a *specific* causal factor in the development of sexually abusive behavior or whether it serves as a *general* risk factor for dysfunctional, antisocial, and/or criminal behavior, of which sexual abuse is just one variant. Although inconsistent, evidence supports the presence of an attachment-related risk factor but, for the most part, not *specifically* or uniquely to the onset of sexually abusive behavior.

It is no surprise to learn that deficits in attachment and social deficits contribute to life difficulties, functional limitations, relational experiences, and social satisfaction in general, as well as contributing to the development of alternative, socially deviant means to establish social connections and acquire socially valued goals. There is similarly no surprise in learning that among offending (sexual offender and non-sexual offender) populations, insecure attachment is far more common than in non-forensic populations, as we have already seen the higher incidence of insecure and disorganized attachment in clinical/psychiatric populations (Chapter 6). Individuals with secure attachment are more rarely found in clinical and forensic populations than in the general population, and we can conclude that secure individuals are comparatively well adjusted and able to tolerate adversity, meet goals, and experience satisfaction more readily than clinical and forensic groups, and thus show less psychiatrically troubled, antisocial, or criminal behavior.

ATTACHMENT LINKS TO ADULT SEXUAL OFFENDERS

The theoretical basis for most of the attachment-related studies of adult sexual offenders is that early attachment difficulties contribute or lead to later difficulty, including sexually abusive behavior, and support is thus sought for this assertion. Nevertheless, most studies have been unable to significantly distinguish among groups of forensic individuals based on their patterns of attachment. That is, sexual offenders do not stand out because of their particular attachment styles or deficits. For instance, in their study of 30 child molesters, 24 non-sexual offenders, and 29 non-offenders, Marshall et al. (2000) conjectured that they would see differences in attachment style between groups. However, they were unable to detect any significant difference between groups, reporting instead "that all subjects (in all groups) reported greater security in their attachments to their mothers than to their fathers" (p. 17).

Even prior to the Marshall et al. (2000) study, Ward et al. (1996) acknowledged a similar conclusion. Using self-report scales to assess romantic attachments in 55 child molesters, 30 rapists, 32 violent non-sexual offenders, and 30 non-violent/non-sexual offenders, their results suggested that although the majority of sexual offenders were insecurely attached, this was also true for all four groups of incarcerated prisoners. They concluded that insecure attachment is likely to be a *general* vulnerability factor, rather than specific to sexual offenders. Similarly, in a study comparing 48 sexual offenders to 16 non-sexual (and non-violent) criminal offenders and 16 non-criminals, Smallbone and Dadds (1998) reported that sexual offenders were significantly less secure than the non-offender group in their attachment, but were similar in attachment to the non-sexual criminal offenders. Even within just the sexual offender group, no significant differences were found with respect to insecure or secure attachment. However, despite finding no differences in attachment style across groups, the study nevertheless found other important differences within the adult sexual offender group. Whereas child molesters reported problematic relationships with their mothers, sexual offenders who had raped strangers experienced difficulties with their fathers, experiencing them as uncaring and abusive.

In their study of a non-offender sample of 162 male undergraduate students who completed self-report attachment measures, Smallbone and Dadds (2000) found that their hypothesis that childhood attachment styles predicts adult attachment styles was only partially supported, as was their hypothesis that insecure attachment in childhood predicts antisocial, aggressive, and coercive sexual behavior. Contrary to their hypothesis, they found that insecure maternal childhood attachment did not predict adult attachment style, and paternal attachment, although a somewhat stronger predictor, also failed to significantly support continuity of attachment over time. Although not strongly correlated, Smallbone and Dadds did find partial support for a connection between childhood insecure attachment and the development of aggressive, antisocial, or sexually coercive ideation. Their most supported conclusion was that avoidant paternal attachment may influence the development of aggressive and antisocial dispositions. However, this was contradicted by their subsequent study (Smallbone & Dadds, 2001), also involving non-criminal under-graduates, which showed that avoidant maternal, and not paternal, attachment was impli-cated in the development of coercive sexual behavior. In this study, insecure attachment was once again partially associated with coercive sexual ideation, but not significantly so when isolated from more global factors of antisociality and aggression. Despite stating that inconsistencies between the two studies are difficult to reconcile, the authors never-theless conclude that associations between insecure attachment and sexual offending stand up to replication. This appears quite optimistic in light of limited support for the position.

In arguing that conclusions like this, and others described, offer *partial* support for a theoretical proposition one may just as easily, or more accurately, argue that they show considerable support for a *lack* of evidence. We see how our conceptualizations and under-lying beliefs about what drives sexually abusive behavior, and the intuitive appeal of the attachment deficit model, seem to shape conclusions drawn from studies that most often do not support the attachment hypothesis. In fact, theorizing aside, much of the data offers little support for attachment as a causative factor specific to sexual offending, even though it seems very clear that attachment deficits are over-represented in criminal offenders in general.

In their study of incarcerated male sexual offenders, Smallbone and McCabe (2003) concluded that, contrary to their expectations, the 48 sexual offenders in this study were no more likely to have experienced insecure attachment than they were to have experi-enced secure childhood attachment, and the frequency with which the sample reported insecure attachment was no greater than in the general population. In fact, in the study sexual offenders reported secure attachment more than they did insecure attachment. Between 31% and 40% reported insecure childhood attachment, which is very much in line with the generally reported 33–38% of the general population that experiences inse-cure attachment. The study did report that in this group, however, insecure paternal attachment was correlated with a history of childhood sexual abuse, and that sexually abused offenders tended towards earlier onset of masturbation. This onset of early sexual behaviors supports the Marshall model (Chapter 11) of early sexualized experi-ences and sexualized coping that sets the pace for continued and behaviorally reinforcing sexualized behaviors, in some people contributing to the development of sexually abusive behavior.

Following an attachment track, Bogaerts, Vervaeke, and Goethals (2004) studied parental sensitivity, attitude towards relationships, and personality disorders in a group of 84 child molesters and a cohort group of 80 non-offenders. Using the Parental Bonding Instrument they found that relational attitude and personality disorders differentiated between the child molesters and the comparison group. The child molesters reported less parental warmth, greater distance from fathers, less safe adult romantic relationships, less trust, and more schizoid, antisocial and narcissistic personality traits than the comparison group. However, the hypothesis that relational attitude would discriminate and predict pedophilic behavior was not proved, and personality disorder contributed as much to the incidence of sexually abusive behavior as did relational attitude. In either case, 80% of the variance was unexplained, and Bogaerts et al. report the inevitability that factors other than relationship attitude (i.e., the presumed attachment link) play a significant role in the development of sexual coercion, including the possibility of an element of psychopa-thy. Hudson and Ward (2000) note also the possibility that interpersonal deficiencies in sexual offenders may reflect a more general psychopathy rather an underlying attachment deficit.

Providing evidence that more closely supports a model of attachment differences specifically in sexual offenders when compared to other offender populations, Marsa et al. (2004), in their study of 29 child sex offenders, 30 violent non-sexual offenders, 30 non-violent offenders, and 30 non-offenders, found that a secure adult attachment style was four times *less* common in the child sex offender group than in any of the other three groups, and child molesters reported more emotional loneliness than other groups. Similarly, although noting that evidence regarding attachment style in adult sexual offenders has been inconsistent, Lyn and Burton (2004) also report that insecure attachment distinguishes sexual offenders from non-sexual offenders. In their study of 144 adult sexual offenders incarcerated in a mid-west US prison and 34 incarcerated non-sexual offenders, they hypothesized that insecure attachment would be associated with the sexual offender group, and attachment status would be associated with the characteristics of sexually abusive behavior. They found that 85% of the sexual offender group were insecurely attached, whereas this was true for only 64% of the non-sexual offender group, and that insecurely attached individuals were 5.5 times more likely than securely attached subjects to be in the sexual offender group. In particular, fearful attachment was significantly associated with having a history of sexual offending, although neither preoccupied nor dismissing insecure attachment was associated with sex offender status. They report that fearful insecure attachment was three to four times larger than expected in a non-offender population, although the preoccupied and dismissing styles matched community norms. However, the hypotheses that attachment style would be related to the *type* of sexual offense was not significantly supported by the data. In a related study, Lyn and Burton (in press) also report that the sexual offenders in their study were more angry and generally more anxious than those in the non-sexual offender group.

Lyn and Burton therefore conclude that insecure attachment status is specific to sexual offending and is *not* characteristic of criminality in general. However, this finding is not in keeping with the general outcomes of almost all of the limited studies on attachment in adult sexual offenders and other non-sexual criminals, which asserts that attachment deficits are likely to be a risk factor for criminal behavior in general, rather than specific to sexual offending. Lyn and Burton recognize that their results contrast with the work of other researchers who report non-significant differences, and also suggest that it is unlikely that a single-factor model can sufficiently describe causes of sexually abusive behavior, pointing to the likelihood of multi-factorial causal models instead. They also note the limitations of their study, particularly with respect to a study population limited to incarcerated offenders who are unlikely to be representative of all sexually abusive men, the voluntary and self-selective nature of the research sample, the reliance upon self-report measures, and questions of honesty and depth in reporting. Still, these are flaws typical, in one form or another, of most of the studies described here.

Weak Support

In fact, aside from the studies of Marsa et al. and Lyn and Burton, although it may well be that attachment deficits or styles are significantly related to the onset of sexually abusive behavior in juveniles or adults, little evidence is available to support what must, for now, remain little more than a theory. The assertion of Ward, Hudson, Marshall, and Siegert (1995) that different types of sexual offenders will be characterized by different types of adult attachment styles has not been borne out, nor has any hypothesized difference between sexual and non-sexual offenders been established. Based on the bulk of the evidence thus far, it seems unlikely that attachment itself is a direct link to the development of sexually abusive behavior or a factor that can discriminate between sexual offenders and others.

The problem in more specifically linking attachment deficits to sexually abusive behavior may be a matter of assessment instruments that are not sensitive enough to detect differences between sexual offenders and non-sexual criminal offenders, or it may be that the very limited typology we have of attachment styles is simply too limited and concrete to distinguish among types of insecure attachment. It may be that a typology consisting of only two or three variants of insecure attachment simply lacks the nuance required to reflect differences in attachment style and is thus incapable of subtle distinction, just as organized or disorganized attachment as a variable is too dichotomous to reflect the continuous and richly gradated subtleties of human attachment behavior, organization, and coherence. It may also be that there really is *no* difference in attachment style between sexual offenders and non-sexual criminal offenders, and attachment difficulties merely serve as early vulnerabilities along a developmental pathway that is weakened from the outset. In this case, as suggested at the conclusion of Chapter 11, it is the quality and interaction of other factors that appear at a later point along the developing pathway, and not attachment at all, that determines the development of behavior that is sexually abusive, non-sexual but criminal, or troubled but non-sexual and non-criminal.

The recent meta-analysis conducted by Hanson and Morton-Bourgon (2004) confirms a multidetermined path to sexual coercion, at least with respect to offense recidivism. In a review of 95 different studies that involved more than 31,000 sexual offenders, the most pertinent predictors of re-offense were deviant sexual arousal, personality disorders, and antisocial rule breaking. On the other hand, an adverse childhood environment (i.e., the sort of early conditions that lead to insecure attachment) was only weakly correlated with sexual offense recidivism, including attachment disruption events such as being separated from parents. Lack of empathy for victims was also not significantly linked to recidivism and, similarly neither low social skills nor loneliness, reported to be common among adult sexual offenders, were associated by the meta-analysis with increased risk. However, of note, sexual recidivism was mildly associated to conflicts in *current* intimate relationships, certainly offering some support for a model that links current sexually aggressive behavior to *current* attachment experiences.

Although unable to discriminate between sexual and non-sexual offenders with respect to attachment style, Smallbone and Dadds (1998) concluded tentative support for the hypothesis that sexual offenders have troubled childhood experiences. As is true with most attachment studies with adult sexual offenders, early childhood difficulties appear to be a general risk factor for later troubled, antisocial, and criminal behavior, rather than sexually abusive behavior in particular. They suggest only that early insecure attachment experiences may place some men at risk for sexually abusive behavior in the context of other factors present in their lives, thus supporting insecure attachment as a general factor, potentiated by other life circumstances. Craissati, McGlurg, and Browne (2002) found support for this position, in reporting that childhood neglect and emotional abuse are somewhat significant in distinguishing between sexual offenders who themselves were victims of childhood sexual abuse, and those who were not, and that the sexually abused perpetrators were more likely to have a broader range of psychosocial difficulties. In their study of 178 convicted child molesters, 46% self-reported a history of childhood sexual abuse, and 82% reported a history of either sexual, physical, or emotional abuse. These figures are in keeping with those generally reported regarding the personal histories of sexual offenders, although Craissati et al. acknowledge the long-standing variability in the reports of prior sexual victimization among sexual offenders, ranging from as low as 17% in some cases. Their study found that early childhood difficulties and maltreatment, however, were present for all subjects in their sample.

Again, the question is not whether sexual offenders were raised under adverse conditions, but what is the difference between the paths taken by sexual offenders and other non-sexual criminal offenders who come from similar backgrounds? In many cases, these two populations cannot be distinguished from one another on the basis of either background factors or attachment deficits, presumed through attachment style.

OTHER DIFFERENCES AMONG SEXUAL OFFENDERS

Leaving direct reflections of attachment aside for one moment, it does seem clear that sexual offenders, as well as other criminal offenders, experience social deficits and difficulties, and further that there *must* be some differences not only between sex offenders and other non-sexual criminals, but *within* sexual offender groups. In particular, evidence does suggest differences between child molesters and rapists. Despite concluding that the sexual offenders in their study could not be distinguished from the non-sexual criminal cohort on the basis of social and intimacy deficits, Ward, McCormack, and Hudson (1997) nevertheless describe the child molesters in the study experiencing a more negative view of themselves than other sexual offenders and non-sexual criminal offenders included in the study. Although not always supported, this is not an unusual finding.

Similarly, although unable to detect differences in attachment across groups, Marshall et al. (2000) also found important differences between the child molesters and other subjects in their study. Whereas neither measures of self-esteem nor coping behaviors predicted membership in either the sexual offender, the non-sexual criminal offender, or the non-criminal group, child molesters were nevertheless characterized by coping styles that were more emotion-focused than problem-focused. Of this, Marshall, Cripps, Anderson, and Cortoni (1999) write "it is clear that child molesters, relative to participants in the other two groups, suffer from low self-esteem and employ dysfunctional (emotion-focused) coping strategies" (p. 959).

This observation about coping style is also found in other studies of adult sex offenders, suggesting that child molesters are distinguished from rapists and other criminal offenders by their use of coping strategies that are aimed at avoiding stressful situations and retreating from proactive solutions. Unlike task-focused coping strategies that tackle stressful situations and emphasize problem solving, emotion-focused strategies are aimed at relaxation, refocusing, and emotionally separating from the stressor. In their study of 25 pedophiles, Kear-Colwell and Sawle (2001) also found that child molesters did not simply have insecure attachment styles, but tended to use escape-avoidance coping strategies that distanced them from stressful interpersonal situations. It must be stated, of course, that such coping strategies are not necessarily related at all to attachment style. Nevertheless, it does allow us to recognize distinctions between and within groups of adult sexual offenders, perhaps not in attachment per se, but in the manner in which these individuals experience and respond to the world. However, although Kear-Colwell and Boer (2000) argue that a link is strongly indicated between pedophilia and insecure attachment, they too acknowledge that there is no evidence of such a causal link, writing that it is not clear why some individuals develop pedophilic interests and others do not. Indeed, this reflects the likelihood that the development of sexual interests *and* sexual behaviors is multifaceted and multidetermined.

EMPATHY, INTIMACY, AND SOCIAL DEFICITS IN ADULT SEXUAL OFFENDERS

It has already been established that although attachment deficits and patterns may be significant in understanding the development of life difficulty, they do not seem to be of special relevance to the specific development of sexually abusive behavior. One may argue that it is *character*, or personality, that is most important, rather than attachment per se, or social deficits. This may be especially true when we consider the particular deficits and strategies that seem common to child molesters, who appear more relationship-oriented than rapists, which perhaps contribute to a personality "type" more than an attachment "type." In this case, attachment contributes to and builds personality, but is far from the whole story. Indeed, Hudson and Ward (2000) note that there are many plausible pathways to sexual offending, including general psychopathy (not considered attachment related), and it is even possible that adult sexual offenders intentionally under-report their social skills in order to justify their criminal behavior.

As we have noted, sexual offenders are thought to suffer from empathy deficits, often considered a significant precursor and maintainer of sexually abusive behavior, as well as being related to and possibly required for the development of intimacy, or close relationships. In an early paper, Marshall (1989) described emotional loneliness as the result of the failure to achieve intimacy (or close relationships), which, in turn, he hypothesized, leads to aggression. According to Marshall, this produces "a tendency to pursue sex with diverse partners in the hope of finding intimacy through sexuality or through less threatening partners" (p. 491), and he describes the absence of deep and intimate relationships in the lives of male sexual offenders. However, quite a few studies have failed to find evidence of particularly low social skills specific to the sexual offender population, including empathy and intimacy, as compared to other criminal groups and, in some cases, non-offender groups. Of this, Hudson and Ward (2000) have written that it is intuitively appealing to consider sexual offenders "being deficient in empathy . . . However, despite the plausibility of this proposition, there has been little clear evidence to support this view" (p. 510).

In fact, like attachment itself, and believed related to and even evidence of attachment, elusive constructs such as empathy, self-esteem, intimacy, and emotional loneliness are often seen to be as intact in sexual offenders as in any other group, although like studies of attachment style among adult sexual offenders, the results of such studies among sexual offenders are inconsistent and inconclusive.

ASSESSING EMPATHY

Although recognizing the role of empathy as a protection against the victimization of others and a lack of empathy as instrumental in the commission of crime, more often than not sexual offenders do *not* appear less generally empathic than others, despite hypothesizing that they *should* as an obvious precursor to sexual aggression. Part of the difficulty with measuring empathy, however, is our failure to fully understand it, or at least what we mean when we use the term.

Fernandez (2002) writes that although empathy is crucial for effective human interaction, we lack a concise definition of the construct or clear approach to measuring empathy. Marshall, Hudson, Jones, and Fernandez (1995) have worked to operationalize the empathy construct, defining it as a complex multicomponent process in which sequentially earlier elements form the basis upon which later aspects of empathy are built and are dependent. In their multistage model, empathy involves first being able to recognize and accurately identify emotion in others, followed by a second stage that involves perspective taking, or the ability to assume another's point of view, emotionally as well as cognitively. The third stage of empathy is affective in nature, requiring the ability to feel the emotional experiences of the other, and have these feelings vicariously replicated in oneself. The final element, built upon the prior stages, involves the decision to respond on the basis of vicarious feelings, in tune with the feelings and needs of the other. Whereas, the last two stages approximate sympathy (Marshall, 2002), all four stages together constitute empathy, moving from emotional recognition to acting in the best interests of the other. These stages involve both cognitive and affective aspects, both generally considered to be central to the construct of empathy, although Feshbach (1997) notes that the relative role of each varies with the situation, age, and personal characteristics of the individual. Of course, in any model involving any level of cognitive sophistication—including that of perspective taking—cognitive development and maturation are requirements, and so empathy is a process that can only fully develop and be experienced in adolescents, and then into adulthood.

Hoffman (2000) considers the key to empathy to be "empathic distress," or the sympathetic component of empathy, as this is the aspect that results in action (or Marshall et al.'s "decision response"). This requires "the involvement of psychological processes that make a person have feelings that are more congruent with another's situation than with his own situation" (p. 30), or the motivational domain that coexists with the cognitive and affective domains that Hoffman identifies as the structural constituents of empathy. Davis (1996) also identifies three constituent domains of empathy, although selecting a perceptual, rather than a motivational, domain in addition to the affective and cognitive domains. In the development of his Interpersonal Reactivity Index (IRI), often used in the assessment of empathy, Davis's model seems to provide the basis for the Marshall model of empathy, involving perspective taking, transposing oneself into the emotional realm of another, sympathetic concern for another, and affective distress, which prompts the response decision.

Hoffman describes empathic distress built upon a metacognitive awareness of others and evoking a metacognitive awareness of oneself acting empathetically. Hence, this model of empathy can be tied to the metacognition identified in attachment theory as an outgrowth of secure attachment, and thus the capacity to understand self and others. Beyond this, Vetlesen (1994) writes that empathy sets up and establishes a relationship *between* self and others, with its focus on the interpersonal rather than the intrapersonal. He describes empathy as the basic human emotional faculty, because he considers it to lie at the heart of all emotional connection with others. One would therefore expect to find in securely attached individuals the development of mature, well-tuned (accurate), and responsive empathy. Conversely, we can expect a diminished or less-developed sense of empathy in less securely attached individuals, as well as in children who have not yet developed the cognitive framework required for elements such as perspective taking. It seems reasonable, then, to use empathy not only as an important concept to measure in its own right, but also, in part, as a proxy measure for assessing attachment.

EMPATHY IN SEXUAL OFFENDERS

Despite expecting to see low empathy in sexual offenders, as noted, sexual offenders do not appear less empathic than other non-sexual criminal offenders, and often no less empathic than the general public. For instance, in a study of 61 child molesters and in a second study involving 29 child molesters and 36 non-offenders, Fernandez, Marshall, Lightbody, and O'Sullivan (1999) found no difference in global empathy between groups, supporting the notion that sexual child molesters are generally not particularly unempathic. Similarly, in their study of 88 convicted sexual offenders, Smallbone, Wheaton, and Hourigan (2003) found no relationship between empathy and sexual offending.

In a study of empathy in both juvenile and adult sexual offenders, D'Orazio (2002) found no difference in measures of empathy between sexual offenders and non-offenders, but did find that juveniles are generally less empathic than adults, regardless of status as sexual offenders or non-offenders. Comparing groups of 30 juvenile sexual offenders, 30 non-delinquent juveniles, 30 adult sexual offenders, and 30 adult non-criminals on a measure of intimacy, D'Orazio found that empathy is a developmentally age-related construct that (potentially) grows only over time and maturity, and that less empathy in adolescents than in adults is a normative feature of adolescence, not related to juvenile antisociality. In addition to finding that adults are more globally empathic than adolescents, supporting the premise that empathy requires cognitive maturity, D'Orazio also found that the sexual offender groups were not assessed as having lower general empathic tendencies than non-offenders. Nevertheless, she found that sexual offenders low in perspective taking engaged in the most severe sexually abusive behavior, as did those who began criminal activity at a younger age. In particular, differences in empathy between adolescents and adults, as measured by the IRI, were most significant with respect to the aspect of empathy involving perspective taking—a cognitive component of empathy.

In a study comparing empathy and self-esteem in 27 incarcerated rapists and 27 incarcerated non-sexual criminals (Fernandez & Marshall, 2003), rapists showed the same or *more* empathy than non-sexual offenders. However, in an earlier study of 34 child molesters, 24 non-sexual offenders, and 28 non-criminals, Marshall, Hamilton, and Fernandez

(2001) studied differences between global aspects of empathy and aspects of empathy specific to victims. They found that the child molesters were less empathic towards their own victims than non-sexual criminals, and displayed more cognitive distortions regarding sexual behavior between adults and children—frankly, not surprising. Whether this represents less empathy and decreased capacity for mentalization, or simply rationalization for behavior of choice, is a matter of opinion. After all, as Hilary Eldridge (2000) has written, "most sex offenders do sexual things . . . because they want to" (p. 315). The fact that the molesters showed less empathy towards their own victims (victim-specific empathy) than they did in general (global empathy), is no surprise, and of course cannot be compared to the non-offender cohort, who have no victims.

Supporting this distinction, however, between global and victim-specific empathy, in his analysis of victim letters written by incarcerated British sexual offenders engaged in treatment, Webster (2002) found no relationship between general empathy and victim-specific empathy, writing that "sexual offenders are devoid of empathy for their victims" (p. 281). The suggestion is that sexual offenders suppress empathy or distort experience in order to maintain sexually abusive behavior, and this may reflect errors in *thinking* more than a lack of developed *empathy*. In fact, Keenan and Ward (2000) suggest that problems with victim empathy, and related or resulting cognitive distortions, may be the result of a lack of mentalization rather than a lack of empathy. As we have seen, a lack of metacognition may itself be considered a failure of the attachment process.

SUPPRESSING HUMANITY

In describing the medical doctors who worked at and experimented upon humans in the Nazi concentration camps, Lifton (1986) describes the phenomenon of "doubling," or the division of the self into two wholly functioning parts, so that each partial self acts as an entire self. He asserts that this psychological mechanism served to allow these doctors to do their inhumane work and yet remain somehow untainted in their "other" lives as normal human beings, behaving immorally yet remaining moral in their own minds. He describes five characteristics of the doubling process, involving not a dissociation but a connectivity between the parts, a coherence and consistency between aspects of the self, a sacrifice of others on behalf of self-survival, the capacity to split off and avoid guilt, and a resulting change in moral consciousness, which he calls transfer of conscience, that occurs outside of conscious awareness.

Lifton (1993) writes that empathy is *always* a selective and situational process, in which we choose to allow empathy to be activated at times and under certain conditions and do not allow its activation at other times. In describing what he calls the "protean" self, he describes a shifting sense of self in response to the perceived environment, in which, as the self shifts and fragments, the capacity for empathy is lost. "Absorbed in its own struggle to hold together, the fragmenting self is unable to be concerned with others, and tends to be unable to mobilize the cohesiveness to perform the empathic act" (p. 206). Focusing on the doubling process, Lifton describes an emotional numbing process that is invoked to allow the self to meet its needs free of guilt, writing that doubling enables the individual to move towards empathy or to return to it after a lapse. Lifton's description, of course, is very much in keeping with a description of sexual offenders who experience global empathy and can maintain a normal life, yet are able to step out of their everyday selves, suspend or detach themselves from empathic experience, and engage in behaviors that victimize and harm others without necessarily destroying their sense of their own worthiness or humanity. They seem to be able to assume the protean flexibility described by Lifton—the ability to assume different selves, without dissociating and losing continuity across the parts.

OTHER MEASURES OF SOCIAL EXPERIENCE

Other than empathy, in seeking indirect evidence of attachment deficits, sex offender researchers have attempted to measure other aspects of social functioning. But just as empathy assessment has shown interesting but inconsistent data, so too have measurements of other social skills that we expect will tell us something about social satisfaction, including satisfaction with self and in relationships.

Despite the assumption that poor attachment will result in lessened self-esteem, in Fernandez and Marshall's (2003) study of empathy and self-esteem in rapists and non-sexual criminals, not only did the rapists report the same or greater level of empathy, they also showed no differences in self-esteem. Similarly, Marshall, Barbaree, and Fernandez (1995) found that child molesters did not differ from a matched community group of non-offenders with respect to social anxiety, under-assertiveness, or self-esteem. On the other hand, in a review of parental attachment, although no significant differences were found in perceived parental rejection between 24 child molesters and 23 non-offenders, Marshall and Mazzucco (1995) *did* find significantly lower self-esteem in the sexual offenders. Despite this, they were unable to link low self-esteem to parental rejection, and thus unable to correlate either construct to sexually abusive behavior.

Fischer and Beech (1999), in their study of 140 child molesters and 81 non-offenders, found significantly lower self-esteem in sexual offenders, as well as heightened emotional loneliness and personal distress, and less victim empathy. In a study of 172 adult sexual offenders beginning treatment in prison and an additional 53 beginning treatment in the community, Thornton, Beech, and Marshall (2004) linked low self-esteem to a higher rate of sexual recidivism, and concluded that low self-esteem obstructs effective treatment participation. They theorize that individuals with low self-esteem avoid novel activities, therefore inhibiting the acquisition of new ways of thinking and the required application and practice associated with consolidating new ideas and behaviors. They surmise also that low self-esteem draws males to sexual relationships that are non-threatening, such as relationships with children, or non-demanding, such as sexual relationships with coerced partners, and in both cases produces a sense of power and competence that is otherwise lacking.

With respect to emotional loneliness, in comparing rapists, child molesters, violent non-sexual offenders, non-violent offenders, and non-offenders, Seidman, Marshall, Hudson, and Robertson (1994) reported that the sexual offenders were lonelier than other groups. But in their study of 55 child molesters, 30 rapists, and 32 violent non-sexual offenders, Hudson and Ward (1997) found no significant differences among offender groups in measures of emotional loneliness, hostile attitudes towards women, or intimacy, although child molesters and non-violent offenders were found to be less angry than rapists and violent offenders. Interestingly, although no significant differences were found by offender type, some differences were found by secure and insecure attachment styles.

Drawn from this same study, Ward et al. (1997) derived 12 relationship-related categories, and found that although sexual offenders experience a number of significant intimacy deficits, these were also largely shared by violent non-sexual offenders and were *not* specific to the sexual offenders. Hudson and Ward (2000), therefore, conclude that the sort of social deficits that interfere with intimate relationships are not specific to sexual offenders but are shared with other non-sexual offenders, and McCormack, Hudson, and Ward (2002) report that early experiences of both sexual and non-sexual offenders are overwhelmingly negative, but not specific to sexual offenders. That is, although the early family life of adult sexual offenders "is characterized by violence and disruptions" (Marshall, 1989, p. 497), the same is generally true for non-sexual violent and often non-violent criminal offenders.

INCONSISTENT DATA

Something must explain these apparent contradictions in results across different studies of the same types of phenomena. One possibility is that the research designs are different, and another that there are differences in instrumentation. Still another is that these results reflect the heterogeneity of the population, and different studies produce different results because sexual offenders are *not* homogeneous in their personal attitudes and qualities. Yet another is that the manner in which we interpret data influences the apparent information yielded by the data.

A good example of data that can be analyzed and interpreted to produce different results can be found in a study of substance abuse in adult sexual offenders and its relationship with intimacy deficits. In their study of 95 rapists, child molesters, and non-sexual violent criminals, Looman, Abracen, DiFazio, and Maillet (2004) found no differences between the two sexual offender groups on any of the measures. However, when the results of the Social Intimacy Scale were computed in a certain way, no differences were found between sexual and violent offenders either, but when computed in a different way, child molesters showed lower intimacy scores than non-sexual violent offenders. This obviously produces mixed results, and confuses the research findings.

Although Proeve (2003) writes that "attachment theory offers a useful perspective for understanding the problems experienced by sexual offenders with intimate relationships" (p. 248), he concludes that "there does not appear to be consistency in findings regarding attachment styles and sexual offending" (p. 258). On a similar note, Smallbone and Dadds (2000) have written that it is premature "to conclude that prevention and treatment of sexual aggression should adopt attachment concepts and respond to their implications; there is insufficient evidence to support such a broad conclusion," although they continue to suggest that "notwithstanding these limitations, these results indicate that childhood attachment may play some role in the development of coercive sexual behavior" (p. 13).

However, given the overwhelmingly inconsistent, variable, and, in the final analysis, uncertain outcomes of similar studies, it is obvious that we are *not* clear of the role of attachment or social deficits in the specific development of sexually abusive behavior.

Indeed, Ward et al. (1997) described "a major conclusion" of their study of 85 sexual and 62 violent and non-violent non-sexual offenders that intimacy deficits in sexual offenders were shared by non-sexual violent offenders and "therefore, were not specific to sexual offenders" (p. 72).

ATTACHMENT AND JUVENILE SEXUAL OFFENDERS

As noted, of the limited work conducted in relating attachment disruptions and disorders to sexual offending, it is clear that almost all has been completed with adult sexual offenders, with very little attention paid to juvenile sexual offenders. However, three groups of researchers have begun work in studying attachment in juvenile sexual offenders, although each of these is in the early stages of data analysis and further development. At this time, Michael Miner of the University of Minnesota appears to be the most advanced in his work, and has published the most in this area, although his work remains in process. Under a grant from the US Office of Juvenile Justice and Delinquency Prevention, Miner and Swinburne-Romine (2004) studied 43 sexual offenders and 44 non-sexual juvenile delinquents, aged 13–17. Although the study is not yet complete and data have yet to be further analyzed, early results, presented in late 2004, suggest that juvenile sexual offenders who molest children (as opposed to those who sexually assault peers or adults) have fewer friends, feel more isolated, associate with younger children, and have more concerns about masculinity than other juvenile sexual offenders or non-sexual juvenile offenders. Although their study is not complete, Miner and Swinburne-Romine do not consider juvenile sexual offenders to be more rejecting of social relationships than non-sexual juvenile delinquents, just less competent, and do believe that there is a link between attachment, social isolation, and sexually abusive behavior. In this conceptualization, sexual abuse appears to be driven by socially isolated, normless behaviors rather than by aggression, at least in those who molest children—mirroring the conjecture of Hudson and Ward (2000) that sexually abusive behavior among adults is often more connected to the need for social connection and the acquisition of social goals than deviant sexuality.

Despite a lack of a juvenile sexual offender typology, as with adult sexual offenders we can recognize a crude and simple three-way typology in which we see: (i) juveniles who sexually offend younger children, (ii) juveniles who sexually assault peers or adults, and (iii) juveniles who engage in both forms of sexual aggression. By far, juvenile sexual offenders fall into the first category, with very few falling into the last group. In fact, juveniles who molest younger children represent *most* of the juvenile sexual offender population, at least in the United States. Whereas juveniles sexually assaulted only 4% of adult victims, they were responsible for 40–43% of the sexual assaults against children under 6 years of age (Snyder, 2000; Office of Juvenile Justice and Delinquency Prevention (OJJDP), 2000). This is particularly sobering when one realizes that over two-thirds of all sexual assaults in the United States are directed against adolescents and children. Thirty-three percent of sexual assault victims are aged 12–17, 35% are below age 12, and 14% are below age 6 (Snyder, 2000); and 39% of all victims aged 6–11, and over 40% of those aged 6 and younger, are sexually assaulted by juveniles. Accordingly, if Miner and Swinburne-Romine's early data have validity, they suggest that much of the sexually abusive behavior of juveniles is the result of social isolation, social inadequacy, and social anxiety. Such deficits can, of course, be linked to the hypothesized role of attachment in the development of self-confidence, self-agency, and self-efficacy or, in this case, the failure of attachment experiences.

In a related study, under a Centers for Disease Control and Prevention (CDC) grant, Miner (2004) is studying 300 male adolescents, age 14–18, identifying attachment relationship risk factors that are unique to juvenile sexual offenders, and those shared by juvenile sexual offenders and non-sexual juvenile offenders. Miner hypothesizes that among three groups consisting of juvenile sexual offenders of children, juveniles who sexually assault peers and adults, and non-sexual juvenile delinquents, all three groups will share insecure attachment, but different variants will discriminate between different groups. Specifically, using Bartholomew's four-category model (Chapter 7), Miner expects juveniles who sexually abuse children to show anxious or fearful attachment, juveniles who sexually assault peers or adults to have dismissing or fearful attachment styles, and non-sex delinquents to show an insecure dismissing attachment style. This hypothesis, of course, mirrors expectations that have been largely unsupported in similar research with adult sexual offenders.

In addition to the attachment question, Miner also expects to find evidence that a high level of hostile masculinity is linked to juvenile sexual offending of peers and adults, whereas low masculine adequacy will be linked to juveniles who sexually abuse children. Here, Miner is addressing issues of masculine security, suggesting that aggressive masculine assertiveness is related to rape and masculine inadequacy is related to child molestation. This hypothesis, too, is similar to ideas about adult sexual offenders, partly addressed also by Malamuth (2003) who describes hostile masculinity as one of the two important, interactional legs that result in sexual aggression.

As described, there has been some modest support for the idea that (adult) child molesters and rapists experience relationships and use coping skills differently from one another, and that child molesters may exhibit different social characteristics than the general population. However, the idea of differences in self-perception and perception of others as key variables in adult sexual offending has not yet been shown to be the case, and with respect to adolescents remains to be seen as Miner's study is still in process. In any circumstances, as should always be the case and in order to validate the data from Miner's work, similar results will need to be seen in cohort populations and in studies replicated by other researchers. Indeed, this is one of the weaknesses in current studies of attachment in adult sexual offenders, and often in other research with adult and juvenile sexual offenders. We either see idiosyncratic research designs that cannot be easily compared to one another, including the use of different instrumentation and the use of different tools for statistical interpretation, or studies are conducted by research teams that attempt to replicate and thus validate their own data, rather than by independent research groups whose views may be considered more objective.

In the Minnesota Survey of Adolescent Sex Offenders (Miner & Crimmins, 1997), data were gathered from 78 juveniles in sexual offender treatment and compared to a group of 73 violent non-sexual juvenile delinquents and a group of 80 non-delinquent youth, both synthetically derived from data collected in 1978 for the National Youth Survey (Elliott, 1994). Miner and Crimmins report that the juvenile sexual offenders did not differ significantly from non-sexual juvenile delinquents in either attitude or behavior, but that the sexual offenders were significantly more isolated from family than non-delinquent youth and more socially isolated from peers than violent delinquents. Miner concludes that preliminary work points to the importance of peer relationships in adolescent healthy and well-adjusted behavior, the possibility that juvenile sexual offenders expect adult and peer rejection, and the centrality of attachment difficulties in the development of sexually abusive behavior. Building on this, Miner and Munns (in press) compared differences in conventional attitudes, normlessness, and social isolation among 78 juvenile sexual offenders (presumably the same sample), 156 non-sexual juvenile delinquents, and 80 non-delinquent adolescents. They found no differences among the three groups on conventional attitudes or family normlessness, and although juvenile sexual offenders experienced more social isolation in school and in their families than non-sexual delinquents, they again did not differ significantly from non-sexual juvenile delinquents. All three groups had similar scores on peer isolation, but peer normlessness was slightly more common among juvenile sexual offenders than either the delinquent or non-delinquent groups.

Overall, Miner and Munns found that juvenile sexual offenders experienced social isolation in all measured contexts but, consistent with other research, are quite similar in this regard to non-sexual juvenile delinquents, as well as in their capacity for deviant social behavior. Nevertheless, they report that sexually abusive juveniles feel more isolated from their peers than non-sexual juvenile delinquents. It is not clear that the evidence supports their perspective, but Miner and Munns conclude that juvenile sexual offenders appear to experience a deeper level of social isolation than non-sexual juvenile delinquents and non-offenders, and suggest that the inability to experience satisfaction in social relationships may turn some adolescents to younger children to meet sexual (and presumably) social needs.

To assess attachment, Miner's CDC and OJJDP studies use Kim Bartholomew's History of Attachments Interview (or Family Attachment Interview), an instrument that bases attachment style on a semi-structured interview that is later analyzed by trained raters. As described, this is the preferred way in which to assess attachment, rather than deriving attachment classification from questionnaire self-reports. Although analysis of interviews is the preferred model for interpreting attachment data and assigning classification in adolescents and adults, it is a more complex and time-consuming process and often not practical as a result. Two additional studies, one conducted by Barry Burkhart of Auburn University and the other by David Burton of Smith College, examine attachment in juvenile sexual offenders using the Inventory of Parent and Peer Attachment (IPPA), among other more general measures of behavior and adjustment. Although the IPPA is a limited self-report instrument that measures security and satisfaction with relationships rather than attachment, the use of the same instrument in both studies will allow for some comparison across studies, at least with respect to the attachment data produced by the assessment tool. Although data have yet to be released for these studies, the use of the IPPA will allow a comparison of the two studies, as well as comparisons to other studies of adolescents (non-sexual offenders) that have used the instrument.

Part of the problem with using the IPPA, however, is that it has not been used to establish a normal distribution, and thus has no cut-off scores that indicate what security in relationships looks like in a non-clinical population. Mark Greenberg, one of the authors of the IPPA, notes that we do not have a reliable sense of where the cut should be, or the ability to distinguish between expected/normative and clinical levels of security/insecurity (M.T. Greenberg, personal communication, November, 2004). Accordingly, unless attachment measures like the IPPA are used in research designs that include non-forensic/ non-clinical populations, we can only reflect upon the incidence of secure attachment within the populations measured. Although both Burton's and Burkhart's studies are able to contrast juvenile sexual offenders against non-sexual juvenile delinquents, neither includes a non-offender adolescent population. In order to compare IPPA attachment/security measures against a general non-clinical norm, then, we can only turn to the general attachment theory literature for a sense of what secure attachment may look like in the general population. Recall from Chapter 6, that 40–45% of non-clinical adolescents may experience insecure attachment, rather than the 33% considered the norm for children and adults.

CONCLUSION: ATTACHMENT AS RISK, NOT CAUSE

As we have seen, the focus of the limited work on the relationship of attachment to sexually abusive behavior is largely geared towards adult sexual offenders and has tended to focus on child molesters in hypothesizing a pathway from attachment deficit to sexual abuse. Even so, despite attractive ideas and some compelling data, at best there is partial and inconsistent evidence to support attachment as a primary cause of sexual coercion. In addition, a critical review of attachment-based research suggests that it is inconsistent, weak in instrumentation, and difficult to replicate across studies. It is also not clear that such studies always have a firm grasp on the ideas of attachment theory, or how to apply them.

Further, the conclusions of many research studies seems to fit the data to theory, rather than either confirming or repudiating theory or developing a grounded theory that allows theory to emerge from the data. Although researchers are frank and honest in describing the weaknesses and unexpected outcomes of studies designed to find evidence for an a priori theory of attachment-driven sexual coercion, almost every study described here optimistically concludes partial support for the theory, sometimes with little justification. It is a credit that research that does not support the hypothesis is not shelved,[1] but study conclusions nevertheless continue to suggest that there is something about the data that supports attachment theory, when in most cases data do not support this conclusion. That is, we have not been able to find a significant distinction between the attachment experiences and classifications of sexual offenders and non-sexual criminal offenders. It is therefore prudent to be cautious in accepting research conclusions that are often not heavily supported by the data, but nevertheless optimistically support the driving theory.

Here, we must bear in mind Lamb's (1987) warning that the design and methodology of attachment research may actually bias results in a manner that supports the attachment hypotheses. Just as, in film, you see only what the director wants you to see, so too in theory-driven research you see only what the theory embraces. This is a special concern if the theory fails to see the whole picture. In any distribution of ideas, information is always biased by the producer of the ideas, even if unintentionally. As important, just as

---

[1] The so-called "file drawer effect," or positive outcome bias, in which there is a tendency to publish research that supports the premise and file away that which doesn't.

the producer of the idea may bias the information presented, so too is information biased by the filter of beliefs and perspectives through which the reader receives and interprets the information. All the more important then, to ensure well-informed readers who exercise critical thinking in all they view.

In fact, with such little work undertaken or completed with respect to adolescents, we are not yet in a position to say whether the research will support an attachment-driven theory in the development of juvenile sexual offending. Nevertheless, there is no compelling reason to believe it will, if we discount our very active desire to support this attractive theory. This is especially pertinent in light of the lack of strong evidence found in similar adult studies, and compounded by the limited instrumentation we have available for recognizing and measuring attachment in older children and adolescents. Accordingly, at this time, although attachment and social deficits seem apparent in juvenile sexual offenders, as they do in adult sexual offenders, they appear more as a general risk factor than a cause of sexually abusive behavior. There is little more we can say at this time about the relationship between attachment and juvenile sexual offending, other than recognizing that suboptimal attachment experience is likely to serve as a predisposing factor and link to the onset of *many* troubled and troubling behaviors in juvenile sexual offenders, including serving as an important factor in the development of sexually abusive behavior.

Attachment deficits are unlikely to be the *cause* of sexual aggression. However, despite our ability or inability to prove attachment as a cause of sexually abusive behavior, it seems an obvious and important target for assessment and treatment in juvenile sexual offenders. Indeed, as Smallbone (2005) has written, there is substantial indirect evidence (and some limited direct evidence) to support the idea that attachment-related vulnerabilities are significant predisposing factors in the development of sexually abusive behavior for some adults and adolescents. In fact, it's not clear to me that we actually have to prove anything more than what we already know. Here, I echo the sentiment of William Lindsay (2004) who writes, "it is pointless trying to determine the percentage of sex offenders with intellectual disability. We know the number is significant and we should focus on the most effective way to provide assessment, treatment and management services" (p. 169). Similarly, I hope the reader by now will be convinced of the role that the attachment experience plays in the development of the individuals who engage in sexually abusive behavior, regardless of its role as cause or contributor.

In the treatment of sexual offenders we must be alert to, take into account, and be able to recognize attachment difficulties and deficits, building treatment settings that create social connections, restore relationships, and improve social skills. We conclude this chapter, then, by describing the assessment and treatment of attachment as a central part of any treatment program for sexually abusive youth, in some ways serving as the *heart* of the treatment. That is, the role of insecure attachment, even if not *the* factor, must be recognized as a contributing factor, not just in the etiology of sexually abusive behavior but in current functioning.

The reader by now has guessed that I like to turn ideas into organizational and flow charts that describe relationships and sequences. Before moving on to the next chapter, then, where we examine developmental factors that contribute to juvenile sexual offending, we look at a more complete model that reflects ideas about attachment and the pathway to sexually abusive behavior discussed thus far. Although it may appear complex, Figure

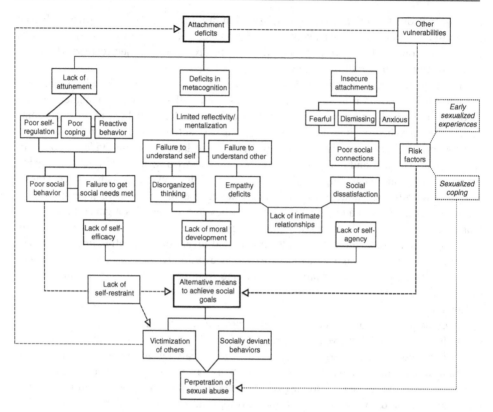

Figure 12.1 A hypothesized pathway from deficits in attachment to social victimization/anti-social behavior, in which one possible outcome is sexually abusive behavior. Additional links to risks for sexually abusive behavior, tied to the Marshall model, are shown in italicized, dashed boxes

12.1 shows three main streams beneath, and subsumed under, the Attachment Deficits heading. *Lack of attunement* reflects elements that eventually contribute to a lack of self-efficacy, whereas the *insecure attachments* stream results in lack of self-agency. Stemming from *deficits in metacognition* is the inability to fully understand self or others, resulting in both disorganized thinking and deficits in empathy, both of which in turn contribute to a lack of moral behavior. These strands of weak self-efficacy, moral development, and self-agency limit the ability of the individual to meet personal and social goals, requiring the pursuit of alternative means for the achievement of social goals, as predicted by strain theory. Such alternative means, when acted upon by other unspecified vulnerabilities and risk factors—which may or may not be directly related to attachment experiences, including the sexualized experiences and coping hypothesized by Marshall—may result in deviant social behavior and victimization of others, with one possible outcome being sexual aggression.

These ideas, and particularly those of self-efficacy, self-agency, and moral development are discussed in the next chapter, with respect to the development of sexually abusive behavior in juveniles.

CHAPTER 13

Antisocial Pathways

By now the reader is fully familiar with attachment theory, both in its complexity and, I hope, also in a more straightforward and concise manner that helps us quickly to recognize patterns of attachment and apply attachment-informed ideas in our work. The reader is also aware of hypothesized links between attachment deficits and sexually abusive behavior, certainly in adults and to some degree in adolescents, both in terms of the etiological role of attachment, and attachment and social deficits as contributors to ongoing behavioral and relationship problems that may contribute to sexual aggression. Despite difficulty with empirical evidence in adult sexual offenders and a lack of any evidence in juvenile sexual offenders, the attachment perspective shows sexually abusive behavior as one possible outcome of a human psychology weakened by a lack of social connectedness, which is particularly relevant if one sees sexually abusive behavior as a crime of relationships rather than a crime of violence.

Regardless of its weaknesses and limitations, the attachment model offers a set of ideas and a framework for exploring and making sense of the development of sexually abusive behavior from a developmental and social perspective. When understood and applied judiciously, attachment theory indeed adds a significant and very useful lens through which to view and interpret behavior, recognize contributing causes and drives, and devise and apply treatment interventions. Such a model, at least on a theoretical level, can be applied to both adult and juvenile sexual offenders. But, as shown in Figure 13.1, there are many influences upon the development of sexually abusive behavior in children and adolescents, in which no single element is likely or believed to produce sexually aggressive behavior. However, the combination of several or more elements, compounded by other factors that it may not be possible to discover or even envision, may come together to form unique combinations for different individuals. "Implicit theories" refer to those ideas that are built into the internal working model, and underlie cognitive distortions, behavioral scripts, and "automatic" thinking.

The current chapter cannot possibly highlight or describe the many factors that have been hypothesized or proven to influence antisocial behavior in children and adolescents, and indeed these have been described in detail elsewhere, with increasing frequency. Among other authors, I have elsewhere described pathways that contribute or lead to juvenile sexual offending (Rich, 2003), and many have already been mentioned in this book. These include difficult, chaotic, disrupted, and often dysfunctional family environments, in which children who at a later stage perpetrate sexually abusive behavior are themselves the victims of earlier or ongoing maltreatment and/or physical or sexual abuse. Starzyk

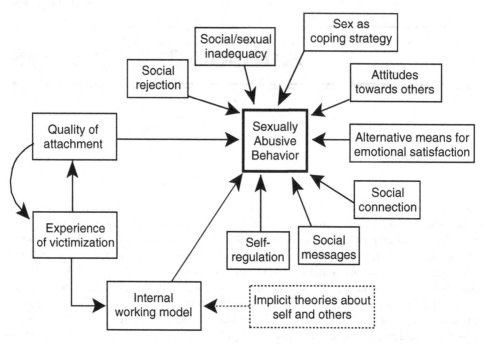

Figure 13.1 The constellation of pressures and influence that affect the development of sexually abusive behavior as an outcome in some children and adolescents

and Marshall (2003), for instance, describe consistent evidence that adult sexual offenders are more likely to have been sexually abused as children than non-sexual criminal offenders and, of course, non-offenders. With respect to juvenile offenders, Burton and Meezan (2004) describe a rate of sexual victimization among a sample of 8,135 juvenile sexual offenders three times higher than that in a cohort of 5,811 non-abusive juveniles, and almost 49% of 1,388 juvenile sexual offenders in residential treatment and 31% of 1,053 juvenile sexual offenders in community-based treatment had experienced prior physical abuse. However, Burton and Meezan acknowledge that no matter how compelling, social learning theory alone—that is, how children learn behaviors and social roles—cannot explain sexually abusive behavior in adolescents.

This chapter, however, explores the influence of antisocial attitudes and behaviors on sexually aggressive behavior, and in particular how antisociality develops and unfolds in the social environment, shaped by the environment and, in turn, shaping attitudes, interactions, and behaviors in the environment.

MASCULINITY IN THE EMERGENCE OF JUVENILE AGGRESSION

Being a male is of special significance as we discuss juvenile sexual offending, as the National Incident-based Reporting System shows that 96% of all sexual offenses in the United States between 1991 and 1996 were committed by males (Snyder, 2000), and the National Task Force on Juvenile Sexual Offending (1993) reported that boys commit 90% of juvenile sexual offenses. In exploring elements that offer insight into why some juveniles engage in sexually abusive behavior, Miner's (2004) hypothesis that aggressive masculine assertiveness is related to rape, and masculine inadequacy to child molestation, points to an interesting perspective about masculinity in general.

In describing the relationship between attachment theory and male criminality, Hayslett-McCall and Bernard (2002) consider the masculine identity to *always* be of concern, in the United States at least. They assert that males disproportionately fail to meet a goal of secure attachment when compared to females, because of culturally normative child-rearing practices that suppress secure attachment in boys, and particularly with respect to the ability to experience dependency and express vulnerability. Consequently, most men, they write, experience themselves as violating standards of masculinity with respect to gender role expectations, and this contributes to aggressive, antisocial and criminal behavior. They suggest, then, that being a male is *itself* a risk for impaired attachment, which is not far from a public health perspective that identifies risk and protective factors that serve to promote or jeopardize social values. For instance, in the report on youth violence issued by the office of the US Surgeon General (US Department of Health and Human Services, 2001), just *being* male places children and adolescents, from ages 9 to 14, at risk for violence, whereas being female in both age groups is considered a protective factor. In her review of psychopathy[1] in juvenile offenders, Saltaris (2002) writes that it is well-known that psychopathy and other behavioral disorders, such as antisocial personality disorder, conduct disorder, and oppositional defiant disorder, are, across the life span, more prevalent in males than in females, reporting that such disorders are five to seven times more common in men than in women.

Hayslett-McCall and Bernard consider antisocial behavior in men to be mediated through *detachment*, which they consider to be an acquired state resulting from a failure of the child-rearing environment. They assert that such an environment produces detached males and is the norm in the United States, and that the masculine role *itself* is a product of suboptimal attachment experiences that are built into child-rearing practices for boys in the US and similar countries. Accordingly, although they recognize that male criminal offending cannot be explained by a single theory, Hayslett-McCall and Bernard believe that antisocial, aggressive behavior, and lack of self-regulation in boys is driven by culturally defined disruptions embedded into the child-rearing environment in which attachment develops. Aside from reflecting on differences between the way that males and females are raised and eventually enculturated (or socialized), this view suggests that it is the attachment process itself that is the cause of the male risk factor (for antisocial and aggressive behavior). In turn, this suggests that attachment experiences for boys are intrinsically linked to the very traits that mark antisociality and conduct disorder, which also underlie the contemporary construct of psychopathy, for which, as already noted, males are at higher risk.

However, 9–14-year-old boys are considered at risk, not because they are male per se, but because they are *statistically* involved in more aggressive and antisocial behavior than

---

[1] As previously mentioned, the reader should remain aware of the distinction between "psychopathy," or the development of significant antisociality, and "psychopathology," or the development of mental health disorders.

girls. No immediate cause for that statistic is necessarily inferred, and, of course, it is pointless to describe being a male as the cause. It may be, as Hayslett-McCall and Bernard assert, that the root of this problem lies in a culturally defined attachment process that creates aggression and detachment in men, or it may be that males are temperamentally prone to aggression and emotional distance. As not every boy grows up to be aggressive or emotionally detached, however, it is unlikely that either element is the cause of male aggression and it is more likely that it is the interaction of both temperament (nature) and attachment (nurture) that produces antisocial behavior in males, but only when exacerbated by other factors along the developmental path. In addition, as psychopathy or sociopathy is relatively rare, even in males, this suggests that factors other than the attachment process must be at work.

HOSTILE MASCULINITY AND EMOTIONAL CONNECTION

Malamuth (2003) describes two pathways to sexually abusive behavior in adult men. One pathway is attachment-related, although Malamuth doesn't classify it as such, involving early abusive home life that contributes to the later development of impersonal and promiscuous sexuality. Malamuth refers to the other pathway as hostile masculinity, encompassing narcissistic hostility to women and a level of social isolation, described by Hunter, Figueredo, Malamuth, and Becker (2004) as a distrust of and anticipated rejection by women, and a subsequent need to control women in relationships.

The model proposes that, when catalyzed by low empathy and nurturance, these two pathways interact to produce sexually abusive behavior. In Malamuth's research, a "self-centered" rather than "other concerned" orientation was the attenuator that made the difference, with its focus on the capacity for empathy. That is, Malamuth proposes that men with traits of hostile masculinity and/or impersonal and promiscuous sexuality do not engage in sexual aggression if high in compassion and concern for others. The self-centered dimension described by Malamuth is reminiscent of the self-focused, negative other view in Bartholomew's categorization of dismissive insecure attachment. Therefore, it is neither masculinity nor hostile masculinity alone, nor for that matter negative childhood experience, that makes the difference, but social connectedness and related social skills. In fact, none of these elements on their own is sufficient to produce sexual aggression; it is the combination of masculinity, negative childhood experiences, hostile attitudes, and attachment deficits that produces the outcome.

In their study of 182 juvenile sexual offenders, age 12–18, Hunter et al. (2004) found that adolescents who sexually abused boys or girls younger than age 12 (average victim age of 6.1) showed greater psychosocial deficits than adolescents who sexually abused females aged 12 or older. As juvenile sexual offenders predominantly assault children (described in Chapter 12, they are responsible for 39% of sexual assault against 6–11 year olds, but only 4% against adults), this suggests that it may be psychosocial deficits that *most* mediate and catalyze other factors, rather than elements such as hostile and egotistical masculinity described by Hunter et al.

Knight and Sims-Knight (2003) add to Malamuth's (2003) model a third pathway of callous unemotionality. They propose that sexual drive and preoccupation results from early childhood sexual abuse (revising Malamuth's sexual promiscuity), and represents one pathway. Antisocial and aggressive behavior, beginning in early childhood and remaining active through adolescence, represents a second path, derived in part from early physical and emotional abuse (in the family) and from the development of callous unemotionality in the individual. The third path of callousness and unemotionality is also the product of early physical and emotional abuse, and together the three paths predict sexually aggressive behavior. Thus, the paths must interact to produce the outcome, and in some respects each pathway is interdependent upon the others; that is, the pathways catalyze, and in some ways act to produce, one another. For instance, callousness acts upon sexual preoccupation to increase the chances that it will lead to sexually aggressive behavior, as well as acting on and contributing to antisocial behaviors that also edge the individual towards sexual abuse. In fact, Knight and Sims-Knight's third path of callous unemotionality seems close in principle and action to the low empathy and lack of compassion that Malamuth conceives as catalyzing his two pathways.

In both models, a lack of empathy/compassion, or callous unemotionality, fuels and catalyzes other experiences and attitudes, coming together to produce aggression, driven, according to Knight and Sims-Knight, by emotional detachment, also a key element in Hayslett-McCall and Bernard's theory of male antisocial behavior. Found in the models of both pathways, an attachment element is thus present and significant, but it is also true that no single element, acting alone, presents as sufficient cause. Consequently, when we add antisociality, early negative experience, and sexual preoccupation and sexual drive (and other, undefined factors) to Miner's model of masculine assertiveness/inadequacy, we evoke a clearer understanding of the interacting factors that can produce sexually aggressive behavior in juveniles.

Nevertheless, these elements do not explain as much as we would like. That is, Knight and Sims-Knight tell us that these pathways are predictive of *general* antisocial recidivism, as well as sexual recidivism, which fits with what we already know about the similarities and difficulties discriminating between sexual offenders and non-sexual criminal offenders. However, they certainly give us a strong handle on some of the major elements that may come together to produce sexually abusive behavior in adolescents already troubled and experiencing disconnections in social relationships.

CALLOUS UNEMOTIONALITY OR SOCIAL INSECURITY?

Whereas a model of callous unemotionality may be a reasonable pathway to hypothesize for adult rapists, it does not fit the clinical presentation of most juvenile sexual offenders. That is, most juveniles who enter treatment for sexually abusive behavior do not appear to be either callous or devoid of emotionality. In fact, just the opposite, they appear to be very emotional, albeit in an emotionally "unintelligent" manner; that is, at times these juveniles do not seem to be in touch with their own emotions or able to control or express them appropriately. To this degree, they tend to be numb to their own emotions, unable to recognize them, and/or unable to maintain behavioral stability. In the first case, this suggests a process that allows emotional avoidance or suppression, in the second a lack of metacognition or reflectivity, and in the third case an incapacity for self-regulation.

As described in Chapter 12, most juvenile sexual offenders are not younger equivalents of adult violent sexual offenders, and in terms of their sexual offenses predominantly assault children. If Miner's assertion about masculine self-image is correct, in which masculine inadequacy is prevalent in juvenile sexual offenders who assault children, this means that *most* juvenile sexual offenders experience these self doubts about their masculinity. This reflects self doubt in juvenile sexual offenders, then, related to both self-agency and self-efficacy, or a general and larger sense of social inadequacy. It also suggests that these boys consider themselves to be inadequate when compared to their imagined or presumed standards of what it means to be a man in society and their evaluations of other males their age. This fits well with Hayslett-McCall and Bernard's (2002) assertion that *most* men experience themselves violating standards of masculinity. These young sexual offenders are more likely high in emotionality and doubt about themselves and how they measure up, than they are the callous and unemotional males described by Knight and Sims-Knight, or the unempathic and uncompassionate male that Malamuth describes. They almost certainly match the "self-centered" orientation that Malamuth describes as pushing hostile masculinity and promiscuous sexuality into sexually abusive behavior, but this is also true for most adolescents, who are generally and age-appropriately self-oriented.

Consequently, we surmise here, that although some of these young offenders will develop into the adult rapists described in developmental models of adult sexual offending, it is a mistake to draw from the adult literature in trying to understand juvenile offenders. What we do seem to have in common for both juvenile and adult sexual offenders is social inadequacy and social isolation, which for some adult sexual offenders turns towards the callous and unempathic pathways described by Knight, Sims-Knight, and Malamuth, as well as poor self-regulation and an impaired or underdeveloped moral code for behavior. Less at play for adult sexual offenders perhaps, in sexually reactive children and juvenile sexual offenders we also see the added element of highly sexualized social messages, and pressure applied by the media regarding the desirable qualities of sex.

PSYCHOPATHY AND DEFICITS IN ATTACHMENT

Remaining with the theme that callousness and unemotionality are instrumental to adult sexual offending, and perhaps juvenile sexual offenders as well, we can turn to literature that suggests that psychopathy, often associated with these characteristics, can be diagnosed in children and adolescents, and in some cases is related to insecure attachment, or non-attachment. However, it is argued here, that although psychopathy, or traits that resemble or prefigure adult psychopathy, may be found in some children and adolescents, such traits are not, in general, a feature relevant to most juvenile sexual offenders (or most conduct-disordered youth, for that matter).

In fact, shallow and superficial affect, inconsideration for others, lack of empathy, and risky lifestyle—which are all considered elements of psychopathy—are normative behaviors in many adolescents. Consequently, Seagrave and Grisso (2002) describe the risks inherent in diagnosing adolescents as psychopathic, a sentiment is echoed by Hart, Watt, and Vincent (2002) who express their concerns about the implications of diagnosing psychopathy in children and adolescents.

Nevertheless, Forth, Kosson, and Hare (2003) describe psychopathy as a stable personality disorder that is first evident in childhood, probably the result of genetic transmission. Careful not to use the youth version of the Hare Psychopathy Checklist

(PCL–YV) to diagnose psychopathy in adolescents aged 12–18, the authors nevertheless conclude that psychopathic traits are observable in adolescents (and children) and may be effectively and accurately measured, although they also report that personality can change during adolescence and between adolescence and adulthood. However, Forth et al. also acknowledge the lack of prospective studies of personality traits conducted in adolescents later diagnosed with psychopathy, noting also that none of the psychological mechanisms proposed to explain adult psychopathy has been thoroughly examined in children or adolescents. Frick, Cornell, Barry, Bodin, and Dane (2003a) note also that psychopathy has not been studied extensively in children and adolescents, and is limited to cross-sectional and retrospective, rather than prospective, studies.

Forth et al. (2003) also link attachment deficits to the development of psychopathy, in some cases, by asserting that the maladaptive and hostile interpersonal style characteristic of psychopathy is likely to be found in children with an insecure and dismissive attachment style (which would be insecure avoidant in a typical childhood attachment classification—the dismissing style is usually reserved for descriptions of adult, and sometimes adolescent, attachment). They thus conclude that "children characterized by a lack of attachment to others are expected to display impulsive, dominant, and nonanxious interpersonal behavior and, eventually, to develop a coercive interpersonal style that is associated with psychopathy" (p. 6). However, although describing avoidant attachment, the authors are not applying attachment theory to an analysis or understanding of the behavior. From an attachment theory perspective, rather than describing behavior reflective of psychopathy, the lack of attachment described by Forth et al. is exactly that behavior expected in insecure avoidant attachment, and is not evidence of a lack of attachment (or psychopathy, for that matter). Thus, as virtually all children are considered to be attached, even if insecurely, Forth et al. are either describing detached avoidant behavior (rather than an actual lack of attachment) or children falling outside of the range of normative insecure attachment, and perhaps into the disorganized range.

The idea that children who are biologically predisposed to the development of psychopathy are unattached may be true, but this represents only a small fraction of the population, and is not apparent in the attachment theory literature. It also cannot be said to characterize juvenile sexual offenders in general. This is additionally borne out by Forth et al.'s study of over 2,400 conduct-disordered juveniles. The heaviest clusters of psychopathic traits were typically found in institutionalized youth, with a mean score of 24 (compared to a cut score of 30, which is the basis for the diagnosis of psychopathy in adults), with a relatively low percentage falling into a category that reflects psychopathy. About 70% of the community-based sample of conduct-disordered youth had PCL–YV scores of less than 4; conversely, less than 20% of the most serious institutionalized youth scored between 28 and 32, about 13% in the 32–36 range, and around 9% with a score higher than 36.

Nevertheless, Forth et al. report that evidence links psychopathy to adverse family histories, such as those common to both insecure attached children and juvenile sexual offenders, and suggest that such histories are developmental antecedents to psychopathy. However, as Saltaris (2002) has pointed out, there is no direct evidence that applying to children the "attachment profiles" and retrospective histories of adult psychopaths can prospectively predict the emergent development of psychopathy in children. Forth herself acknowledges the lack of prospective research with this population, as do Frick et al.

(2003a), with studies limited to retrospective designs. In fact, the use of retrospective studies, as previously described, may lead to conclusions that are incorrect, and Smallbone (2005) has noted the obvious limitations of retrospective designs typically used to study the development of sexually abusive behavior in children and adolescents.

However, if psychopathy *is* a phenomenon linked to early history, then this suggests it is *developmental* rather than temperamental, in which sociopathic traits and behaviors essentially develop over time and through harsh and difficult life experiences. On the other hand, if psychopathy is temperamental, or *genetic*, unfolding into an environment in which, dependent upon environmental conditions, it may or may not develop into a full blown psychopathy, then it is not derived from early attachment experiences. In this case, the unattached personality that characterizes psychopathy is the product of temperament, rather than of experience. Here, predispositional genetic traits set the course for both attachment deficits (or unattachment, as psychopathic theory suggests) *and* psychopathy, neither of which, in this model, is experience based. Further, as Saltaris (2002) points out, although positive attachment experiences may mediate and dampen the development of innate psychopathic tendencies, these very same dispositions will inhibit or severely limit the ability of the child to form attached relationships in the first place. From this perspective, then, attachment deficits have little to do with the development of psychopathy, at least insofar as it is considered temperamental and/or biological.[2]

CALLOUS UNEMOTIONALITY, PSYCHOPATHY, AND SEXUALLY ABUSIVE BEHAVIOR

Paul Frick also believes that callous unemotionality (CU) characterizes certain children, and especially those who exhibit severe forms of impulsivity and conduct disorder prior to adolescence, and that CU in children marks a path towards adult psychopathy. Like Forth, he avoids and warns against labeling adolescents and children as psychopaths, but makes it clear that he is measuring early signs of psychopathy in children. Indeed, the instrument developed for this purpose, the *Antisocial Process Screening Device*, was formerly known as the *Psychopathy Screening Device*. Frick et al. (2003b) describe CU traits falling into an affective domain that includes absence of guilt and unemotional presentation, and an interpersonal domain that includes manipulation of others for self-gain and failure to show empathy.

There seems little doubt that Frick and Forth have correctly identified a significant subset of troubled children who demonstrate unusually severe behavior. It is also clear that early onset and severe conduct disorder in children is prognostically of greater concern than adolescent-onset conduct disorder, with respect to a continued trajectory of troubled behavior through adolescence and into adulthood. However, it is not clear that the behaviors and psychology they describe are consistent with either callousness or unemotionality. For instance, Frick et al. describe these children as behaviorally and emotionally unregulated, which does not match their description of these same children as emotion-

---

[2] Although many use the terms "psychopath" and "sociopath" interchangeably, Robert Hare considers psychopathy to be genetic and biological in origin, whereas he sees sociopathy as determined by social forces and developmental experiences (for instance, Hare, 1993).

ally constricted or limited in their display of emotion. On the contrary, these children are recognized, in part, *by* their high levels of emotionality and behavioral dyscontrol rather than shallow or absent emotion. In addition, we already recognize that empathy is less developed in children and adolescents than in adults, and is a concept that is difficult to measure, even in adults. To equate a lack of empathy or limited displays of empathy in children with callousness may simply reflect our lack of understanding, or our overstatement, of what it means to be "empathic" during childhood and adolescence.

Nevertheless and quite distinctly, Frick does describe a definite subset of children as less moral, less empathic, and less connected than their peers, even within a conduct-disordered cohort (Frick et al., 2003b). Further, as does Adele Forth, Frick considers these children to potentially be constitutionally different from their peers, reflected in part through the early onset of their severe behaviors. If Frick and Forth are correct, then these are children whose affect and behavior are driven by psychopathic processes that make them "similar to adults with psychopathy" (Frick et al., 2003b, p. 256). Indeed, although they appear reluctant to say it, and are cautious and equivocal in their descriptions, these theoreticians clearly support the idea that psychopathy does appear in childhood, and the children described are, in effect, young psychopaths. In fact, if psychopathy is innate and not developmental, then it must be dispositional in children and adolescents, long before emerging as adult psychopathy.

However, although intending to describe early psychopathic traits, Frick and Forth are also describing children affected, as partly suggested by Forth, by early attachment difficulties and ongoing life experiences. In this case, the behavioral and emotional traits that Frick and others consider to represent callousness and lack of emotionality may distinguish these children from others because they reflect more severe attachment difficulties, including disorganized attachment, rather than psychopathy. That is, the significant lack of self-regulation, limited metacognition, poorly developed morality, and social disconnection experienced by these children may be developmental responses to early experiences, rather than manifestations of innate psychopathy. If unchecked, these developmental (rather than dispositional) traits may yet lead to the callous unemotionality that marks adult psychopaths, as these children harden through adolescence and into adulthood. In this scenario, psychopathy may be a developmental phenomenon, in which adult psychopaths are made, rather than born. This more closely fits Hare's description of sociopathy, however, as a developmental rather than predispositional phenomenon, although others make no such distinction between the terms.

Nonetheless, although recognizing the impact and influence of *external* developmental events in the shaping of personality, Frick is asserting that the CU traits he and his colleagues (Frick et al., 2003a, 2003b) describe in children are ultimately precursors to, or a rudimentary version of, psychopathy and are temperamental traits that reside within the child. As already stated, in this event, as dispositional traits, the significant behavioral and emotional dysfunction described as callous unemotionality cannot be considered an aspect of disordered attachment, although no doubt such traits are fostered and amplified by poor attachment experiences. However, in such a model, the dispositional traits described by psychopathy theory are more likely to have affected and shaped the attachment experience than vice versa.

Meloy (1992) holds a very clear view of psychopathy as a severe disorder of attachment that lies along a continuum. At one end he describes psychopathy as a disorder of profound detachment and, at the other, as a disorder of extreme attachment, involving an intense, pathological, and intrusive bond. However, he is referring to a level of dysfunction of extreme proportions, considering severely pathological forms of attachment at the heart of erotomania (sexual stalking), violence, and murder. These connections between psychopathy and violent attachment (as he calls it) cannot be said to represent the juvenile sexual offender, or even most adult sexual offenders. They must be reserved for extremes in which Meloy's psychopathic disorders of attachment are more likely driven by other forms of psychopathology, and not the disrupted childhoods that typically give rise to insecure attachment.

In fact, although many juvenile sexual offenders have a history of conduct-disordered behaviors that are not sexual in nature, and are far more likely to get into future trouble for non-sexual rather than sexual behaviors (Weinrott, 1996), most do not come close to a definition of psychopathy or antisocial personality disorder. In writing that approximately 50% of juvenile sexual offenders may be diagnosed with a conduct disorder, France and Hudson (1993) also imply that approximately half may *not* be conduct disordered, let alone psychopathic. In their series of 24 studies that included over 1,600 juvenile sexual offenders and 8,000 non-sexual juvenile delinquents, Seto and Lalumière (in press) conclude that although many juvenile sexual offenders are conduct disordered, they generally score lower in conduct-disordered behavioral problems than non-sexual juvenile delinquents. This was especially true of juvenile sexual offenders who assault children, who, as noted, represent the majority of sexually aggressive juveniles. Seto and Lalumière suggest that it is in the *lack* or reduced level of conduct-disordered behavior that we see a substantial difference between juvenile sexual offenders and non-sexual juvenile delinquents.

Accordingly, if we follow this line of reasoning, we recognize that elements of psychopathy, including callousness and unemotionality, are limited to a small subset of the population and are not relevant to the majority of juvenile sexual offenders. We also recognize that it is the *non*-conduct-disordered behaviors and causes in which we should be interested. These are more likely to help us to distinguish the vast majority of juvenile sexual offenders from other children and adolescents, and better define treatment interventions.

SEXUAL OFFENDING AS A DISORDER OF ATTACHMENT

Unlike other crimes that have victims, sexual offending, and perhaps especially among juveniles, appears in many cases to be directly connected to having a relationship of some kind, rather than simply victimizing another individual. That is, in many crimes the criminal act itself is required for some other instrumental gain, such as acquiring money, but is not the specific goal of the criminal behavior. In such a case, for example, the reason for actual or threatened violence is to get something that is wanted and not necessarily for the sake of violence itself. When violence *is* the instrumental purpose, it is usually related to crimes of passion, revenge, domination, or sadism of some kind.

However, in sexual abuse the instrumental purpose *is* to engage in a sexual act with another person, and thus to engage in some form of relationship. As described in Chapters 11 and 12, for some sexual offenders the sexual abuse itself constitutes a form of social/intimate relationship and moves sexual offenders closer to relationships, however distorted, in which the intention is to engage with someone in a social relationship or derive some perceived or imagined social benefit. In these situations, as Hudson and Ward (2000) have written, despite the socially deviant behavior, the sexual abuse is intended to meet social needs that are themselves not necessarily deviant. This may be true of many adult sexual offenders, but appears particularly relevant to juvenile sexual offenders, many of whom are socially isolated, experience themselves as socially inadequate and low in masculine adequacy, and develop many of their sexual attitudes through early maltreatment, including abuse, and/or the media and its usually attractive depictions of sexual behavior, as well as through hard core depictions of sexual behavior depicted in easily accessible pornography.

In the simple typology shown in Figure 13.2, one can discern four forms of sexual abuse:

1. *Unattached/no relationship*, in which the victim is a pure object of sexual desire, and in which no relationship is implied or sought.
2. *Sadistic relationship*, in which the victim is forced to engage in a very direct and distorted relationship with the perpetrator.
3. *Victim as object of social connection*, in which the victim represents a connection to larger social relationships or social competencies.
4. *Victim as object of affection*, in which there is a clear intention to engage in a genuine relationship with the victim, which implies some level of intimacy on the part of the perpetrator.

If these categories of sexual abuse are laid along a continuum, at one end we see no attachment at all, as in the non-relationship of psychopathy, whereas each of the other three forms represents disturbances in attachment, but not unattachment (although detachment may be required on the part of the offender in order to engage in the behavior).

Shown in Figure 13.3, separating type 1 and 2 sexual offenses from types 3 and 4 is an arrow pointing towards disconnected, remorseless, affectless, and unattached psychopathy at one end of the continuum. In the other direction, the arrow points towards connected, socially incompetent, socially inappropriate, but attached pathology at the other. In the case of types 1 and 2, although they may vary in attachment, they nevertheless both lie at the psychopathic end of the scale, and, consequently, intervention and treatment are

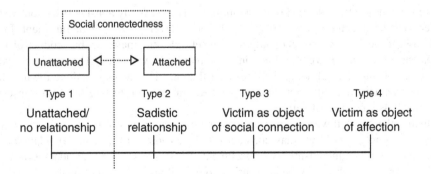

Figure 13.2 Typology of sexual offenses: from unattached to attached

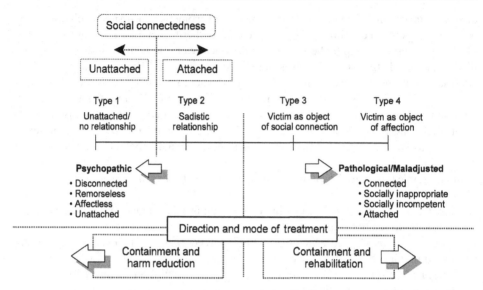

Figure 13.3 Typology of sexual offenses, from unattached to attached, and implications for containment and treatment

likely to be quite different from treatment interventions applied to types 3 and 4 offenses. The dividing line thus separates treatment into two forms: *containment and harm reduction* at one end, and *containment and rehabilitation* at the other.

We recognize that the behavior of our clients has lapsed into sexually abusive behavior for any number of reasons, but certainly we hold here that social connection and social adequacy are included among those reasons. However, when we consider sexual crimes along an attachment-related typology, such as that shown in Figure 13.3, virtually every child we treat will be seen to fall on the containment and rehabilitation, rather than the containment and harm reduction, side of treatment.

CONCLUSION: PATHWAYS TO SOCIAL CONNECTION

When we consider the role of callous unemotionality in sexually abusive behavior, we can either consider it as an aspect of psychopathy or of developmental maladjustment. In the first case, if we consider psychopathy as a genetic development, or the product of temperament, we are not traveling along an attachment pathway at all. The condition exists as a predisposing trait, although it is possible that attachment may mediate the development of psychopathy, with secure attachment serving as a protective factor and insecure attachment as a catalyst of sorts.

On the other hand, if we recognize callous unemotionality as a *signal* of antisocial development, and not a *cause*, we may consider it to be a sequela of insecure avoidant attachment, *en route* to adult dismissive attachment. What starts out as an adaptation to an environment in which it may be appropriate to be callous and unemotional develops into a dysfunctional pathology. Either way, as Hunter et al. (2004) point out, although emotional callousness and aggressive behavior may result from the individual's perception, and even accurate perception, of effective and adaptive behavior within his or her subculture, it can be surmised that such attitudes do not bode well for the individual's functioning within the larger social environment.

Whether developmental or temperamental, antisocial behaviors are linked to a lack of morality, limitations in empathy, and a lack of connection to social values and, indeed, to the larger society itself. These result from and contribute to a self-centered perspective and reduced sensitivity towards others, creating further vulnerability for an increasing attachment gap, continued antisocial behavior, and opportunities for the victimization of others. In the next chapter, we continue to explore developmental pathways related to attachment, by examining the development and role of empathy, morality, and social connection.

CHAPTER 14

Essential Elements: Empathy, Morality, and Social Connection

The previous chapter discussed the role of antisociality, including exaggerated masculinity, callousness, and emotional disconnection, as links to aggression, violence, and victimization, and particularly sexual aggression. Underlying antisocial behavior, however, and perhaps stemming from the same source, are the development of skills and elements essential to social functioning and social relatedness.

This chapter focuses on three specific aspects of juvenile development, clearly related to the growth of attachment and its sequelae: empathy, morality, and social attachment, their interrelationship, and the implications of these intertwined strands in an attachment-informed understanding of sexually abusive behavior in children and adolescents.

THE DEVELOPMENT OF EMPATHY

It is not a far stretch, of course, from callousness to lack of empathy, of which we have spoken (Chapters 12 and 13). Most simply, empathy is described by Feshbach (1997) as an interaction in which one person experiences and shares the feeling of another. However, more than just being able to recognize and share the emotions of another person, empathy involves cognitive, emotional, and motivational elements.

Described as a multistaged process, empathy is considered to involve both objective perspective taking and elements of subjective sympathy. That is, we must be able to cognitively and objectively recognize and correctly identify emotional states in others, feel a subjective affective response within ourselves produced by the experience of the other, and be motivated by the "empathic distress" (Hoffman, 2000) evoked within us by the experience of the other to the point of making a choice to reach out and help. This final element of empathy is identified by both Hoffman (2000) and Marshall (2002) as key to the decision to help.

For the most part, research suggests that empathy is not only a multidimensional model, progressing in stages, but also not a stable trait that is unvarying under different conditions. In fact, sexual offenders appear to possess the same sort of global, or dispositional, empathy as non-sexual criminal offenders and even non-offenders, and it is only in victim-specific empathy that they differ. Even here, however, sexual offenders are not essentially different from non-sexual criminal offenders, as one must be able to switch off or simply not feel empathy in order to victimize another person. This is where callousness and unemotionality, of course, come into play. In non-offenders, who, by definition, have no victims, we cannot assess the equivalent of victim-specific empathy, except to say that almost everyone is able to suppress empathy at times, or we would face what Hoffman (2000) describes as "promiscuous empathy."

Further, D'Orazio (2002) finds empathy to be developmentally age-related, in which adolescents experience less empathy than adults in general, and limitations in empathy in adolescents are more normative than they are a feature of juvenile antisocial behavior. Hence, it is a mistake to consider the nature of adolescent empathy in the same terms as adult empathy, or to map ideas about empathy deficits in adults onto adolescents and children. In fact, among adults and adolescents, even in the suppression or absence of victim-specific empathy, we may not be describing a lack of empathy at all, but actually describing the effects of cognitive distortions that allow victimization to occur.

In describing empathy as the basic human emotional faculty that predisposes people to develop concern for others, Vetlesen (1994) describes it as always *other*-directed, rather than self-concerned. Hoffman (2000), too, describes empathy as an emotional response that is "more appropriate to another's situation than one's own" (p. 4), or having feelings that are more related at that moment to the perspective or experience of someone else rather than one's own experience. Similarly, Rogers (1980) describes empathy "dissolving alienation," and connecting the individual to others. In relating empathy to self-exploration, Rogers is to some degree also describing metacognition, or the capacity to recognize ideas and feelings both within oneself and within others, as is Hoffman, who describes in those who reach out to help, a metacognitive awareness of the fact that they are responding empathically.

It may be more relevant for us to consider empathy in juvenile sexual offenders, then, as not simply the capacity to recognize emotion in others and care about it, which may be limited in all adolescents (remember D'Orazio's finding that adolescents are generally less empathic than adults), but to also feel *connected* to others. Hence we can recognize empathy in adolescents as a measure of social connection and belonging, rather than a lack of sympathy and concern for others. In this case, limited empathy in adolescents, compounded by other factors, may be reflected, not so much in a lack of concern for others, but in a sense of disconnection, alienation, and normlessness, described below in terms of connection and attachment to society and to social values. The risk, if we think of empathy in adolescents in adult terms, is that we may indeed conclude that we are seeing callousness and unemotionality, rather than a developmental task in process.

In terms of the development of empathy, Feshbach (1997) notes that when infants and very young children become upset due to the distress of another child, it is sometimes considered a demonstration of empathy. Although uncertain of the age at which empathy clearly emerges, she notes that it may be present in a rudimentary form even at birth. Liam Marshall (2002) writes that infants seem able to recognize distress in others, becoming distressed themselves, described by Hoffman (1976) as empathic distress, and this capacity seems to have some congenital basis. This suggests that the roots of empathy, at least, lie in early childhood, or the capacity to have feelings evoked in one's own self through the emotional experiences of another. Hoffman (1976, 1987) describes empathy as an innate process, developing from early infancy through distinct stages until empathy becomes a complex cognitive-affective skill, rather than an indistinct reaction to others as it is in the empathic distress experienced by infants. In mature empathy, self-oriented empathic distress is transformed into a sympathetic concern *for* the other, rather than a distress for one's own condition (Hoffman, 1976).

EMPATHY AND ATTUNEMENT

Rogers writes that people learn to become empathic by being with and learning from empathic people. Of course, this means having the experience of being understood by another person. In a model of early attachment, this means parents and this is certainly in keeping with ideas about attachment and early child development proposed by Schore (1994, 2001a), Stern (1985/2000), Siegel (1999) and others who write of the attunement, connection, and understanding that exists between infant and mother. Feshbach (1997) describes the capacity of the empathic parent to understand and share the child's perspective and emotional experience as integral to socialization, and Kohut (1977) described "defects in the self" resulting mainly from empathic failures in the parent (p. 87). In this vein, Davis (1996) writes that the emotional quality of family relationships is important to the development of empathy within children, and that secure attachment is associated with behaviors that reflect empathic concern for others. Conversely, he writes that in abusive families the capacity of empathy in children is diminished.

We recognize empathy, then, as a requirement for socially connected human experience in which one is seen, understood, and cared for by others and in turn is able to see, understand, and care about others. Developed throughout life, from an attachment perspective, empathy initially unfolds through the attuned relationship between infant and mother, and later develops further through the broader experience of the goal-corrected attachment partnership and family life populated with multiple attachment figures. As the child develops, the capacity for a more mature and complete empathy is shaped by emotional experience and facilitated by cognitive development. In this regard, empathy is tied not only to the experience of being understood and cared about by others, but also to the theory of mind, or metacognition, and the ability to experience the cognitive and emotional states of others—and care about *them*. Limitations in metacognition, and hence limitations in empathy, not only contribute to the callous unemotionality described by Knight and Sims-Knight (2004) as central to sexual aggression, but are central to Fonagy's (2001a; Fonagy et al., 1997a, 1997b) model in which lack of metacognition allows and even fosters antisocial behavior (Chapter 4).

Hence, in treatment, the unfolding and realization of empathic states is critical, both in terms of the client feeling empathically recognized and understood and experiencing empathic concern for others. Nevertheless, for latency age children and adolescents, we must recognize that empathy is still in its earlier form. Requiring the development of perspective taking for a higher level of empathy, developing around age 12–15 with the onset of Piaget's formal cognitive operations, empathy, as we have to come to understand it, is really in its formative stages during adolescence. It is, therefore, the capacity of empathy to connect us to others and thus avoid alienation, rather than the sympathetic qualities of mature empathy, that are of the greatest relevance as we examine the development and experience of empathy in adolescents. We are especially interested in the relationship of empathy to the development of a higher level of moral decision making and behavior.

At the same time, key to the capacity to victimize others, as described in Chapter 12, we are also able to suppress empathy. Lifton's (1986, 1993) description of the Nazi doctors and the doubling process speaks to this, as does Marshall's comment that "quite clearly, sexual offenders do not display sympathy toward their victims during their offending behaviors, and their most marked deficits in empathy are toward their own victims" (2002, p. 15). However, Hoffman (2000) writes that although empathy is the glue of society, we *must* be able to suppress what he calls "promiscuous" or "diffuse" empathy in order to function as a society. His point is that we would otherwise be emotionally overwhelmed, incapable of ever turning away from others in distress or never able to act in our own best interests if this meant not acting in the best interests of another. It is the relationship between empathy and morality that allows empathy to be suppressed without victimizing or abusing others: "Empathy's limitations are minimized when it is embedded in relevant moral principles" (Hoffman, 2000, p. 216).

We move, then, from understanding empathy as a product of and requirement for attachment, to recognizing it as a prerequisite for the moral development that will allow empathy to be embedded and experienced in the structure and principles of social rules. Figure 14.1 provides a simplified overview of the process by which empathy develops, from its most primitive and innate state to the multistage process of mature empathy, showing its relationship to social attachment, metacognition, and moral development as it develops over time.

FROM EMPATHY TO MORAL DEVELOPMENT

Hoffman (2000) describes the cognitive dimension of empathy as the controller of the affective experience, in which empathic concerns for others translate into and become congruent with social moral codes. In a similar voice, Vetlesen (1994) writes that empathy is a precondition for moral decision making, and that perceptions of morality are built on the experience of empathy for others. These authors see empathy and morality merging, in which empathy builds the groundwork from which moral identity emerges. Morality is the attitudinal and behavioral equivalent of empathy.

THE MORALIZATION OF ATTACHMENT

Stilwell, Galvin, Kopta, and Padgett (1998) describe moral development incorporating social values, as well as the experience of attachment and its transformation into moral behavior. Stilwell's model integrates emotional, cognitive, and behavioral systems into a dynamic mental model of conscience, passing through five stages prior to age 18, incorporated into five domains of conscience. In the first stage, prior to age 7, *external* conscience involves an external locus of moral behavior, subsequently passing through the developmental stages of *emotional, personified,* and *confused* consciences, with the internalization of morality developing from childhood until mid-adolescence, until the development of an *integrated* conscience around age 16. Each stage contributes to the

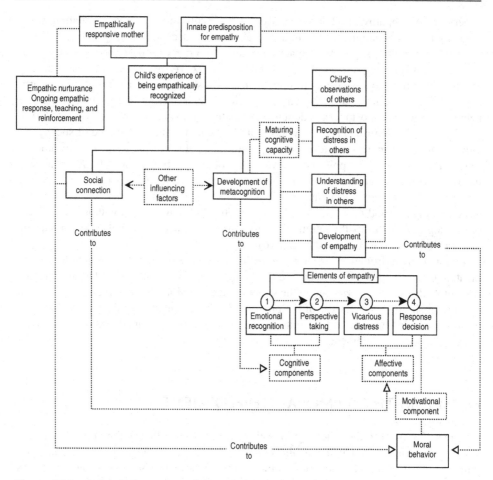

Figure 14.1   A simplistic version of the attachment base of empathy, the empathic process, and the relationship of empathy to social connection, metacognition, and moral development. The solid lines represent direct connections, while the dashed lines represent contributing or background processes

development of four domains that underpin the development of moral attitudes and behavior: (1) moralization of attachment, (2) moral–emotional responsiveness, (3) moral valuation, and (4) moral volition.

Stilwell's model largely involves the transformation of attachment and social experiences into the values, attitudes, and beliefs that underlie relationships and behaviors, resulting in a moral conscience. Linked to neurological and cognitive growth and maturation, she writes that neural development provides the substrate for moral development, which is impaired or impeded by both neurobiological impairment and psychopathology. However, even under normative conditions, morality must be nurtured, which Stilwell reports first occurs during early attachment relationships, and includes expanding relationships with other family members, adults, and friends, and within the social organizations and institutions in which children are raised and grow to adulthood. Conversely, the development of moral identity is negatively influenced by parental abuse and neglect, maltreatment, psychological loss, and traumatic experience—all related to the development of secure attachment.

Stilwell's *moralization of attachment* domain is tied directly to the experiences of early attachment and ongoing human relationships, and represents the foundation for social conscience and the moral domains that later develop. Attachment, described by Delson (2003) as "the linchpin of moral development" (p. 25), establishes the base for what is right, how to act, and what others expect, and thus sets the pace for future moral development. In these circumstances, breaches of trust and the loss or disintegration of trusted relationships erodes the moral meaning attached to relationships (Stilwell, Galvin, Kopta, Padgett, & Holt, 1997). The domain of *moral–emotional responsiveness* involves emotionally driven attitudes and values which regulate behavior, in which moral motivation is based on further developing ideas about right and wrong, influenced and amplified by relationships. These include positive and negative experiences in early attachment, including the capacity to engage in reparation and "moral restoration" following moral transgression. *Moral valuation* essentially means attaching meaning and value to moral decisions and behaviors, involving obligations to others and to social authority. It also means becoming part of something larger, and hence involves social connection with higher behavioral ideas and moral values. In traumagenic circumstances, however, value attached to moral behaviors may be negatively affected and behavioral decisions may become survival driven more than relationship driven. Under severe conditions, this may result in a loss of meaning and a sense of anomie (social normlessness). Finally, the domain of *moral volition* includes the development of "doing things right," even when no-one is looking, and thus involves self-regulation and a higher level of intentional moral behavior. However, in the absence of moral nurturance or when it is weak and lacks meaning, when incentives for cooperation are seriously damaged, or when the individual experiences uncertainty and insecurity about the future, moral and behavioral dysregulation develops in place of self-regulation. These four domains are synthesized into what Stilwell et al. (1997) describe as a fifth "supradomain," that of *conscience conceptualization*, or consciously derived ethical decisions and behavior embedded within the mental structure of each individual (Stilwell & Galvin, 1985).

Stilwell's model of moral identity is very much attachment-based, and comprises elements virtually identical to those found in the attachment model. To this end, she defines moral delay, arrest, and deviancy as developmental disruptions, interruptions, or derailments that result from disruptions in attachment, neglectful parenting, or trauma (Stilwell, Galvin, Kopta, & Norton, 1994). Hence, moral identity may be considered to be the equivalent of attachment style, ranging from secure and organized to insecure and disorganized. In all cases, moral development is contingent upon the relational and social environment from which all experience is derived, and in which the capacity for self-agency and self-efficacy is engaged and tested. Moral identity is the equivalent of the agentive mind, described by Fonagy (2004) as central to our ability to evaluate behavior, form our sense of selfhood, and act on our own behalf. Stilwell's description of moral nurturance mirrors that of empathic development, and is dependent in part upon the provision of ongoing empathic responses and guidance provided by primary attachment figures, as shown in Figure 14.1. These ideas reflect the relationships between attachment, the development of selfhood, the development of empathy and moral identity, embodied in self-image, or self-in-society.

MORAL IDENTITY AND ATTACHED RELATIONSHIPS

Moulden and Marshall's (2002) description of "social intelligence" is a description of an amoral metacognition that influences social behavior. They describe the capacity to monitor self and others, predict the consequences and results of behavior on other people, and self-regulate personal behavior to meet goals. Writing that "social intelligence requires the person to be adept at recognizing emotional responses in others and to be good at seeing things from the other person's perspective" (p. 63), Moulden and Marshall describe social intelligence as neither prosocial nor antisocial. It is moral identity and value that thus transform social intelligence into prosocial behavior, and it is the absence of morality that contributes to intentional and planned antisocial behavior. In turn, Gilligan and Wiggins (1987) comment that it is attachment and socially connected relationships that create an awareness in the child of being affected by and having an effect on others, recognizing and becoming attuned to moral relationships through attachment.

Gilligan and Wiggins are critical of theories of moral development that overlook the implications of attachment, which they assert heavily influence the way in which the child comes to understand how to behave towards others and how others feel—metacognition, in effect, about human relationships. They note that childhood experiences provide the groundwork for care and justice, both criteria for moral thinking and behavior, and that the themes of inequality or equality and attachment or detachment underlie all human relationships: a "relationship-focused perspective on morality leads us to see experiences of equality and of attachment as critical to the growth of moral understanding" (p. 296). Most strongly, connecting the attachment experience to human growth and behavior, Gilligan and Wiggins insist that moral under-development does not reflect a lack of moral knowledge, but the absence of the attached relationships that are necessary for making moral decisions.

THE ACQUISITION OF MORALITY

Like empathy, "morality" is not a single-staged or single-element construct. It has affective, cognitive, and motivational elements, and involves separate but intertwined elements of moral attitudes, thinking, decision making, and behavior that, like virtually all other aspects of child human development, matures in stages. These come together and form Stilwell's domain of "conscience conceptualization," with a level of advanced and self-aware conscience possible only as a result of earlier developmental experiences. Although moral development and advancement are partially and substantially the result of social experience, they are nonetheless predicated by neural and cognitive development, another example of nature and nurture working together to produce a result, rather than one over the other.

Recognizing that moral sense and moral action (affective and behavioral components) are based upon social relationships, and particularly those of early childhood and parental relationships, Kagan (1984) describes the cognitive underpinning as recognition and eventual acquisition of social standards, beginning by about age 18 months. By the second year, children are both aware of violations of standards and can anticipate the expected feelings of others under different particular situations (an early form of metacognition and perspective taking in the development of empathy), and by age 3 are capable of reversing roles and experiencing emotions linked to moral behavior (Emde, Johnson, & Easterbrooks, 1987).

Emde et al. describe two streams of moral development occurring in early childhood, involving the emergence of empathy and the internalization of prohibitions through social referencing.[1] They report that the internalization of empathy and moral behavior is promoted through parental behavior, guidance, and induction, resulting in what they refer to as the moral emotions becoming consolidated into the child's level of self-awareness by age 4. They thus link empathy, morality, and self-awareness (what we might also call metacognition) as strands of the same developmental weave, falling into Bowlby's relational phase of clear-cut attachment (age 6–36 months) and the stage of cognitive development identified by Piaget, during which intentional behaviors and object awareness develops. When events do not coincide with the expected and normal appearance of events, the child's ability to recognize and respond to behavioral and interactional standards and expectations becomes driven by anxiety (Kagan, 1984), contributing to the dysregulation described by Stilwell.

This uncertainty is reflected in the first of two factors that, Stilwell et al. (1994) report, regulate moral behavior, in which anxiety and affect directly influence moral–emotional responsiveness, or the capacity of emotions and values to regulate and motivate moral behavior. The second factor, psychophysical homeostasis, involves a reduction in anxiety and a return to emotional comfort resulting from engagement in moral behaviors that meet social expectations, thus relieving anxiety and restoring emotional and physical comfort. These two factors, involving anxiety and anxiety-reduction, represent an affective-cognitive blend that serves to foster and maintain prosocial, or moral, behavior, described by Turiel, Killen, and Helwig (1987) as central in guiding and organizing social life.

Indeed, Kagan (1984) and others report that anxiety-provoking elements are crucial in developing and maintaining morality. He writes that standards serve as a base for comparison with others and correct behavior, and that failure to adhere to an expected social standard results in *guilt*, followed by *shame* when others become aware of the transgression. These are emotionally uncomfortable elements that he considers central to adherence to moral standards.[2] On the other hand, he writes that adherence to standards, when recognized by important others, provides a source of motivation in assuring the child of its goodness, or value. Dunn (1987) similarly considers that distress, anxiety, shame, or fear aroused by transgression of social standards is crucial, not only as forces that drive and shape morality, but for the development of social understanding. She writes that negative

---

[1] Social referencing involves the development of social behavior and understanding through the ability to read, understand, and take cues from another in any given social situation. In itself, it is both a form of metacognition as it requires an understanding of the mind of others, and a mechanism for what we might even call "social metacognition" as it requires the ability to understand, through the cues and behaviors of others, how the "mind" of society works.

[2] Kagan (1984) suggests that psychopathy is an appropriate description of individuals who commit serious moral transgressions, unaccompanied by feelings of remorse or guilt.

emotions are required to prevent antisocial and destructive behavior, and describes family standards and the manner in which rules are violated, disputed, and resolved within the family as instrumental in forming the child's sense of moral understanding.

Kagan (1984) describes both empathy and morality as essential to the socialization of behavior. He writes that the child's acquisition of standards is facilitated by the recognition of feelings and thoughts in self and others, mediated through the development of empathy. He thus makes moral development contingent upon the development of empathy. We see, then, how morality can be conceptualized as the operational counterpart of empathy, in which empathy is expressed through the effects of decisions and behaviors on others.

MORAL DEVELOPMENT: FROM RULES OF MORALITY TO MORAL SELF

Piaget believed that moral development is based on respect for and acceptance of social rules and conventions, and a sense of justice derived from values about equality, responsibility, and reciprocity in human relations (Likona, 1976). Addressing both dimensions, that is the internalization of rules and attitudes about them, Piaget asserts that "all morality consists in a system of rules, and the essence of morality (lies) . . . in the respect which the individual acquires for these rules" (1932/1997, p. 13).

Piaget (Piaget & Inhelder, 1969) described two stages in the cognitive development of morality, which were later expanded to six stages by Kohlberg in his well-known model. Piaget's first stage of *heteronomy* is based on a moral realism, in which the child's morality is based largely on external control. Decisions about behavior are subordinated to what the child believes the parent wants and expects, hence the development of standards is based upon the parent–child relationship, or at least the child's interpretation of parental expectations. The importance of adhering to values transforms into a duty to adhere to standards, and introduces the idea and builds the groundwork for an objective and subjective conception of personal and social responsibility. With cognitive and emotional growth, this morality of constraint develops into an increasingly *autonomous* morality that recognizes and acts upon the best interests of others as well as self, or a morality of cooperation. Attitudes and decisions are based upon mutual respect, reciprocity, and a sense of justice, rather than external authority, mandates, or sanctions. Piaget describes the more advanced autonomous morality of cooperation developing after the age of 12, culminating in the ability to fully understand and, in effect, codify, rules, based on cognitive developments, with the capacity for formal cognitive operations, and increasing perspective taking, abstraction, and hypothesis formation.

Kohlberg (1976) refined Piaget's model, expanding it into six stages of moral judgment, collapsed into three overarching primary levels, within which the second stage is a more advanced and organized form of that level of moral development. As the capacity to move from one stage to the next is significantly influenced by the development of cognitive and reasoning skills, it is not possible for an individual to achieve a higher stage of moral development than his or her cognitive level will permit. However, a more developed cognitive level does not necessarily imply that the individual has achieved or will mature into a higher stage of moral development. That is, not all individuals will operate at a higher level of moral functioning, despite a cognitive capacity that allows higher moral reasoning.

Kohlberg's first two stages are subsumed under Level I *preconventional* morality, or Piaget's heteronomous stage, between about age 3 and age 10. This level of moral development is characterized by adherence to standards that are largely independent of self, defined by others in authority, with a movement towards a recognition, acceptance, and greater understanding of those standards, and therefore internalization, of social rules. Kohlberg associates this stage not only with children, but also some adolescent and adult criminal offenders suggesting, of course, that people in this stage, regardless of cognitive capacity, never move beyond external sanctions and never accept or internalize social rules. Stages 3 and 4 are collapsed into Level II *conventional* morality, or moral judgment and behavior shaped by conformity to prevailing social and peer values, helping to maintain, support, and justify that order. Stages 5 and 6 involve Level III *postconventional* moral judgment, which, according to Kohlberg, most adults do not acquire until after age 20, if at all. This level of moral development involves ideas about morality that are based on principles of equity and justice that are not necessarily tied to prevailing social conventions and, in the case of stage 6, beliefs about ethical principles that Kohlberg describes as universal, and not therefore tied to the social order.

Like Piaget, Kohlberg recognized the significance of the personal values and meanings that are attached to social rules; in fact, it is the establishment of meaning that makes it possible to move from one level to another, rather than just biological and cognitive growth, which helps to explain why everyone does not move from one level to the next. He describes three different relationships between the individual and social rules, and therefore describes individuals at Level I as *preconventional* people (of any age) who experience rules and social expectations as external to themselves, and are bound to them only insofar as there are external mandates and sanctions. Level II individuals are characterized by Kohlberg as *conventional* people who have identified with, internalized, and accepted social rules as part of themselves, and Level III individuals are *postconventional* people who have achieved a level of differentiation from the set rules and expectations of others, defining their own values and principles.

Kohlberg explains that in addition to the requirement for a level of cognitive development commensurate to each moral stage, stages of *social perspective* are also key to and foster moral development. Although related to morality, social perspective does not address issues of fairness, equity, and choices as right or wrong. Instead, it embodies how the individual sees and understands others, an analogue to the metacognitive skills of attachment theory and the perspective-taking capacity of empathy. Kohlberg's first four stages are those of moral *judgment* rather than *behavior*, and he describes a horizontal sequence of steps, moving from logic to social perspective taking to moral judgment, culminating in the act of moral *behavior*, which he suggests is fully possible only at stage 4 of moral judgment. He writes "to act in a morally high way requires a high stage of moral reasoning. One cannot follow moral principles (of stage 5 and 6) if one does not fully understand or believe in them" (1976, p. 32).

By now it is clear that in a model of attachment and social relationships, the capacity for moral and emotional growth is fostered or inhibited by the development of empathy, metacognition, and social connection, as well as the experience of self-agency and self-efficacy, and the capacity for self-regulation.

THE INDUCTION OF MORALITY

Returning to the idea that moral behavior is required for social order, and that guilt serves the social order by acting as a disincentive for violating social standards, Hoffman (2000) describes avoiding guilt as a prosocial motive to avoid harming others. He defines "empathy-based" guilt as a dystonic and tense feeling that results through experiencing empathy with another who is in distress, and awareness of being the *cause* of that distress. In describing guilt as a prosocial motive, Hoffman reports that reparation to the victim and/or helping other people helps to restore emotional equilibrium and motivates future prosocial behavior. This is congruent with Stilwell's second factor of moral–emotional responsiveness, in which reparation and healing restore psychophysiological stability and therefore promote future morally appropriate and responsive behavior.

However, Hoffman also reports that empathy-based guilt is felt only when individuals have internalized a moral standard and are aware of the violation. This means that the individual must have achieved a level of moral judgment and awareness in which: (i) the rules have been internalized, (ii) the transgression is recognized by the violator, and (iii) the transgression is of concern to the violator. In addition, in order for guilt to serve as an inhibitor of antisocial behavior and a prosocial force, Hoffman notes that the individual must have the mentalizing capacity to reflect upon harm caused, impact upon others, personal motivation, and personal responsibility. This again reminds us of Fonagy et al. (1997a, 1997b) who describe a lack of mentalization not only allowing antisocial and criminal behavior to occur, but also in some cases contributing to and even causing such behavior. Fonagy (2001b) writes that certain types of violence are associated with moral disengagement that results from failed mentalization. Also described in Chapter 4, he hypothesizes that this contributes to: (i) a lack of self-awareness and clear social identity, (ii) an inability to anticipate the psychological consequences of behavior to others, (iii) the capacity to treat others as objects, and (iv) the ability of the individual to rationalize behaviors that make acceptable, and even justify, antisocial behavior.

Hoffman (2000) defines morality as a network of empathic emotions, cognitive representations, and behavioral motivations that includes *principles* about social interactions, *norms* regarding social behaviors, *rules* about acceptable behavior, *knowledge of socially correct behavior*, and *internalized personal culpability* for behaviors that have hurt or helped others. Like other theorists, he considers this internal network to be contingent upon social experiences and socialization, with special respect to ongoing parental interventions around discipline and what he refers to as moral induction. Altruism in the child is enhanced when he or she is raised in a supportive and caring family that openly communicates thoughts and feelings, and models a sense of moral concern for the welfare of others and the effects of one's own behavior (Hoffman, 1976). But, although non-disciplinary parental behavior contributes to moral development in the child, especially by providing social role models and demonstrating and reinforcing empathy for others (see Figure 14.1), Hoffman writes that parental discipline is the key to the internalization of moral values and the necessary development of guilt. Describing several forms of non-physical parental discipline, Hoffman (2000) defines disciplinary interventions as corrective opportunities through which children learn about harm they have caused to others, whether by intention or accident, and experience guilt as a result. He describes *induction* as the means by which parents teach their children about the perspective and distress of the other person and the child's actions as the cause, resulting in the induction of a moral code into the child.

Hoffman concludes that empathic morality is a universal attribute in people, but that it neither develops nor operates in a vacuum. The development of morality, in conjunction with and building upon the development of empathy, occurs in the social environment, both in the early child-rearing/family environment and the larger social environment. Describing morality as fragile, Hoffman states the obvious requirement for positive social experiences and social role models that nurture and reinforce the natural proclivity for empathy and moral development. This is exemplified in Shweder, Mahapatra, and Miller's (1987) social communication theory of moral development, which describes the effects of cultural beliefs and ideology on the development of morality in children, imparted through the context of family life and routine social practices of everyday life. The premises of moral thinking and behavior in any given society are thus expressed through culturally institutionalized behaviors, both teaching morality to children and helping them to make sense of everyday social life. As with chaotic and dysfunctional families, societies with contradictory or confused moral values or practices are likely to contribute to a moral vacuum, confused or inconsistent morality, or amorality in their children.

SOCIAL BONDS AND SOCIAL VALUES

Piaget (1932/1997) recognized that social morality is not a homogeneous packet of values, mores, norms, and rules, because society itself is not "just one thing." Instead, as Piaget writes,

> society is the sum of social relations, and among these relations we can distinguish two extreme types: *relations of constraint* [italic added], whose characteristic is to impose upon the individual from outside a system of rules with obligatory content, and *relations of cooperation* [italic added] whose characteristic is to create within people's minds the consciousness of ideal norms at the back of all rules. (p. 395)

The larger social context in which child rearing and child development occurs is not just an important, but passive, backdrop to the development of attachment, but *itself* is an active ingredient in attachment. We have already seen that culture has something, and probably much, to do with the development of attachment (Chapter 6); but, in addition, the individuals within society become attached to the norms and values of their societies, and build these into their identities and character. Hence, ethnic stereotypes have some meaning in that individuals from within those cultures, along with all of their cultural peers, embody some, or many, of the values, behaviors, mannerisms, and beliefs of their culture thus forming links to their peers, as well as their society. Attachment as we understand it, must also be understood from the perspective of society, not just as the backdrop against and within which relationships with attachment figures form. Social attachment is an entity in its own right, building and giving identity, shaping attitudes and behaviors, and providing cues and directives for the acquisition of selfhood, the role models by which selfhood is compared and defined, and social lessons learned. In this conceptualization, the social environment is not simply a passive entity but an active player in the development of secure identity and prosocial behavior, just as it is in the case of troubled and socially deviant behavior.

With this in mind, we can presume that individuals who may be considered to be securely attached, are also attached to the norms, values, and social rules of their society. We have already seen that this is not necessarily the case for juvenile sexual offenders who Miner and Crimmins (1997) describe as socially isolated and normless, yet no different from other youth with respect to their desire to achieve socially acceptable goals (Miner & Munns, in press). As we have seen, this is a pathway to deviant social behavior as an alternative means for goal accomplishment when conventional social means are beyond the capacity of the individual for one reason or another (for instance, see Figure 12.1, Chapter 12).

In exploring school performance, Libbey (2004) examined the relationship between academic success and the experience of students with respect to their sense of attachment to their schools. Regardless of different terms used to describe this sense of school belonging, including school attachment, bonding, connection, and engagement, and different measures used to assess each construct, Libbey found that school success was often related to a sense of belonging, having a voice, positive peer relationships, engagement in school activities, teacher support, and a sense of safety. Catalano, Haggerty, Oesterle, Fleming, and Hawkins (2004) defined school bonding as close and affective attached relationships with peers and faculty, an investment in the school environment, and doing well socially and academically. They write that such bonds are produced by opportunities for involvement, recognition of effort and success, and the teaching of social, emotional, and cognitive competencies. Like Libbey, they conclude that school bonding contributes to academic performance and social competence. Once strongly established, Catalano et al. report that school bonding inhibits behavior that is inconsistent with the norms and values of the school, and reduces problems with antisocial behavior. In their meta-analysis of 66 studies, Hawkins et al. (2000) grouped predictors of risk for youth violence into five domains (individual, family, school, peer-related, and community). In addition to describing low levels of parental involvement and poor family bonding as predictors of risk (in combination with other risk factors, and in the absence of protective factors), they also identify low bonding to school as a risk factor, noting that connection to school served as a protection against youth violence.

As described briefly in Chapter 4, anomic theory is derived from the work of Emile Durkheim (1893/1997, 1897/1951), which asserts that attachment to social values and norms, or social attachment, leads to prosocial experiences and behaviors. Conversely, a lack of social values and the experience of normlessness, or anomie, significantly contributes to personal dysfunction and social problems, including crime. With respect to its contributions to criminal behavior, Agnew and Passas (1997) write that anomic theory focuses on a breakdown in the capacity of society to regulate individual behavior. Theories of social normlessness assert, then, that without a coherent social structure and consistent social norms, individuals unattached to or alienated from society may engage in deviant behaviors in order to get their goals met, many of which are legitimate social goals even though they are acquired through illegitimate means.

SOCIAL VALUES AND SEXUAL BEHAVIOR IN CHILDREN AND ADOLESCENTS

From the perspective of control theory, without the control of social attachment, in a normless society individuals are unrestrained from engaging in antisocial behaviors. In strain theory, individuals who have no sense of attachment to social norms and institutions lack the means to tolerate social stress and the means to gain social goods, and thus socially deviant behavior is required as the only means to achieve socially desirable goals. Rather than freeing the individual to engage in antisocial behavior, as social control theory asserts, Agnew and Passas write that the breakdown in social regulation creates *pressure* for individuals to engage in deviant behaviors as a result of their inability to meet their goals through legitimate means. Jerome Kagan (1984), too, considers that social conditions contain *causal* power. He writes that our society insists, with increasing frequency, that individuals are not responsible for many of their actions, and that modern western society is increasingly tolerant of moral and ethical violations. This, he asserts, leads to the experience of children and adults alike, in which they find no-one who will disapprove of many of their behaviors, thus decreasing the likelihood that they will experience shame or guilt for their behaviors.

The idea that society itself, rather than just the unique experiences of individuals, contributes and defines the way in which attitudes and behaviors develop offers a very compelling perspective, and particularly with respect to juvenile sexual offending and sexually abusive behavior in children. Indeed, this perspective is endorsed in this book, in which social conditions give rise to and catalyze the very behaviors we are attempting to rehabilitate. The social environment, *completely independent of the individual*, is thus a significant contributor to the sexually abusive behaviors we seek to understand and treat. In this context, socially desirable goals and behavior include the acquisition of sexual knowledge, sexual experience, and sexual control, related commodities that are highly valued by our society. The value and importance of the sexual commodity is reflected both in the quantity and frequency of sexual messages in our media, and in the histories of many of these children who have themselves been the victims of sexual abuse or have been exposed to sexual pornography and other sexual images. The message in either case—whether delivered through the use of sex in the media or the imposition of sexual abuse in their own lives—is clear. Sex is desirable, and endows special properties onto those who engage in and control it, including power, adulthood, masculinity, special knowledge, pleasure, and prestige. Indeed, Prendergast (1993, p. 6) has written that

> society is preoccupied with sex and uses sex to prove everything, especially manhood. Both boys and girls are affected by this factor, especially as they enter adolescence. Boys develop the need to prove their manhood. What they see on television . . . portrays sex as the ultimate proof of reaching adulthood and being accepted as normal and healthy.

For troubled children and adolescents, sex may appear as a remedy for what ails them, whether that be a loss of personal control, a lack of social competence, sexual and/or masculine insecurity, or a failure to otherwise find satisfaction or success in social relationships. As Fagan and Wilkinson (1998) have pointed out, stolen goods have value that exceeds any material value they may have, symbolizing the criminal's ability to dominate another person, to take what he or she wants, and gain deference. Although they are discussing robbery, the point is nonetheless well made and quite applicable here.

Miner's (2004) assertion that masculine attitudes may be tied to juvenile sexual offending, and especially his reference to masculine inadequacy, fits well when we consider the role that taking what you want sexually and living out a sexual dream, however inappropriately, may play in helping to dissolve and ameliorate social distress. Theories of normlessness, then, are easily applied to understanding sexually abusive behavior as a means for acquiring a social goal that is clearly advertised by society as valuable, legitimate, *and* normative, by individuals who are not otherwise able to accomplish such goals. Unattainable goals are created when society fails to set limits on individual goals or specifically encourages their pursuit, and when individuals are either not capable of achieving those goals or are not attached or committed to society or its agents (for instance, family, peers, school) in a way that makes such goals achievable, or puts them into perspective (Agnew, 1997).

For children and adolescents who aspire to such goals, who are also emotionally and/or behaviorally troubled and who lack connection to the agents of society, the only way to accomplish otherwise unattainable goals is through social deviance. For a recipe for sexually aggressive behavior, add to the ingredients of insecure attachment, social inadequacy, poor judgment, lack of metacognition, and limited self-regulation, the ingredient of sex, delivered through the selling of sex in the media and/or the sexual abuse that many juvenile sexual offenders have previously experienced. Now we may be more easily able to recognize how attachment deficits can interact with social messages to produce sexually inappropriate behavior in children and adolescents who have little connection to prosocial norms.

Indeed, Passas (1997) tells us that whenever the guiding power of conventional norms is weakened, high rates of deviant behavior can be expected. In circumstances of weakened norms and limited social attachment, people commit deviant acts whenever an opportunity is offered in order to meet perceived needs. As people relate to reference groups to which they would like to belong, from which norms frequently emerge, Passas asks: To what extent does the prevailing culture encourage "non-membership" reference groups (that is, attractive groups to which anyone can belong), such as those presented in the sexual media? In particular, he asks how the media affects the adoption of reference groups as normative by young people in society.

In fact, many teenagers rank the media as their major source for sexual ideas and information, and there appears a strong link between exposure to sexual content in the media and sexual beliefs and behaviors (Brown & Keller, 2000; Kunkel, Cope-Farrar, Biely, Farinola, & Donnerstein, 2001). Mediascope Press (2001) reports that the media portrayal of sex as normative contributes to teen sexual behaviors, and Brown and Keller write that "the clash between the media's depiction of sexual relationships and the real-life experiences of youth contributes to their difficulties in making healthy sexual decisions" (p. 255). They noted also that "the media saturated world in which children live is a world in which sexual behavior is frequent and increasingly explicit" (p. 255). Similarly, Mediascope writes that sexually seductive messages embedded in the media provide little to no support for an actual understanding of sexual feelings nor help to define responsible sexual behaviors, and such messages contribute to both confusing and contradictory beliefs and behavior in adolescents.

SOCIAL CONNECTION AND ATTACHMENT

The Commission on Children at Risk (2003) describes a crisis in American childhood, based upon a lack of social connection, both to other people and to constructs such as morality and personal meaning. The Commission considers this to be the result of a break-down in social institutions, such as that described in anomic theory. Their perspective is that the task is to re-connect children, not just to peers and adults in the community, but to society itself, writing that "a great deal of evidence shows that we are hardwired for close attachments to other people, beginning with our mothers, fathers, and extended family, and then moving out to the broader community" (p. 14). Directly linking social attachment to moral development, and hence social behaviors, the Commission describes moral behavior stemming from attached relationships as much as the acquisition of rules. Taking the position postulated by attachment theory, they conclude that we are genetically predisposed to connect with others and form attachments, and that our sense of right and wrong originates largely from a biologically primed need for attachment. Moral behavior stems as much from relationships as from the acquisition of standards and rules, thus, the failure to form secure attachments necessarily means the failure to form a strong moral code.

RISK AND PROTECTION IN THE ENVIRONMENT AND WITHIN OURSELVES

Human behaviors do not spring out of nowhere, and are usually not without purpose or reason. To this end, Shonkoff and Phillips (2000) write that human development is shaped by the ongoing interplay among sources of vulnerability and sources of resilience. Although "some developmental pathways follow trajectories or patterns that are deeply ingrained and thus less amenable to influences that may deflect them in a positive or neg-ative direction" (p. 30), human development is nevertheless influenced between and among elements that influence or actually increase the possibility of problems and those that buffer against risk and therefore increase the possibility of a positive outcome. We have already read of the balance described by Werner and Smith (1992, 2001), in which the presence of protective factors can ameliorate or counteract the effects of high-risk conditions.

In Chapter 13, the public health model describes risk factors for violence in children and identifies males at risk for the development of violence between ages 6 and 14, just because they are males. Besides being a boy aged 6–14, which is something we can do nothing about, there is the number and combination of risk factors that increases the prob-ability of violent and antisocial behaviors (Hawkins et al., 2000), which we *can* do some-thing about. In the development of violence in children, the public health perspective also implicates as sources of risk or protection many of the elements identified by attachment theory as factors that promote or inhibit secure attachment in children. In its report on youth violence, the US Surgeon General (US Department of Health and Human Services, 2001) described a series of factors, shown in Figure 14.2, that address many of those same issues, also identified in this chapter as sources for the development of empathy and moral-ity, as well as connection to the larger society.

However, rather than focusing on the many variables that constitute risk or protective factors, Rutter (1987) tells us that the focus of attention should be on the *processes* and mechanisms that operate at critical life junctures, and particularly those that serve as pro-tection against risk. He describes classes of protective factors as: (i) those that limit expo-sure to high-risk situations, (ii) those that reduce the likelihood of uncontained reactions

Risk factors	Protective factors
• Being male • Antisocial attitudes • Low socioeconomic status • Antisocial parents • Poor parent–child relationship • Low parental involvement • Harsh, lax or inconsistent parent discipline • Broken home • Separation from parents • Abusive or neglectful parents • Family conflict • Poor or absent parental supervision • Weak social ties • Antisocial peers	• Being female • Positive social orientation • Perceived sanctions for transgressions • Warm, supportive relationships with parents or other adults • Parent's positive evaluation • Parental monitoring • Close family relationships • Prosocial parental values • Parent self control • Appropriate sanctions for poor behaviors • Respectful parents • Prosocial peer group

Figure 14.2 A partial list of risk factors for violence and proposed protective factors identified by the office of the US Surgeon General (US Department of Health and Human Services, 2001)

that result from exposure to risk, (iii) those that increase self-efficacy through the development of secure relationships, and (iv) those that provide opportunities for success. However, Rutter suggests that "protection does not reside in the psychological chemistry of the moment" (p. 329) but is, in the end, established in the psychology of individuals and how they deal with life and the events and relationships by which it is defined. Once again, then, we are taken back to the internal working model as the psychoneurological interpreter and container of such experience, in which individual psychology resides.

CONCLUSION: REHABILITATING SOCIAL CONNECTION

Early consciousness coalesces out of the experiences of the infant and very young child. The elements present in that early universe, contained in these experiences, also coalesce, and are embedded into early consciousness as the material from which mental representations of the world are built, and which continue to influence relationships and behavior throughout life. These early experiences, therefore, are the primitive forerunners of personality and social functioning, including the way that we experience, process, and express empathy, morality, and social connection. In considering these three important aspects of human development, interaction, and connection, we also recognize their foundations in, and relationship to, the early attachment experiences that shape our view and experience of ourselves and others, and the relationship that exists between us. Although we may never fully recognize those factors that result in juvenile sexual offending, and which distinguish it from other forms of antisocial behavior, in our assessment and treatment of sexually abusive youth it is these three elements of empathy, morality, and social connection that we should bear in mind.

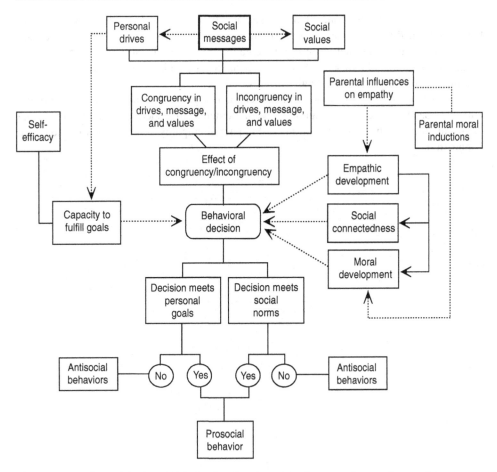

Figure 14.3 A model of social behavior, involving the impact of empathy, social connection, moral development, and self-efficacy on decision making and the ability to meet personal goals and social norms

In describing adolescent sexual risk-taking, Kirby (2001) writes that "a remarkably simple conceptual framework" (p. 276) may partially explain the disparate findings and ideas about adolescent behavior. He writes that the norms of the social reference group and the connectedness of the individual to that group, as well as the interaction between these constructs, are central elements in understanding behavior: "consistent with the social norms-connectedness framework . . . the norms of the individuals or groups with whom adolescents are connected or with whom they interact affect adolescents' sexual behavior" (p. 277).

What then, might be the results for insecurely attached children with social skills deficits who are constantly exposed to sexual behavior, ideas, and imagery in their developmental/learning environment, whose capacity for understanding, judging, and acting upon ideas is weak, who live in a society with confusing and contradictory norms and values, and who are *not* strongly connected to a social reference group? In fact, it seems likely that it is from this group that most juvenile sexual offenders emerge. It seems equally likely that it is the combination of these elements, acted upon by still other social or personal forces, that results in sexually abusive behavior in children and adolescents, and not the impact of a single or even small cluster of elements.

Synthesizing the ideas described in this chapter, Figure 14.3 illustrates prosocial and antisocial behavioral choices as an outcome of elements embedded in self and in the social environment, including the interactions and impact of empathy, moral behavior, and social connection.

CHAPTER 15

The Neural Self: The Neurobiology of Attachment

Fago (2003) writes that it is essential for those who work with children and adolescents to broaden their understanding of developmental neurology. In fact, it is not possible to adequately discuss attachment without considering the neurological processes of attachment, or the manner in which, as a psychological and social experience, attachment is reflected in the physical processes of brain development and functioning. This is especially pertinent when we recognize that attachment is, after all, considered as a biological process. Hence, before proceeding to discuss the elements and implications of attachment-informed treatment, it is pertinent to review attachment and its neurobiology.

However, this chapter cannot be, nor is intended to be, a primer on brain anatomy. This is far beyond the scope of the book, as well as my skills and knowledge, and there are many excellent books, chapters, and articles that address and describe neurobiology, for the layperson as well as the scientist. These contain exciting and fascinating ideas, but are also complicated and difficult to follow, sometimes presenting subtle differences and sometimes overt contradictions regarding the neural topology and structure, the role of brain processes, and brain development and functioning in general.

I write this chapter as a layperson, of course, doing my best to understand how the brain works and how it can contribute to our understanding of attachment and attachment-related behaviors in children and adolescents, as well as what we might target for change in the brain as we consider treatment of attachment deficits in juvenile sexual offenders. In some cases, when we see certain erratic and disturbed behaviors in kids, it may be that we're seeing the behavioral outcome of right brain processes that experience the world in a spatial, emotional, non-language based, and global manner in which everything is responded to at once, without discrimination or cognitive processing. In other cases, when we see youths whose behavior seems devoid of emotional content, we may be seeing a cognitive, left brain strategy for addressing internal (neural) events and meeting needs, in which there's very little emotional understanding, depth, or context to balance or inform cognitive decision making. In either case, we're probably seeing a lack of bilateral integration of left and right brain processes, and therefore seeing kids who are "half formed," so to speak. In an attachment-informed model of neurobiology—or perhaps that should be a neurobiologically informed model of attachment—we can recognize neural development and functioning as a product of attachment experiences, and attachment and other social behaviors driven by neural development. This chapter explores and discusses some of the ideas most relevant in developing an understanding of the relationship between developmental neurology and attachment.

NATURE AND NURTURE: THE ASSEMBLAGE OF ATTACHMENT AND NEUROLOGY

As described, it is the grounding in biology that makes attachment theory unique among theories of psychology and child development. From the biological perspective, attachment is simply an evolutionarily evolved process to ensure species survival, and is thus as much a part our biology as that of any animal. From this perspective, the internal working model is not merely a psychological phenomenon, but a physical entity, hardwired into neural circuits and reflected in neurochemical and electrical activity within the central nervous system. It is thus a neurobiological structure, the result of synaptic processes, out of which human cognition and behavior emerges, resulting in LeDoux's (2002) description of our "synaptic" self, or how our brains become who we are. Siegel (2001) describes the pattern and clusters of synaptic firing as, "somehow creat(ing) the experience of mind" (p. 69). He writes that "integration" reflects the manner in which functionally separate neural structures and processes cluster together and interact to form a functional whole—in this case, ourselves.

Because neurobiology affects behavior, behavior results in experience, and experience effects changes in neurobiology, we recognize that everything we do and experience has an internal neurobiological and external behavioral counterpart. Everything is physical at the neural level, including emotion and thought, but the physical activity of the brain is translated into non-physical cognitive and emotional mental processes. In turn, these result, and are expressed, in behavior and social interactions, which stimulate cognition and affect, and are transcribed back into the brain through resulting synaptic activity and the encoding of experience in neural memories.

To this end, the Commission on Children at Risk (2003) writes that in the nature versus nurture debate, there is no "versus" at all. The argument over whether our personality, relationships, and behavior are determined by in-born temperament and genetic disposition (nature) or the social environment (nurture) is misleading because it is not one or the other, but a harmony produced by these two interacting processes. "It is time to reconceptualize nature and nurture in a way that emphasizes their inseparability and complementarity, not their distinctiveness: it is not nature *versus* nurture, it is rather nature *through* nurture . . . Nature is inseparable from nurture, and the two should be understood in tandem"(Shonkoff & Phillips, 2000, p. 41).

As we explore the ideas in this chapter, bear in mind that any separation between internal events and external events is artificial. That is, for every external event involving human behavior or the five physical senses of perception, there is an equivalent neural event. One might argue that neural processes mirror, integrate, and respond to external events brought into the central nervous system by physical perception, or equally that human behavior is merely the reflection and outcome of the responses and firing of neural chemical and electrical processes. However, either description is superficial because external behavior is not possible without being triggered by a neural event, and every perceived external event triggers a neural process. Figuring out which comes first is a meaningless chicken and egg exercise, because one cannot exist without the other. As far as we know, every neural process results in physical behavior, whether it be the production of blood platelets, breathing, walking, or talking, which in turn acts back upon the brain to maintain or change its present processes. Similarly, every emotional experience is the result of neural activity, and emotional experiences influence and direct neurobiological processes. Behavior, emotion, mood, and thought are but reflections of neurobiology, and neurobiology is affected and reshaped by behavior, emotion, mood, and thought.

There is at all times, then, a level beneath the exterior at which our behaviors, thoughts, and emotions are the result of synaptic firing and patterns. Accordingly, as shown in Figure 15.1, our psychological and behavioral states are defined and shaped by neurobiological processes (nature) which are themselves shaped and defined by the experience (nurture). Of this LeDoux (2002) writes "people don't come preassembled, but are glued together by life . . . What's interesting about this formulation is not that nature and nurture both contribute to who we are, but that they actually speak the same language. They both ultimately achieve their mental and behavioral effects by shaping the synaptic organization of the brain" (p. 3).

Brain development is associated with experiences in the environment that trigger and produce neural activity. Whether the experiences are positive or negative, neural activity occurs, responding and adapting to those experiences. Adaptations that we consider positive are those that result in neural developments that enhance our ability to function effectively in the world. Conversely, neural adaptations that we consider to be negative impair our capacity to function optimally with respect to prosocial relationships and behaviors.

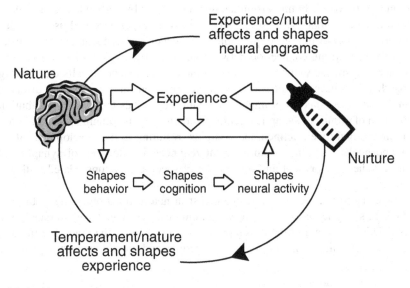

Figure 15.1   Nature and nurture

In the latter case, maladaptation,[1] or negative adaptivity, is most associated with unresolved stress, produced by events experienced by the brain as traumatic. Accordingly, it is not possible to discuss brain development in light of attachment processes without relating poor attachment experiences to stress and trauma that involve neurological stress responses, and in which enhanced neural and psychosocial functioning is possible only when the source of the stress is resolved. Indeed, Restak (2000) writes that large portions of the brain are devoted to fear and stress responses, "simply because survival is at stake" (p. 138).

INTERACTIVE NEUROLOGY: THE BRAIN AND THE SOCIAL WORLD

With respect to the biological process of attachment, the Commission on Children at Risk (2003) asserts that the processes by which we form social attachments and remain attached are biologically primed and discernible in the structure of the brain, and that the provision or absence of nurturance in early childhood development directly affect the development of brain circuitry.

This chapter focuses on four primary aspects of neurology pertinent to attachment and the treatment of attachment-related pathology. The first is that, although the brain is primed for attachment, neural processes develop and unfold over time in concert with the environment, and are both receptive and adaptive. As Spear (2000) has noted, "biology is not destiny, and is modifiable by social behavior and other experiences" (p. 447). That is, the morphology of the brain, including the shape and volume of its structural components, is formed, modified, and reshaped by environmental stimulus and input. As the brain develops, its structure is, in effect, shaped, sculpted, and reshaped by the environment, notably through the processes of *pruning* and *parcellation*. The overabundance ("exuberance") of cells found in the young brain is trimmed down (pruned) by early adolescence, limited to those neural circuits that are most actively defined by experience and use, and strengthened by the process of long-term potentiation in which the frequent activation of certain synapses forms a strong connection between neurons. This makes it more likely that the same synaptic response will occur more and more easily. Hence, "cells that fire together wire together," creating networks of synaptic connections and the shaping of neural circuits in the brain. Related to pruning, parcellation describes the loss, redistribution, and consolidation of groups of synaptic circuits. Cultivated by the pruning process, brain areas become increasingly well defined and complex, resulting in the development of cortical regions and nuclei (ganglia) comprising interconnected collections of synaptic circuits, allowing for the development and dominance of specific functions related to that region of the brain.

This takes us to the second point of interest in neural functioning. The ability of the brain to form synaptic connections, or neural circuits, describes what we mean by neural plasticity. This refers, not to the development of new areas of the brain, but the development and strengthening of new synaptic connections and possible morphological changes

---

[1] Technically, we are not describing maladaptation, but just adaptations that we consider to have a negative outcome for psychosocial functioning.

in brain volume, and particularly in the hippocampus, one of the few areas of the brain in which new neural cells continue to develop throughout life. Through treatment, we can hope to take advantage of the ability of the brain to form, not new structures, but new neural circuits and synaptic connections. Here, we hope to develop the capacity for a different level of brain functioning in which formerly less active areas are brought into use, and the neural "net," or the manner in which the brain integrates simultaneous activity across the brain and across both hemispheres, is thus strengthened. It is this process to which we refer when we say "brain-based learning." However, given the fact that the brain is sculpted by its environment, for better *or* for worse, we appreciate Shonkoff and Phillips's (2000) warning that "plasticity is a double-edged sword that leads to both adaptation and vulnerability (p. 194).

One might argue that external experience entering the brain is emotionally neutral. It is through neural structures, and probably those most associated with the limbic system, that emotion is not only attached to experience, but woven and integrated into experiences that are processed and interpreted by the brain, and subsequently stored as memories, inseparable from their emotional valence (or force). These mental experiences form the basis of cognitive scripts, schemata, and plans and influence the way in which we think, feel, and behave. Thus, the brain is not only shaped to some degree by its environment, but also through its expression in affect, cognition, and behavior; the brain, in turn, affects and colors all future experience and, thus, the environment itself. The third aspect of concern is the interactive brain, or the manner in which environment shapes the brain and the brain shapes the environment. With neural structures that add meaning and emotion to environmental information, we end up with a brain that is not just a neutral receiver, but an interpreter of experience and a shaper of its environment. We see again, the inseparability of nature and nurture.

Finally, we are interested in the consolidation and amalgamation of social experiences into emotional and memory systems, which, in effect, constitute the autobiography of the mind. We are, of course, particularly interested in the effects of the attachment experiences on the early brain, and its direct and indirect affect on and interaction with neurological development. Allan Schore and Daniel Siegel, in particular, are very much of the mind that attachment experiences are intimately involved, and furthermore necessary components, in healthy and well-functioning neural development. Siegel (2001) writes that when "certain suboptimal attachment experiences occur, the mind of the child may not come to function as a well integrated system" (p. 70).

THE USE-DEFINED BRAIN

All models of human psychological functioning and consciousness recognize that the internal world is developed through interactions with the external world, and that the external world is absorbed and re-created in a neural form within the brain. We thus recognize that the morphology and the structures of the brain are influenced by and respond to the environment and its inputs. The brain that develops is an adaptation to, and to some degree a reflection of, the external world in which the individual carrying that brain lives.

This interaction between the external physical world and the internal mental world allows individuals to develop an interactive neurobiology that is tuned and responsive to the external physical world, and in turn acts upon that external world. In this respect, neurobiology, as experience-*expectant* and experience-*dependent*, is shaped by and tied to a larger social reality. Elbert, Heim, and Rockstroh (2001) describe the impact of social experience on neural development as significant. The functional organization of the brain is substantially influenced by social and emotional experiences that occur early in life, affecting maturation of the brain and the development of intellectual and emotional functioning. Although they write that "the structural and functional organization of the brain is shaped in the course of development" (p. 192), the results of a dynamic interplay between experience and developmental stages, they nevertheless note also that the impact of experience on the neural development is not confined to very early periods. Shonkoff and Phillips (2000) also describe brain development contingent upon expected biosocial experiences that organize and structure essential neural systems. This aspect of neural development is "experience-*expectant*" because normal brain growth relies on exposure to expected and predictable environmental events. Throughout life, however, new and unique experiences also help to trigger brain growth and refine existing brain structures; these are "experience-*dependent*" neural developments because they rely on idiosyncratic life experiences to contribute to individual differences in brain growth. Brain development, therefore, "depends on an intimate integration of nature and nurture throughout the life course," according to Shonkoff and Phillips (p. 54).

The idea of the use-defined brain is reflected in the already described idea that repeated brain activity results in the formation of strong synaptic connections (cells that fire together), as well as the processes of kindling and priming described in Chapter 5, the likely result of repeated early experience or adaptation to early conditions synaptically sculpted, or hardwired, into neural circuits. In kindling, usually associated with forms of brain damage, affected areas of the brain are easily triggered into activity (seizures, for instance), with each episode exacerbating damage to and making more likely further easily triggered activity in that portion of the brain. Priming refers to the tendency of the brain to easily recall frequently repeated events and experiences that are stored in memory, with little effort. Like kindling, priming requires little stimulation, as the brain, through prior repeated experience, has become geared to respond and react in a particular manner. In effect, this is a form of brain autopilot, which has its pluses and its minuses as brains can be primed to easily recall and engage in behaviors that are prosocial and rewarding, or those that are antisocial, counter-productive, and self-defeating.

Siegel (2001) describes five ways in which synaptic connections may be altered during the course of development: (1) pruning that strengthens, weakens, or eliminates already present connections, (2) experiences that serve to form new synapses, (3) short-term memory needs that result in short-lived synapses, (4) the effectiveness and efficiency of neural connections as influenced by the development of the myelin sheath that surrounds axons, and (5) the introduction of stressful experiences or the absence of expected experiences that foster growth may lead to the elimination of synapses. The brain is not just use-defined in a manner that promotes positive functioning, but conditions that are stored in memory systems and promote brain development and activity can just as easily stimulate dysfunctional behaviors; hence, plasticity as double-edged. Noting that the maturation and development of neurological functioning are substantially influenced by social and emotional experiences, Elbert, Heim, and Rockstroh (2001), like Shonkoff and

Phillips, note also that neural learning experiences may be beneficial or, under adverse, abusive, or neglectful conditions, disadvantageous.

The use-defined brain results in not just priming, long-term potentiation, and synaptic circuits, but also morphological changes. Maguire et al. (2000), for instance, found that posterior hippocampal[2] volume in London cab drivers was larger than in non-cab drivers, supporting their hypothesis that the rear area of the hippocampus is linked to spatial navigational skills. But of more interest here, as London cab drivers must learn and memorize a vast amount of information in order to acquire their licenses, the study supported the conclusion that change in hippocampal size is a direct result of the learning experience, indicating "the possibility of local plasticity in the structure of the healthy adult human brain as a function of increasing exposure to an environmental stimulus" (p. 4402). However, morphological changes can work both ways. Bremner, Innis, and Charney (1995, 1996) describe an 8% reduction in the volume of the right hippocampus[3] in combat veterans who experienced post-traumatic stress disorder, compared to the average adult brain. They conclude that stress-related chemical processes are implicated in the destruction of neurons in the right (but not left) hippocampus, resulting in damage to short-term memory and fragmented memory storage often associated with PTSD. Stein, Koverola, Hanna Torchia, and McClarty (1997) found a similar result in their study of women who had been sexually abused as children, in which they also found significant reductions in hippocampal size compared to non-abused women. However, unlike Bremner et al., in the Stein study, it was the left hippocampus that showed reduced volume, and not the right, illustrating how little we know about the brain. Although both groups assert that stress is correlated to reductions in hippocampal volume, their findings are inconsistent with one another.

Further, Teicher (2002), although also reporting underdevelopment in the left hemisphere of the brain, did not find any reduced hippocampal volume in his study of sexually abused young adults, and neither did DeBellis et al. (1999b) in their study of maltreated children. In fact, DeBellis found *increased* gray matter (increased neural formations) in the left hippocampus. However, like Teicher, Bremner, and Stein, DeBellis et al. conclude that stress is associated with adverse brain development, and particularly stress associated with childhood maltreatment.

It is possible, of course, that reduced hippocampal volume found in the Bremner and Stein studies was not the result of stress at all but the result of other factors, such as co-morbid substance abuse as suggested by DeBellis et al. (1999b). It is also possible that smaller hippocampal volume may have been a premorbid condition dating back to childhood or adolescence which, rather than resulting from, may have *contributed* to greater susceptibility to post-traumatic experiences in these subjects. This is especially pertinent given the contrary findings of both studies, with respect to the laterality of hippocampal damage, as well as Teicher and DeBellis's inability to replicate the condition. However, it seems certain that the enlarged hippocampi of the cab drivers in the Maguire study *were* the result of their environmental experiences, as it is unlikely that these individuals chose to become cab drivers just because they had good navigational memory. Accordingly, we can agree, with some reservations, that environment affects neurological development.

---

[2] The hippocampus is considered key in the storage of memory, as well as spatial navigation, and, as part of the limbic system, is also related to instinctive behaviors and emotional experience.

[3] All structures in the brain are bilateral—that is, there are two of every thing, except the pineal gland.

THE ROLE OF ATTACHMENT IN NEUROLOGICAL DEVELOPMENT

Schore (2002) writes that the etiology of trauma is now best understood in terms of, not the event itself, but what the individual brings to the traumatic event, as well as how the individual processes the experience after it has occurred. His assertion is that it is personality, rather than the external event, that is specifically associated with the ways that individuals cope or fail to cope with stress. In this conceptualization, forged from the interaction between the brain and the external environment, the *experience* of reality and the external world is determined as much by personality as it is by actual physical events or interactions in the external environment. What we bring to the experience is as important as the experience itself. Personality, then, is not merely passively shaped by its environment but has a hand (so to speak) in shaping the nature of that environment, as well as its own responses to the environment.

Schore (2001b) writes that the events of early infancy, including especially interactions within the social environment, are "indelibly imprinted" into the neurological structures of the early maturing brain. The child's first relationship, typically and most naturally, the mother–child relationship, acts as an imprinting template and permanently molds the child's capacities to enter into all later relationships. In a use- or experience-dependent model of brain development, early experiences and relationships shape the development of personality and, in addition, the capacity of the individual and the capacity and course of neurological development. Through this brain–environment interaction develop emotional and social vulnerabilities, as well as the development of resilience, or resistance against any possible future psychopathology. The process is not merely emotional/psychological, however. Instead, the interactions, or the synchrony and attunement, of the two brains (child and caregiver) catalyze and form neurological pathways in each brain that make it clear that the relationship between "mind and body" is not merely a philosophical idea but an actual phenomenon. In describing the first two to three years of life as the most sensitive period for neurological development, Balbernie (2001) asserts that if such development is disrupted by abuse, neglect, or significant disruptions in attachment, damage may be indelible with respect to its effect on the growth of the orbitofrontal cortex setting a "stamp on the rest of the life" (p. 237). She echoes Schore (1994), who asserts that the early experiences in an attachment-limited environment result in the imprinting of insecure attachment patterns into the central nervous system, and that over the first 18 months of life, "the infant's transactions with the early socioemotional environment indelibly influence the evolution of brain structures responsible for the individual's socioemotional functioning for the rest of the life span" (p. 540). The quality of the infant's relationship with its parents, writes The Child Psychotherapy Trust (Balbernie, 2002), "has a physical effect on neurological structure of the child's brain that will be enduring" (p. 2).

Schore (1994, 2001a, 2001b, 2002, 2003), Siegel (1999, 2001), and Rolls (1999), among others, highlight the orbitofrontal region of the brain, and particularly in the right hemisphere, described by Schore and others (for instance, E. Goldberg, 2001; Maté, 2000) as so interconnected with the limbic region of the brain that it can be considered the associational cortex, or convergence zone (LeDoux, 2002), of the forebrain. Because the orbitofrontal cortex is linked to so many important areas of the central nervous system, including the hypothalamic and autonomic nervous systems, it plays an essential role in adapting emotional and motivational processes. This frontolimbic cortex connects and is linked to a series of essential functions, including arousal reactions, homeostatic regulation, drive regulation, modulation of excitatory influences, and the suppression of heart rate, behavior, and aggression, and is thus connected to both the sympathetic and parasympathetic components of the autonomic nervous system.[4] The orbitofrontal region of the cerebral cortex is involved in social and emotional behaviors, the regulation of physical and motivational states, and in the regulation of emotional responses, as well as executive and decision-making functions. Schore and Siegel assert that this cortical structure is critically involved in attachment processes.

In keeping with attachment theory in general, the essential task of the first year of human life is the creation of a secure attachment bond of emotional communication between the infant and the primary caregiver. For this to occur, the mother must be, not only psychologically, but also biologically attuned to the external and internal states of arousal in her child. Facilitated by the psychobiologically attuned relationship between mother and child, mutually responsive (or sympathetic) processes occur in both parties, including physical responses of the sympathetic and parasympathetic nervous systems and, from Siegel's perspective, direct communication between the emotionally based right brains of both parties. Thus, the mutual relationship introduces involuntary nervous system changes in both parties, in synchrony with one another and in which both bodies, and brains, interact almost as one. Siegel (1999, 2001) asserts that in a secure and well-tuned relationship, this brings about developments in the central nervous system of the child, building the neural framework that establishes a base for the future developmental trajectory of the brain, and all that this implies. Thus is the attachment experience "hard wired" into the brain. From this perspective, Schore (2002) writes that attachment is the outcome of the child's genetically encoded biological predisposition and the particular caregiver environment, representing the regulation of biological synchronicity between individuals. Imprinting, the learning process that mediates attachment, is defined as synchrony between sequential infant–maternal stimuli and behavior.

An early history of mistuned or poorly attenuated mother–child interactions heads the neurobiological attachment system along a different trajectory. With a history of traumatic interactions, the infant/toddler is exposed to a primary caregiver who triggers, and is unable to or does not repair, long-lasting dysregulated states (Siegel, 1999). These negative states lead to significant biochemical alterations in the maturing right brain, and because they occur during the brain growth spurt in early childhood development, long-lasting *states* become *traits*, and are thus embedded into the core structure of the brain and, hence, the evolving personality (Schore, 2002).

NORMATIVE BRAIN DEVELOPMENT

In the report of the Committee on Integrating the Science of Early Childhood Development, Shonkoff and Phillips (2000) write that growing up in an abusive, neglectful, or

---

[4] Both part of the autonomic nervous system, mediated by the transmission of acetylcholine and norepinephrine throughout the body, the sympathetic system is responsible for the increased heart rate and physical excitation present in "fight or flight" responses, and the parasympathetic for "rest and digest" processes that slow the body down, conserve and restore energy, and reduce heart rate.

dangerous environment, or, in their words, a toxic environment, present clear risks for healthy brain development. They write that healthy brain development involves the development of brain cells and their migration through the early years to areas in the brain where they belong, the development of synaptic connections between neurons, and the development of glia[5] nerve cells, representing "an elaborate interplay between gene activity and the surrounding environments both inside and outside the child" (p. 185).

During important neurodevelopmental periods, sometimes called sensitive or critical periods in brain development, specific opportunities for the development of neural structures are available, most typically in early childhood and until about age 3. Of this, MacLean (1978) writes that if neural circuits of the brain are not brought into play at certain critical times of development, "they may never be capable of functioning" (pp. 340–341). By age 2, normal adult brain morphology and structure are apparent in the child, with the major fiber tracts that connect the spinal cord and lower brain to higher functioning brain areas developed by age 3. During this period, from birth on, and even prenatally, the brain is producing an overabundance of neurons. The brain is highly plastic and susceptible to influences upon its future development, both in terms of brain-*expectant* experiences or the absence of those experiences, and brain-*dependent* experiences that will help determine neural development.

Schore (1994) describes the brain developing in discrete, but interactive and dynamic, sequential stages in which neural maturation in each stage brings about a transition to the next, moving to higher and more complex levels of neural organization. Neurons, or brain cells, are connected to one another through their branches of axons (output fibers) and dendrites (input fibers) which form synaptic connections with other neurons, forming a neural network throughout and within the brain, with as many as 15,000 synapses per neuron by the time a child has reached aged 2 or 3, or as many as 85% more than the adult brain, with about 250,000 neurons created per minute during the earliest and more prolific production periods, just before and after birth (LeDoux, 2002). With about 100 billion neurons in the average brain, each neuron is connected to an average of 10,000 other neurons (Siegel, 2001). In addition, non-neuron glia cells which surround neurons and synapses, playing an important maintenance function, may also be key in the development and strengthening of synaptic connections, as well as the formation of memory and neural repair (Fields, 2004). By age 6, the brain has reached about 95% of its adult size (Giedd, 2002), although neuron projections into the cortex continue to thicken into late childhood and early adolescence. Schore (1994) describes neurons developing fully only when stimulated through sensory input, which in turn are required for the adequate development of neural systems involved in the regulation of arousal functions. In a model in which frequently used synapses develop clear and definite neural circuits, the stability and strength of these synaptic connections are determined by the frequency of their activity.

Over time, due to the overproduction of neurons and synapses in early childhood, the pattern of synaptogenesis includes the pruning of excess synapses by early adolescence, bringing the number of synapses down to adult levels by as many as 30,000 pruned synaptic connections per second during periods of pre-adolescent and adolescent development.

---

[5] Glia cells, or neuroglia, are considered to help to develop, support, and improve communication among neurons, but have recently been considered to have much more significance in the brain, in terms of increasing the neural capacity of the brain.

This represents a decline in almost 50% in synaptic connections by the end of adolescence, at about age 20, compared to pre-adolescent synapses (Spear, 2003). Giedd (2002) reports that both advances and changes in neural development are the result, not of the development of synapses, but of their refinement and sculpting through synaptic pruning. It is the effect of experience on these systems that influences hard-wired connections or the pruning of cells, in adverse circumstances possibly leading to irreversible formations. *Experience-expectant* synaptogenesis refers to situations in which an expected experience plays a necessary role in the developmental organization of the nervous system, and normal brain growth relies on these forms of environmental exposure. Deprivation of these essential forms of environmental input can permanently compromise behavioral functioning. *Experience-dependent* synaptogenesis, in contrast, refers to idiosyncratic experiences that occur throughout life, fostering or impeding new brain growth and refining existing brain structures, varying for each individual.

Neurochemical-receptor systems are also instrumental in how the brain alters its physical structure. The neurochemical systems of the brain are open both to input from the environment and to events occurring in the other parts of the body (other than the brain). The response to abnormal (non-normative) stress experiences caused by external events or interactions, or the failure of the caregiver to resolve or repair high-stress situations, can result in the brain being flooded, in essence, with neurochemicals that can cause cell deterioration and cell death, thus contributing to the reshaping of the brain in direct and indirect response to environmental conditions, including response to the caregiver. Stress can thus have a powerful influence on the health and development of the brain, and the entire body. Stress releases a cascade of neurochemicals, producing immediate change in the state of the body (including the central nervous system itself) and puts on hold other essential physical processes. Many of these neurochemical changes take place in the same neural structures that regulate the autonomic nervous system, and involve the development or use of energy, as well as regulating stress responses in the rest of the body. This can produce a hyperstimulating, kindling effect in the amygdala, a hypersensitization of the fear–stress circuits of the brain, and resulting hormonally driven changes in behavior.

Teicher (2002) reports that the trauma of abuse in children induces a cascade of effects, including changes in hormones and neurochemical transmitters that mediate development of vulnerable brain regions. In accordance with Siegel, he writes that childhood abuse is associated with diminished integration of the brain hemispheres. In his study of abused and neglected boys, he reports that parts of the corpus callosum, the integrative and connecting tissue between the neural hemispheres, was significantly smaller than in the control groups.

ABUSE AFFECTED NEURAL DEVELOPMENT

As noted, the hippocampus is a significant structure in the limbic system of the brain, serving as an important mediator in the formation, storage, and retrieval of explicit/ declarative memories, and important as a gateway in allowing new information to be stored and processed as long-term memory. As described, unlike other researchers who found reduced hippocampal volumes among adults who had suffered significant trauma,

Teicher (2002) was unable to replicate this finding. He suggests, however, that reduced hippocampal size may result from prolonged abuse over time, showing abnormalities (such as reduced size) only as individuals age into their mid-twenties as the hippocampus is one of only a few brain regions that continues to create new neurons throughout life and may, thus, show more gradual change. DeBellis et al. (1999b) echo this idea, suggesting that continued replenishment of cells in the hippocampus through to age 30, or neurodevelopmental plasticity, may mask trauma-related damage in younger people. However, DeBellis et al. (1999a) do conclude that "overwhelming stress of maltreatment experiences in childhood is associated with alterations of biological stress systems . . . (affecting) the developmental processes of neuronal migration, differentiation, synaptic proliferation, and may affect overall brain development" (pp. 1267–1268).

Teicher concurs. In his study of 15 psychiatric patients, aged 6–15, with a history of physical or sexual abuse, he (Teicher, 2002) found reduced volume in the size of the left amygdala, correlating with feelings of depression, irritability, and hostility, also suggested by prior studies. In his 2000 article, Teicher reports reductions in left hemispheric regions, including the cerebellar vermis[6] and the amygdala[7], but not in right side structures. He found that the right hemisphere of subjects was more developed than the left, and that left hemispheres appeared arrested in physical development. Teicher reported that abused patients had increased left hemisphere abnormalities and verbal deficits, and diminished right–left hemisphere integration. He thus concluded that a constellation of brain abnormalities are associated with childhood abuse, including deficient development and differentiation in the left hemisphere, deficient left–right hemisphere integration, underdevelopment of the corpus callosum (the connective tissue and pathway between the two hemispheres), and abnormal activity in the vermis.

Creeden (in press) writes that adverse neurobiological development can have five effects. (1) Limbic irritability, or a priming effect of emotional hypervigilance, can result in a tendency to interpret social cues and interactions as threatening, resulting in the activation of the sympathetic nervous system. (2) Fearful anticipation learned by the amygdala may automatically override and exclude the use of other learning which might otherwise result in more appropriate and less reactive behavioral responses. (3) Diminished bilateral integration limits the opportunity to effectively assess and respond to environment stimuli, learn and adapt new problem-solving responses, and process stressful experiences. (4) Stress-related reductions in hippocampal capacity, in conjunction with limbic priming, may create difficulties in central processing and behavioral responses. (5) Limitations in metacognition make it unlikely that the individual will be able to consciously recognize reactive and non-processed emotional responses, and responses are therefore likely to be emotionally processed and reactive rather than reasoned and reflective. Creeden (2005) suggests that avoidant attachment styles may be the result of left brain pathways that "over-modulate" emotional input, resulting in a rigid and limited cognitive transformation of emotional stimuli, whereas ambivalent anxious

---

[6] The vermis, the middle strip between the two halves of the cerebellum (part of the hindbrain at the lower back of the brain, sitting just above the brainstem), is involved in the regulation of neurotransmitters that stimulate left and right hemisphere processes.

[7] The amygdala is implicated in the emotional content attached to and embedded into memory, and the interpretation of incoming sensory information and initiation of appropriate responses, including fear responses.

styles are related to the "under-modulation" of affect, resulting in an immediate and intense behavioral response to stimuli that promote anxiety.

THE STRESSED BRAIN

The neural circuitry of the stress system is located in the early developing right brain, the hemisphere that is dominant in the control of vital functions that support survival and the human stress response, and the hemisphere most active and dominant during the first two years of life. Further, even beyond the dominance of the right hemisphere during infancy and early childhood, stress-coping strategies begin their maturation *in utero*, before the child is born, in biological preparation for the physical reality of survival outside of the womb. Infants under 2 years show higher right than left hemispheric volumes, although the volume of the brain increases rapidly during the first two years and, as noted, by age 2 the development of adult brain structures and interconnecting fibers are apparent. During this first two years, attachment experiences are thought to directly influence the experience-dependent maturation of the right brain. These include experiences with a traumatizing caregiver, typically presumed to negatively impact the child's attachment security and ability to develop stress-coping strategies and self-regulatory skills.

Specific events or environments that are actively traumatizing or fail to prevent trauma produce stress, and may result in extensive pruning (cell deterioration or death) of the higher limbic connections of the orbitofrontal, cingulate, and amygdala systems via the "kindling" process, by which brain areas are repeatedly and easily activated and over-stimulated. Further, such pruning "sculpts" neural networks in the postnatal brain, according to Schore (2001b), and establishes vulnerability to later disorders of affect regulation. Researchers at McLean Hospital (2003) found that adult rats exposed to a social stress during adolescence showed a decrease in hippocampal structure, suggesting that social stress during adolescence causes either a loss of synapses or a decrease in the synaptophysin protein clustered at presynaptic terminals that is associated with learning and memory. They thus assert that exposure to significant adolescent stress may adversely affect the development of synaptic connections in the adult hippocampus, explaining why abuse or neglect may be associated with a decrease in the size of the hippocampus in adulthood.

Stress refers to the physiological changes that occur in the brain and body when there is the physical or emotional perception of threat, induced by actual events in the environment or by anxiety. These changes include changes in levels of neurochemical transmitters and resultant hormonal secretions that directly and often immediately bring about physical, cognitive, and emotional changes, and suspend and divert energy away from other neural and physical activities. These neurochemical and electrical changes are initiated in some of the same areas of the brain implicated with emotion and memory storage, such as the hippocampus, which are eventually bathed in hormones such as noradrenaline and cortisol. At a saturation level, these deactivate the sympathetic nervous system and activate the parasympathetic nervous system, thus reducing tension.

The hippocampus may be particularly susceptible to damage from prolonged stress because it develops slowly, and is one of the few brain regions that continues to grow new neurons after birth. Further, it has a higher density of receptors for the stress hormone cortisol than almost any other area of the brain, and cortisol is therefore drawn to this region. Nevertheless, excessive exposure to stress hormones may affect the morphology of and possibly kill neurons within the hippocampus, possibly resulting in the reduction in hippocampal volume described. This is of importance because the structure is particularly important in the body's response to and regulation of stress, working through the hypothalamic–pituitary–adrenal (HPA) system which triggers the release of corticotrophin-releasing factor (CRF) and adrenocorticotropic hormone (ACTH) that stimulates and later deactivates the body's "fight or flight" mechanism. However, in stress systems that are frequently activated, excessive quantities of and frequently produced stress hormones such as cortisol may have a damaging effect on neural structures, thus causing damage or premature cell death and morphological change. As areas like the hippocampus and amygdala are thought of as centers of stress control, memory, and emotion, these functions may be damaged or affected as a result of constant stress or the failure to reduce or regulate stressful situations.

The vermis, located at the back of the brain just above the brain stem, modulates the production and release of norepinephrine and dopamine, and, like the hippocampus, gradually develops over time, continuing to create neurons after birth. With a high density of stress hormone receptors, it too may be affected by exposure to stress hormones. Associated with several major psychiatric disorders, the vermis may also play a central role in mental health. Overproduction of norepinephrine and dopamine, both regulated by the vermis, can produce psychiatric symptoms, as well as attention deficits. Whereas, the dopamine system has been associated with a shift to left hemisphere-biased (logico-language) processes, the introduction of norepinephrine shifts brain processes to a right hemisphere-biased (non-verbal and emotional) state.

Stress also suppresses production of granule cells which continue to develop after birth, and allow neuron axons to transmit impulses back and forth between the outer surface of the brain and the cerebellum. Another result of stress may be the alteration or suppression of GABA (gamma aminobutyric acid) receptors in the amygdala, which regulate neuronal electrical stimulation, and reduced GABA production or function may allow the development of excessive electrical activity within brain regions. Unlike glutamate, which is a major excitatory neurotransmitter in the process of arousal and stimulation, GABA is its major counterpart, playing an important role in stress reduction and the calming of the arousal state.

Finally, in this model of stress-induced neurobiological damage, the brain never fully develops an integrative connection through the corpus callosum between the right and left brains. In a neurobiology that may be right brain dominated in the neglected or abused child, non-verbal language and rapid emotional responses to stress-arousing conditions are processed by the less logical right brain without benefit of the vertical, or sequential, language and logic-based processes of the left brain. The same is true for the insecure ambivalent child who is emotionally bound, failing to mediate right brain affect with left brain cognition. In the insecure avoidant child, just the opposite may be true, in which emotional responses and behaviors are modulated through logic, language, and cognitive strategies without the benefit of the emotionally oriented and perceptive right brain. The non-integrated brain described here, and by Schore, Siegel, Teicher, and others, fits well with the insecure attachment model typical of attachment theory.

Early abuse negatively affects the development of the right brain as a whole, considered primary in the process of attachment and dominant in affect regulation and stress modulation, thereby creating a potentially weakened template for the physical and emotional coping system. Whereas the left hemisphere is specialized for logical and language-based thinking and expression, the right hemisphere is designed to process non-language-based spatial information, visual cues, and emotional experiences, and particularly negative or anxiety-provoking emotions. From the perspective of Teicher's and similar studies, this suggests the dominance of right brain processing in individuals who have suffered ongoing neglect. This adaptation results in the dominance of non-language and right brain logic systems that use parallel processing systems to rapidly evaluate and respond to perceived environmental cues, without the fully developed capacity of the slower and sequential, logicolanguage-based processing system of the left brain.

ATTACHMENT AND THE STRESSED BRAIN

In a significant way, then, the development of the brain is tied up with stress, the absence of stress, or the ability to resolve stress, and the absence of a nurturing caregiving environment is antithetical to this neurodevelopmental need. Inadequate caregiving produces or fails to resolve stress because it is directly responsible for stress through active abuse or neglect, because it fails to recognize or protect the child against stress, or because it is unable to prevent or repair stress and soothe the child. In each case, inadequate caregiving not only fails to provide the nurturance and guidance required for the development of self-regulation on a neural level, but contributes to the activation of the stress axis and the development of stress-related neural circuits and related behavioral sequelae.

Therefore, as noted, it is difficult to discuss the neurobiology of attachment without considering physical processes within the brain and body that are triggered by stress. These either facilitate effective stress reduction, and hence promote self-regulation, or produce a frequent state of anxiety experienced at the neural level that must be constantly managed. In the case of anxiety-provoking attachment, the sympathetic nervous system is frequently mobilized, all physical resources are channelled to manage the stress, other physical and mental processes are effectively placed on hold, emotions associated with anxiety and vigilance shape and color the storage *and* recollection of memory, and right brain processing is the order of the day, failing to contribute to bilateral integration. In the case of attachment-derived security, however, the brain is able to manage and allocate its resources, remaining in a secure state of mind and thus experiencing a state of relative calm and relaxation allowed by the parasympathetic nervous system, allowing the body and mind to develop in a manner that we consider to reflect positive adaptation, rather than the adaptation to adverse conditions postulated by both Teicher (2002) and Crittenden (2000a, 2000c).

THE ADAPTIVE BRAIN

As described in Chapter 6, Pat Crittenden (2000a, 2000c) argues that all forms of organized attachment are *adaptations*, and it is the adoption of an attachment pattern that doesn't match the environment that makes it unhealthy. In a similar vein, Takahashi, Nowakowski, and Caviness (2001) report that repetition and overlearning of specific operations in early childhood results in enlarged volumes in related areas of the cortex. Thus, they write that the brain is effectively "built" by its specific experiences in the environment, as an *adaptation* to the environment.

The conclusion is supported by Teicher (2002) also, who considers the neurobiological effects of early trauma, resulting in underdevelopment of left brain regions and neural biases to right brain processes, to be *adaptations* to unsafe external environments, rather than *malformations*. Although starting with the hypothesis that early stress is a toxic agent that damages normative brain development and leads to psychiatric difficulties (Teicher, 2000), Teicher (2002) instead concluded that the brain is designed to respond to and be shaped by experience. In response to ongoing maltreatment and/or trauma, or other adverse conditions in the environment, the shift to right hemisphere-dominated brain processing and its rapid, self-protective responses, is an appropriate *adaptation* to an adverse environment, rather than evidence of malfunction or damage. Teicher asserts that appropriate nurturance and the absence of intense early stress permits neurodevelopment that is non-aggressive, emotionally stable, social, and well integrated across both hemispheres, enhancing our social ability to build complex interpersonal structures and realize our creativity. However, in response to the behavior and attunement of the caregiving environment, "stress sculpts the brain to exhibit various antisocial, though adaptive, behaviors" (p. 75).

ATTACHMENT AND THE ASSOCIATIONAL CORTEX

Schore (1994) asserts that for the infant, the very act of unresponsive parenting represents a stressful environment, leading to stress responses as described and high sympathetic nervous system arousal and increased cortisol levels. Thus, insecure attachment contributes to stress-induced neurological experiences, which play a part in shaping the dynamic brain and establishing the substrate for later brain development.

Schore has also clearly described attachment as very significant in the development and integration of basic and higher functions in the right orbitofrontal cortex. He considers this region instrumental in regulating the sympathetic and parasympathetic systems, linking the hypothalamus, which is central in the regulation of bodily functions; the thalamus, a central system for the relay of sensory and motor control signals systems throughout the brain; and the hippocampus and amygdala, both heavily associated with memory, emotional control, and fear arousal and regulation. The orbitofrontal cortex, and particularly the right side, is implicated with stress, arousal, and emotional regulation.

The brain is divided into two hemispheres, connected by the nerve fibers of the corpus callosum with all structures, except the pineal gland, reproduced bilaterally (that is, one in each hemisphere), with four primary divisions of the forebrain, or cerebrum, shown in Figure 15.2: the temporal lobes (one on each outer side of the brain), the parietal lobes (sitting below the crown and to the mid and rear of the skull), and the occipital lobes (sitting at the back of the brain). The frontal lobes, the largest part of the primate brain, occupy as much as 38% of total brain mass (Allen, Bruss, & Damasio, 2004), and are considered the evolutionarily newest part of the brain, responsible for much of higher order human (and primate) intelligence and executive functions of the brain. The cerebellum is

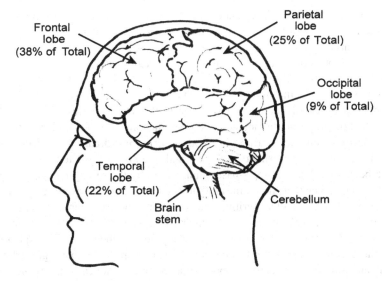

Figure 15.2 Major divisions of the brain
(percentages of size: Allen, Bruss, & Damasio, 2004)

located at the back of the brain, beneath the occipital lobe, part of the most primitive (i.e, early evolutionarily developed) hindbrain, responsible for the maintenance of essential life functions, but also involved in complex planning and executive functions of the brain, including cognition and information processing (Geidd, 2002; Restak, 2000). Deficits in executive function have been implicated in compromised organization, planning and anticipatory activities, self-regulation of emotion and behavior, control of physical responses, self-monitoring, and behavioral flexibility, and are reported as prevalent in attention deficit/hyperactivity disorder and pervasive developmental disorders that lie along the autistic spectrum (Fago, 2003).

But it is the frontal lobes in particular that are considered the seat of planning and human awareness, and especially the prefrontal cortex and orbitofrontal cortex (which is some-times considered a separate division of the frontal lobes and sometimes an element of the prefrontal cortex), and is strongly associated with the development of empathy, morality, and insight into self and others (Allen 1995; Amen, 1998; Balbernie, 2001; Goldberg, 2001; MacLean, 1978; Schore, 1994, 2001b). As described, the orbitofrontal cortex is con-sidered to be a center of neural communication and connection and known as the associ-ational cortex, and sometimes the "limbic frontal lobe," because it is linked to so many important areas of the central nervous system. It is described by MacLean (1978) as "the only neocortex that looks inward to the inside world" (p. 340), and by Goldberg (2001, p. 36) as the region that allows the "inner perception" that is the critical prerequisite for con-sciousness. The orbitofrontal cortex, located behind the forehead and just above the eyes, at the front edge of the frontal lobes, is heavily implicated by Schore (1994) in the devel-opment of all higher cognitive functions, in the integration of attachment experiences, and as the neural region most directly affected by attachment processes. He particularly impli-cates the right orbitofrontal cortex.

Schore (2001a, 2001b, 2002) considers attachment experiences to be directly consolidated in the right orbitofrontal cortex. He describes evidence that adverse social experiences during early development result in permanent alterations in neural processes, and
create permanent physiological echoes in the limbic region, and especially the orbital pre-
frontolimbic system (as Schore, 2001b, describes it). This is of particular importance as
we try to make sense of the dysregulated behavior that can be associated with insecure
attachment, and especially disorganized attachment, as Schore describes the most far-
reaching effect of early trauma, neglect, and poor attachment as a neural inability to regulate the intensity of emotion. In keeping with descriptions already provided, this means
that neural connections are primed to expect and quickly respond to stress, resulting in
automatic behaviors that are stress-based and driven by the highly charged sympathetic
nervous system, rather than the calm and slower paced parasympathetic system. Siegel
(1999) mirrors this exact idea, writing that children who experience severe emotional
deprivation during the first three years of their lives, when the right brain is most dominant, are at risk for losses in the structural development of their right hemispheres, especially in the region of the orbitofrontal cortex. The proposal is that right orbitofrontal
development is limited by negative or poor attachment experiences; that the neurology of
the prefrontal cortex is shaped by early experience, and attachment in particular; and, of
great importance, that early experiences become embedded into the neural structure and
protoconsciousness of the orbitofrontal cortex, and hence the internal working model.

BILATERAL INTEGRATION AND ATTACHMENT STYLES

The amygdala, which is a center for processing and responding to anxiety and fear, as well
as the hippocampus, is linked through the cingulate gyrus[8] to the orbitofrontal cortex which
coordinates input from and communication between the limbic system and neurochemical and glandular functions responsible for further activating the brain and body. If
"trained" through long-term potentiation to react to fear without further cognitive processing, the limbic orbitofrontal cortex will not provide the higher level of affect control,
cognitive processing, and executive functioning of which it is capable. Instead, most of
its functions will be controlled by the right brain, rather than bilaterally coordinated and
integrated with the logicolanguage-based left orbitofrontal cortex. Considered the domain
of emotion-based processing, the right hemisphere is also the hemisphere most associated
with negative emotions (Borod & Madigan, 2000; Gainotti, 2000). This is because the
earlier developed right brain seems to be geared for survival, which is why it is physically
larger and more present in processing experience and determining behavior during the first
two to three years of life.[9] The right brain is more globally orienting, assessing tracts of
information simultaneously and processing them non-verbally, based on their emotionally

---

[8] The cingulate gyrus provides a connection between the decision-making capacities of the frontal cortex, the emotional
functions of the amygdala, and, through its extension into the hippocampus (which connects to the hypothalamus through the
fornix), neural centers of physical movement. The cingulate gyrus thus plays an important role in attention and concentration,
emotional excitation, and motivated behavior, and is described by Restak (2000) as a "supervisory system important to consciousness" (p. 70).
[9] Similarly, Siegel (1999) writes that the development of the sympathetic nervous system is dominant during the first year of
life, with the parasympathetic system developing more during the second year.

arousing qualities. The right brain processes information at once and in parallel fashion, with many neural computations occurring at once. This is in contrast to left brain processing, which is more cognitively, logically, and language based, and not only processes more slowly than the right brain but does so in a linear or serial manner, algorithmically.

The emotional experiences of both the right and left brains are mediated through the finely grained, detail conscious response provided by the left brain (Cahill, 2003). Because the left hemisphere plays a critical role in processing and controlling the emotions of the right brain (Gainotti, 2000; Maté, 2000), the risk in unilateral right brain processing is an affective, cognitive, and behavioral response rather than the reflective decision-making process allowed through bilateral (left–right hemisphere) functioning.

Alone, the left hemisphere understands words without emotional context, content, or meaning. Equally, without the logicolanguage processing capacity of the left brain, right brain functioning must be non-verbal and without logical explanation, responding to stimulus without reflection (Siegel, 1999). The left-brained person operating without bilateral integration is likely to be incapable of the theory of mind required for smooth social functioning; the unintegrated right-brained person develops a quick understanding of action and context, but is likely to respond reactively rather than reflectively. These are clear descriptions of avoidant insecure (unintegrated left brain, cognitive) and anxious insecure attachment (unintegrated right brain, emotional) attachment.

ATTACHMENT, ATTUNEMENT, AND NEUROCHEMICAL BONDING

Schore (2001a, 2001b, 2002) describes the attunement of the attachment process, through face-to-face contact between mother and child, as not only reducing anxiety-produced stress and thus regulating neurochemical processes, but also teaching the skills of self-regulation to the child, in effect through right brain-to-right brain non-verbal communication. According to Siegel (1999), the emotional state of one individual is transmitted and communicated to another through face-to-face contact, contributing to the developing child's capacity for theory of mind. The attuned-attached relationship produces calming and affiliative pair-bonding hormones in both parties, such as oxytocin—a neuropeptide unique to mammals—which also appears to alleviate separation distress and other emotional processes, and is associated with positive social interactions, prosocial behavior, and maternal nurturance (Carter et al., 1997; Giovenardi et al., 1997; Insel, 2000; Panksepp et al., 1997).

Whereas oxytocin is implicated in social bonding for females, male social bonding seems to be related to the neuropeptide vasopressin, which is structurally similar to oxytocin. Although oxytocin is estrogen-related (and vasopressin production and effect is facilitated by androgens), the neuropeptide is also produced in males, and Beech and Mitchell (2005) observe that oxytocin may underlie certain aspects of attachment and associated behaviors. Oxytocin in some ways appears to produce behaviors counter to those of the stress (HPA) axis, lowering the effects of sympathetic adrenal tone and stimulating metabolism, relaxation, and behavioral calm, "constituting an antithesis to the fight–flight response" (Uvnäs-Moberg, 1997, p. 158). In fact, Panksepp et al. suggest that any neurochemical factor that serves to reduce separation-distress may promote social attachments by creating a "secure emotional base" in the brain (p. 85).

Vance (1997) notes that is obvious that secure relationships serve as the primary antidote for fearful or painful experiences. He writes that the release of oxytocin in response through emotional and physical contact not only promotes the exclusivity of relationship bonds, but explains why childhood distress and juvenile aggression often abate as a result of *specific* relationships, such as close maternal or other intimate relationships, rather than general social relationships. LeDoux (2002) writes that although neither oxytocin nor vasopressin has been proven to underlie attachment, both the closely connected amygdala and hypothalamus contain receptors for both neuropeptides and it is therefore tempting to think of them forming synaptic circuits crucial for pair-bonding. Conversely, although recognizing that the role of oxytocin in human attachment remains speculative, Insel (2000) writes that *reduced* oxytocin is often found in psychiatric conditions characterized by a lack of attachment, such a schizophrenia and autism.

ATTACHMENT, SELF-REGULATION, AND NARRATIVE COHERENCE

Schore (2001b) describes the development of attachment as an interactive and synchronous regulator that allows for the bioregulation of emotion in each person. Conversely, he writes, negative attachment experiences induce a pruning of neural axons that inhibit bilateral integration between the orbitofrontal cortices, representing the early expression of alexithymia.

Schore (2002) describes the essential task of the first year of human life as the creation of a secure attachment bond. This is developed through emotional communication between the infant and parent, shaped by the interaction of the infant's psychophysiological predispositions and the attachment environment that results from maternal care. When two right brain systems communicate and interact in this manner, the created resonance plays a fundamental role in brain organization and the development of regulatory processes of the central nervous system (Schore, 2001a). During sequences of interaction between an attuned mother and infant, synchronous psychobiological events occur within both, that work to shape the development of the right orbitofrontal cortex and other brain structures in the infant, as well as promoting psychological developments, including metacognition, empathy, and self-regulation.

Van der Kolk (1987) also writes that disruptions in attachment during infancy may lead to lasting neurobiological change, resulting in hyperactivity or underactivity of neural systems. He suggests that lack of attunement between mother and child results in poor self-regulation, and disrupted attachment bonds may cause extremes of under- or over-arousal, resulting in lasting psychobiological changes. Siegel (1999), similarly, proposes that when mutual resonance between the right brains of mother and child are absent during the first three years, underdevelopment of the child's right hemisphere may result. As reflectivity, or metacognition, is probably dependent upon right hemisphere functioning, Siegel suggests that the child is therefore unlikely to adequately develop the capacity to understand self, resulting in the lack of coherency found in the Adult Attachment Interviews of insecurely attached adults.

EMOTIONAL LEARNING AND MEMORY, AND BEHAVIOR: THE CONDITIONING OF THE BRAIN

Siegel (2001) describes memory as the process by which experience is neurally encoded, and which shapes present and future functioning. It is tied to the physical development of the brain and its capacity for different types of memory systems during different developmental stages (see chapter 4), with explicit memory developing sometime during the second year and self-aware (autonoetic) memory sometime after age 3. Prior to this, the infant has only procedural or implicit memory available, due to the lack of the hippocampal development before the first birthday.

No matter how formed or how available to consciousness, memory and emotion are intimately tied together. That is, memory, and particularly conscious memory (memory that is available for conscious recall), is encoded and stored with emotional valence attached, and emotions shade and configure memory, both in storage and in recollection. The greater the emotional arousal during the original memory, the more likely is emotion to shade the memory when recalled. Hence, eye witness accounts are often unreliable because they reflect emotion as much as fact. Here, the amygdala, injecting affect, and the hippocampus, associated with the storage of memory, are linked to one another in, not just the encoding, storage, and recollection of memory, but *how* memories are stored and retrieved with respect to affective meaning. This is of special importance as the amygdala is central to the linking of perceptions of the external world with affect, cognitive decisions, and hormonal bodily functions (Adolphs & Damasio, 2000). Restak (2001) notes that consciousness "takes a back seat" and is uninvolved in fear-generated neural and physical responses played by the preemotional and precognitive fear and stress response system activated by the amygdala. Hence, he writes that as the amygdala encodes our memories for fear, everything we can learn about the amygdala and its connections throughout the brain is relevant to our understanding of stress (Restak, 2000).

In fact, the amygdala plays a crucial role in emotional learning, on an unconscious and conscious level, capable of responding differentially to emotional stimuli that have not entered explicit memory, and may never be available for explicit recall (Morris, Öhman, & Dolan, 1998). Similarly, Gläscher and Adolphs (2003) describe the role of the amygdala in both conscious and unconscious processing of emotional stimuli, and the control of autonomic neural and physiological responses. Adolphs and Damasio (2000) also describe the importance of the amygdala in emotional and social behaviors, and particularly those related to fear and aggression, and write that the amygdala is essential to the retrieval of socially relevant knowledge, and the recognition of accurate social judgments of other individuals on the basis of their facial appearance.

Morris et al. (1998) write that when shown an angry face for less than 40 milliseconds, the right (but not left) amygdala shows a neural response, suggesting that the amygdala can discriminate based upon visual recognition of images that have previously acquired behavioral significance, and that the response is lateralized. That is, *right* amygdala processing suggests a lack of conscious awareness in which emotional visual stimuli presented to the right hemisphere produce autonomic responses, compared to the *left* amygdala which is more closely associated with increased awareness of the stimuli. In their study of brain-damaged patients, Gläscher and Adolphs (2003) found differences between the functioning and role of the left and right amygdala, concluding that the right amygdala is involved in global processing and autonomic responses to stimuli, whereas the left amygdala "decodes" and contributes to a cognitive evaluation of the stimuli that can be used to plan more purposeful and self-aware behavioral responses. Carr, Iacoboni, Dubeau, and Mazziotta (2003) also describe the limbic system as critical for emotional processing and behavior, and its interactions with the neocortex as critical for interpreting and understanding behavior. In their experiments with facial recognition, they also conclude that the left amygdala is associated with an explicit awareness of observed emotional content and the right amygdala with a non-explicit awareness of emotional content. Writing that empathy plays a fundamental social role, allowing experiences, needs, and goals to be shared among individuals, they suggest that an empathic resonance in the right amygdala, induced by observation and actual physical imitation of others, is the basis for a form of empathy grounded in physical experience and processed by the amygdala, which subsequently imbues the experience with emotional affect that is stored in memory.

THE EMOTIONAL BRAIN

Although not necessarily well defined, in which its constituent structures are not always clear or universally agreed upon, the limbic system is often referred to a major emotional center of the brain. Named for the ring or boundary it forms within the deep brain and around the corpus callosum, the limbic system is described by Restak (2000) as the center of emotional experience. Part of the midbrain that includes the thalamus and hypothalamus, the limbic system is conceptualized as the "old mammalian" brain, evolutionarily older than the forebrain.[10] The "deep limbic" system, including the thalamus and hypothalamus, as defined by Amen (1998), is responsible for imbuing perceived events with emotional tone and color, identifying events as important, the storage of emotionally charged memories, emotional motivation, social bonding, and emotional sexual drive: "The emotional shading provide by the deep limbic system is the filter through which you interpret the events of the day. It colors events" (p. 39).

Emotions are described by Damasio (1999) as complex, biologically determined collections of chemical and neural responses, all of which have a regulatory role to play, and all of which can be engaged automatically and without conscious deliberation. Damasio (2003) additionally describes emotions as a natural means for the brain to evaluate and make decisions about the environment. LeDoux (1996) also describes the largely automatic nature of emotions, programmed by evolution to provide non-conscious responses to significant situations. He conceptualizes emotions developing as behavioral and physical specializations that allowed evolutionary survival to our primitive ancestors. Damasio (2003) writes that emotions become *feelings* only when they enter consciousness, and are experienced on that level. Similarly, Ochsner and Schacter (2000) describe emotion as the means by which the significance of stimuli is appraised, resulting in the storage and retrieval of memories whose emotional valence allows immediate and automatic behav-

---

[10] Perry and Marcellus (1997) describe the "bottom-up" structure of the brain, from brainstem, through the midbrain and limbic system, to the outermost and evolutionarily newest cortex. The lower regions represent old brain and most basic life support functions, whereas the evolutionary progression of the brain provides increasingly more complex functions, including those of emotionality, thinking, planning, and self-awareness.

ioral responses. They write that the amygdala is responsible for stamping emotion into memories stored through the hippocampus.

Both the amygdala and hippocampus are capable of learned associations that allow the anticipatory organization of events (Tucker, Derryberry, & Luu, 2000), in part to ensure the regulation of the internal state of the individual so that it can be prepared for the event and a specific reaction (Damasio, 1999). As noted, the amygdala is an essential point of integration between cognitive representations, affective significance, and physical response (Carr et al., 2003; Gainotti, 2000; Gläscher & Adolphs, 2003), and Ochsner and Schacter (2000) write that "emotion . . . influences the nature and distinctiveness of what is encoded and stored and therefore strongly determines what information is potentially available for subsequent recall" (p. 174). Thus, given the automaticity of emotion, related behavioral response, and a brain primed for constant stress, we can recognize how the amygdala–hippocampal complex may anticipate and produce behaviors suited for adverse conditions, rather than the prosocial behaviors produced by a securely attached brain.

Given the description of the processing properties of the left and right hemispheres, it is clear that there is a risk of reactive emotional responses without left brain mediation. In fact, given the bilateral nature of the amygdala itself, Cahill (2003) notes that the right amygdala tends to assess global aspects of the environment, whereas the left amygdala is more finely tuned. In a right brain environment, such as the environment described by Schore, Siegel, and others, limited in development and bilateral integration by attachment failure, we would expect to see disproportionate and unprocessed defensive emotional reactivity to environmental stimuli, and particularly those perceived as threatening or otherwise stressful. Of this Maté (2000) writes, "of all environments, the one that most profoundly shapes the human personality is the invisible one: the emotional atmosphere in which the child lives during the critical early years of brain development" (p. 55). It is this emotional environment, and the "individual units of experiences" of which it comprises, that Hofer and Sullivan (2001) describe as "something like a network of attributes in memory, invested with associated affect" that become neurally integrated into the internal working model that lies at the heart of attachment theory and the treatment of attachment deficits (p. 608).

THE ADOLESCENT BRAIN

Giedd (2002) reports a second wave of neural development somewhere around age 11 or 12, involving the extension of axons and dendrites in the orbitofrontal cortex, thus thickening the prefrontal cortex. Despite the early exuberance of neuron development and synaptic connection, he writes that enormous dynamic activity in brain biology also occurs between ages 3 and 16, and Siegel (2001) notes that the brain remains plastic or open to continuing environmental influences throughout life.

However, as described, researchers at McLean Hospital (2003) assert that stressful events experienced during adolescence can lead to enduring changes in adult brain structure through its effects on synaptophysin protein and/or loss of hippocampal synapses. Hence, we remember that the blade can cut both ways, reshaping the brain in ways that we consider to be positively and prosocially adaptive, or negatively adapted in ways that promote social inadequacy and antisocial behavior.

In describing the psychobiology of adolescence, Spear (2000) describes multiple behavioral, emotional, and social changes during adolescence, as well as physical, cognitive, and neurological development. Stress is experienced differently by adolescents and adults, partly because of the changing nature of the lives of adolescents and the demands and expectations placed upon them. Spear (2003) describes stress accented by a greater emotionality in adolescents compared to adults, including a greater sensitivity to negative emotions and depressed mood. Yurgelun-Todd (2002) reports also that adolescents experience more emotional responses than adults, but have not yet developed the prefrontal capacity to accurately identify or process emotions.

Although refuting the adage that adolescents are hormone driven, Spear (2000) nevertheless suggests that greater sensitivity to stress and related neurochemical, hormonal, and physiological processes contributes to behavioral and mood problems in adolescents. She writes also that adolescents are more susceptible than children or adults to neurological reward systems that drive and reward certain types of risk taking and exploratory behavior. She notes that during adolescence, brain hemispheres begin to develop the capacity to more effectively process information independently of one another, and that synaptic pruning during adolescence cuts back on excitatory and easily aroused neural circuits, leading to a reduction in the amount of excitatory stimulation reaching the cortex. Through pruning, parcellation, and normative neural developmental processes, the prefrontal cortex is reshaped during adolescence, experiencing a reduction in volume although, as Geidd (2002) notes, it thickens in axon and dendritic extensions that lead into and out of the cortex. The amygdala continues to be of great importance during adolescence, more active in frontal lobe processing than in adults (Spear 2000, 2003) and in its processing of emotional and stressful stimuli, suggesting again the greater dependence of the adolescent brain on emotion and emotional recognition than the adult brain. She describes the adolescent brain in transition, differing anatomically and neurochemically from the adult brain.

Spear's description is of the optimally adaptive adolescent. Nevertheless, her description helps us to understand the adolescent brain in terms of its evolutionary and ideal movement into a more complex and dynamic period of neural activity. From this activity, we see the more complete development of both hemispheres, the capacity for bilateral integration, and a calmer and less easily aroused and excited brain, resulting in a well-formed adult brain capable of adult responsibilities, relationships, and behavior. She helps us to understand adolescent behavior as not just willful, but a complex result of social, neural, and hormonal interactions.

THE NEURAL SELF

We recognize that the development of selfhood is embedded into the central nervous system, tied intimately to emotion, cognition, and, in effect, the internal working model. However, although it is possible that the seat of self-awareness may well lie in the right orbitofrontal cortex as Schore and others suggest, it is more likely that consciousness is holistically contained within the entire neural net rather confined to a single region. Although Restak (2000) describes the language-based left hemisphere as "determining" consciousness more so than the right brain, he also notes that no single brain area is responsible for consciousness, which is not an entity but an active process resulting from the interaction between many components of the brain. In either case, we understand the brain as more than just the container of our experiences, a responder to the environment, or the driver behind behavior. We instead visualize the brain, body, and mind as an integrated system in which *internal* experience is the result of *external* experience, mediated by neurobiological processes that arise independently of the environment. Here, attachment and biology connect on a neural level, triggering automatic, and almost autonomic, responses to current stimuli based on prior neurally learned experience that has become burned into and part of the brain through priming, pruning, and parcellation.

In a neurobiological model, the origins of attachment involve attuned and mutual interactions between the mother and infant, in face-to-face, body-to-body, and, Siegel and Schore would say, right brain-to-right brain contact. This stimulates neurochemical and electrical transmissions and impulses within the child's central nervous system. These stimulate or result from hormonal release, the firing of neurons across synaptic terminals, the creation of synaptic connections, the chemical and emotional encoding of memory, and the development of the neural self. In this neural self—the neurobiological embodiment of the self-in-society—we hope to instill a view of self as efficacious and capable and a view of others as responsive and worthy, and to whom we feel connected.

It's the interaction between two brains, or two personalities, that allows one to affect the other in such a manner. Although in many ways this may sound mysterious, and even mystical, it's no more mysterious or mystical than the way in which the brain interacts with the world and internalizes experiences in general. In this case, we are simply describing the way that the brain of an infant interacts with its mother and other beings, and is just another version of the internal (neural)–external (environment) interaction, which re-creates internal events within the brain of the receiver in response to events in the environment.

CONCLUSION: THE CHANGEABLE BRAIN

We do not understand the brain, although our vistas are just beginning to expand. With the reality of more and more sophisticated and relatively easily accessible functional brain scans that can actually view the brain in action, rather than just mapping its structure and topography, we are increasingly able to see how, where, and when different parts of the brain engage in different environmental circumstances. In fact, functional scans allow us to recognize the direct interaction between environmental events and stimuli and the internal neural response. No doubt we will learn much more about how the brain works in the immediate years to come, and why it works the way it does. In the meantime, however, much of our theory about brain development is based upon studies and observations that are unclear or uncertain, and in some cases contradictory. For instance we do not fully understand the differences between left and right brain function, and particularly the difference between the operation and function of structural components that are reproduced in both sides of the brain, or the interrelationship between the left and right brain versions of the same component.

In addition, in many cases, our assumptions about neurobiological processes associated with attachment are based on studies of non-human mammals, including voles and rats, although it is not clear that human biophysical processes work in the same manner, including pair bonding and affiliation. It is also not clear, given the description of the neurobiological attachment process in humans, why it is that every attachment-deprived child is not heavily right brain oriented, or why some insecurely attached children develop left brain capacities over right hemisphere processing. On the face of it, this leads us to conclude that many factors must be at play, other than attachment processes alone. Be warned, then, that just as we find attachment theory less than complete, and we recognize weaknesses and gaps in theories of sexual offending, so too do we find brain theory to be a developing but incomplete science, that rests as much on theory as on fact. Nevertheless, our knowledge of the brain is clearly developing. Although we don't have a complete understanding of how neurochemicals such as serotonin, dopamine, and norepinephrine work, we do know that the same neurotransmitters work differently in different parts of the brain and central nervous system. Similarly, although we do not fully understand how pruning and parcellation work, or when, how, and in what circumstances brain plasticity is most active, we recognize that new neural paths develop later in life, as in elderly stroke victims, for instance, who apparently develop new neural pathways for speech and movement. We also know that the adolescent brain undergoes dynamic neurobiological change, and we know that cognitive capability leaps at more-or-less defined developmental points, and that cognitive, affective, and relational skills can continue to expand with neurological and cognitive development.

Restak (2000) describes the brain changing from moment to moment, "a dynamic rather than a static structure," more like a fluid and dynamic weather map than a static geographical map. "Moreover," he writes, "this dynamism extends over our entire life span. Whether we are one day old or 100 years old, our brains are undergoing dynamic changes all the time. Each daily activity shapes the brain, sculpting it into a different form depending on the nature of that activity" (p. 56). Although we cannot undo previously developed neural processes, through the promise of brain plasticity we have the opportunity to modify existing neural pathways, condition currently developing synaptic connections, and influence the development of yet-to-be-formed neural circuits. This is most likely to occur, not through our words, but through the provision of experiences recognized on a neural level and which the brain colors with emotions and integrates through practice. This is what we mean by brain-based learning, focused on attunement, stress management, nurturing relationships that stimulate the attachment circuits of the brain, and the enhancement of left–right brain integration and processing.

In different people, different parts of the brain "light up" in response to the same stimuli. For example, cues that are known to activate emotional areas of the brain in most people light up language-based areas in the brains of other individuals. As a result, we know that different people have brains that function in different ways. But given the relationship between nature and nurture, it is not clear whether the differences are the *cause* of different ideas, attitudes, and behaviors in different people or the *result* of different experiences. This returns us to a chicken–egg debate. However, we can be certain that ensuring a healthy social environment in which that brain develops, functions, and interacts gives us the best possible chance to produce healthy people. What we have, then, is an understanding of how external experience, including early attachment and ongoing social experience, interacts with the brain to shape neural processes and the manner in which the brain responds to and shapes its environment. By changing that environment, we can hope, in conjunction with the brain's plasticity, to change the way the brain experiences and functions in the world.

CHAPTER 16

Understanding Attachment-informed Treatment

We recognize that the roots of attachment form in infancy and early childhood. This is true whether we accept adolescent and adult attachment as essentially the same in genotype and phenotype as attachment in infancy and childhood, or we subscribe to the idea that attachment passes through stages to change in appearance, function, and purpose (Chapter 5). Similarly, in either case we recognize that attachment is only a factor, and not the whole ball of wax, in shaping character. It is influenced by and influences many other factors that are both endogenous and exogenous to the individual, forming a developmental pathway from childhood to adolescence.

In any case, regardless of the depth and influence of attachment as a central factor, attachment and social relatedness patterns are well formed by late childhood, and the greatest opportunities for developing secure attachment, providing direction, and producing emotionally healthy and secure individuals lie in early childhood. Providing an attachment-based therapy for juvenile sexual offenders, and indeed any older child or adolescent, is like playing catch up. Building secure attachment, avoiding insecure attachment, minimizing risk factors, and ensuring protective relationships and experiences from infancy through mid-childhood is thus preventive. Conversely, attempting to undo the effects of insecure attachment and exposure to risk, and to provide protective factors and experiences that rebuild or re-establish attachment in later life, is interventive, involving rehabilitation and reconstruction. If we accept that the template for attachment and social connection is neural, as well as social and psychological, we also recognize the difficulty lies in undoing the effects of prior experience and building a new experience of attachment and relatedness. This is especially true when we also recognize the nature of sensitive developmental periods in neural, emotional, and personality development, including the development of hard-wired representations of self and others, cognitive schemata and behavioral scripts, brain morphology, and the capacity for metacognition, empathy, and moral conscience.

It is clear that although we can begin to identify many of the factors and specific pathways that affect and influence sexual behavior in children and adolescents, and we can develop ideas of how to prevent problems, it is much more difficult to treat or rehabilitate behavior for which templates have already been formed and stored in schemata, regardless of whether or not we can conceptualize the pathway that led to that behavior. The bad news, then, in playing catch up is that we have much to overcome at a time during which the brain is preparing to take on a more adult form (adolescence).

On the other hand, adolescence is a time when brain morphology is not fully developed by any means and continues to change and take on its adult form, perhaps even more than during earlier periods of development. In addition, it is during adolescence that the brain is able to assume a perspective and engage in cognitive operations that were not formerly possible, and it is during adolescence, in combination with cognitive development and experience, that empathy, moral development, personal identity, and social affiliation begin to coalesce into their adult forms. Prior to adolescence, perspective taking, empathy, morality, and social relatedness are vague and rudimentary, although they clearly provide the foundations for the character, behaviors, attitudes, and social interactions of the adolescent. Nevertheless, although it may be true that the most critical period for the formation of attachment and early security of self is established in early childhood, late childhood and adolescence continues to offer strong opportunities for the acquisition of identity formation, social connectedness, and social skills and values.

If we consider the plasticity of the brain as a critical factor, we also recognize that change, new learning, and synaptic growth continue throughout life. It is certainly easier for a young child to acquire a new language or learn a musical instrument than for an adolescent or adult, but adolescents and adults can nonetheless also learn new languages and learn to play the piano, although different neural processes are most likely at work in older brains, and it may take far more practice and exposure to different and more stimuli and reinforcers. We also recognize, from the work of Emmy Werner and Ruth Smith (1992, 2001), that even past age 21 (and beyond), people can and do continue to change, and especially with the assistance of others who can provide protective resources for them.

It is true that rehabilitation is quite a different process than prevention. At the same time, however, while primarily engaged in the *rehabilitation* of juvenile sexual offenders, we are also engaging in the *prevention* of adult sexual offending. If we understand the path that leads from juvenile sexual offending to adult sexual offending and elements along that path, such as the development of callous unemotionality, hostile masculinity, social alienation, and other social inadequacies and antisocial attitudes, then we are engaging in the prevention of behaviors that, for some juvenile sexual offenders will otherwise later emerge as adult sexual violence against other adults and children.

THE ECOLOGY OF EXPERIENCE: THE INTERACTIONAL ENVIRONMENT

Before discussing the treatment and rehabilitation of attachment deficits, it is important to first understand the context in which both human development, learning, and treatment occur and within which they unfold. In the case of attachment-informed treatment, we are not simply treating attachment as dispositional, or residing within the individual, but as the result of the interaction between the individual and his or her environment.

In fact, we can understand human attitudes, behavior, relationships from the perspective of a human ecological model in which all development reflects transactions and interactions, not just between people and other people within their immediate environment, or between people and the environments in which they live, but between and within differ-ent environmental layers. Such a model recognizes that human experience, interaction, and development are shaped by multiple forces, both distal and proximal, and sometimes by forces acting in the present, sometimes simultaneously with one another, and some-times over extended periods of time. Here, we recognize that external (exogenous) shaping forces shift and change over time, as do the events and actors in that environment, and that internal (endogenous) forces change as well, with the maturation of the central nervous system and the acquisition of learning. In some cases the external forces lose relevance over time due to the developmental maturation of the individual, or they lose their effect *because* of changes in internal shaping forces.

The attachment pathway is woven into an ecological system of human and environ-mental subsystems in which a myriad of interactions occur at multiple points within and across subsystems that shape and affect outcome. Human development thus occurs within a complex and multiply nested, multiply interacting, and mutually transactional environ-ment, in which it is not possible to understand individual behavior without understanding the interactional nature of that environment. In the ecological environment described by Bronfenbrenner (1979) and depicted in Figure 16.1, individuals live within subsystems that are subsumed by and nested within larger subsystems, through which they commu-nicate and interact with other individuals, organized agents of society, and society itself, and in which different parts and systems of the human environment are in constant touch with one another, within and across different nested levels. Without reference to the larger ecological system that surrounds the individual, Bronfenbrenner considers it impossible to fully understand human interaction. This is as true for sexually abusive behavior as for any other behavior, and requires a more complex view of the individual than just a linear view that sees the individual developing and passing through life affected only by his or her immediate social environment.

Elliot, Williams, and Hamburg (1998) describe the ecological–developmental approach as a framework by which human development is recognized as not occurring in isolation, but in social contexts. These contexts are interactive, not just between people, but between and across systems, and they influence and shape behavior and, in turn, are influenced and shaped by individual behavior. Bronfenbrenner considers four concentric and increasingly larger environmental subsystems, beginning with the individual's immediate environment,

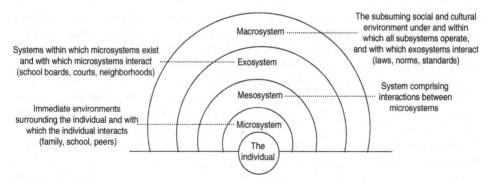

Figure 16.1   Bronfenbrenner's (1979) model of human ecology

to be nested one within the other, as in Russian Dolls, with the individual at the center. Each is a complete environmental system in its own right, but each interacts with and is affected not just by the immediately larger system in which it is nested, but by systems at every level. That is, systems, from the individual at the center to the outermost level of the larger society, interact and transact constantly with one another, with influence operating in parallel, rather than linear, fashion. The ability to understand human development, including the interplay between attachment and behavior, thus requires an understanding of the individual affected by all levels of the ecological system.

The first level involves the individual and other individuals who have a direct or indirect effect on him or her, representing a *microsystem* of interactions and transactions. This might include family and peer relationships, interactions in school, and so on. The individual is also influenced by the *mesosystem*, or the system that exists between two or more microsystems in which the individual is actively affected by the interaction, and this might include transactions between family and school, and the family and social services. In effect, the mesosystem is a system of microsystems. The larger *exosystem* involves environments that do not immediately affect the individual, who is not an active participant at this level, but they nevertheless have a shaping influence on the individual's life at the microsystem level. This includes activities, for instance, of the school board, or the court system, or the corporate headquarters of a television news corporation. The outermost and largest system, the *macrosystem*, refers to the surrounding culture and includes the norms, standards, laws, values, and ideologies that shape the world in which the individual lives and interacts with others at the microsystem level, and the interactions at and between every other subsystem at each level.

Bronfenbrenner's ecological model is dynamic both with respect to individual and system interactions, and changes over time. He describes *ecological transitions* that involve changes in systems, such as school enrollment, graduation, marriage, and parenthood, and also a temporal set of influences called the *chronosystem* that reflects changes and influences on human interactions over time, recognizing that systems do not remain static over the course of human life.

LEARNING AND THERAPY IN THE TRANSACTIONAL ENVIRONMENT

Within this ecological environment, learning is interactional and transactional as well, described by Vygotsky (1978) as transactional experiences in which development not only paves the way for learning to occur, but is actually shaped by the learning that takes place. That is, although learning is sparked by developmental processes, the direction of further development is shaped, in part, by the learning that occurs.

This is as true for learning that occurs during treatment, as for learning that occurs in school or in life. The capacity to learn in treatment is initially very much influenced by factors outside of the treatment environment (described below as extra-therapeutic factors), but the further development of treatment is dependent, in part, upon the learning that occurs as a *result* of the treatment.

Vygotsky conceptualized learning taking place at the individual's actual developmental level and at the cusp of the next developmental leap. This is the point at which the learning tasks of prior developmental levels have been accomplished, and is at the edge of the *zone of proximal development*, defined by developmental processes that are in the process of maturation and learning capacities that are ready to be enacted, although still embryonic. Vygotsky writes that prior learning experiences produce this zone through human interactions and stimulation rather than through learning alone, and new learning occurs in a manner that always stretches a child just beyond his or her current level, but always within the proximal learning zone. For Vygotsky, learning *creates* the zone of proximal development, because it stimulates internal developmental processes that might otherwise lie dormant. Once internalized, learning experiences become part of the child's developmental history and pathway, and thus set the pace for the development of the next proximal learning zone.

Although effective learning is dependent on the developmental process, in turn it creates or limits opportunities for further development. Thus, what and how the child has learned sets the trajectory for future development and learning. Just as we must recognize that multiple interactions occur between environmental systems, and we must intervene at multiple levels to alter trajectories, we must also work to create new opportunities for learning, and new proximal learning zones. Bringing us back to the internal working model, Vygotsky depicts a dynamic that he believes is present throughout the entire span of a human life, in which every aspect of the child's learning appears first on the social level, and then on the psychological level: "first, *between* people (*interpsychological*), and then *inside* the child (*intrapsychological*)" (p. 57). This, of course, returns us, as will always be the case with attachment theory, to the internal working model as the container of past experience, the holder of emotional schemata and cognitive scripts, and the shaper of future behavior.

As we discuss an attachment-informed therapy, we are talking of treatment that aims at accessing and modifying that internal working model, and creating zones of proximal learning, within which the potential for new learning (the "buds" of development, as described by Vygotsky) is immediately ahead. This is the point at which—built on the current (or actual) developmental level—tasks that the child can accomplish today only with assistance, can be accomplished *independently* by the child tomorrow. Treatment must thus be paced, and always on the boundary between the actual and proximal learning zones, never too far ahead or treatment will fail, and always informed by and aware of proximal learning capacity.

ATTACHMENT THERAPY OR ATTACHMENT-INFORMED THERAPY?

As described in Chapter 9, there really is no mainstream "attachment therapy" in the sense of a specific model of therapy or set of therapeutic techniques directly attached to a school of therapy. In fact, there is no such school of treatment, and the closest thing we have is a lens of "attachment theory" that we can apply to clinical populations.

The form of therapy that *is* known as "attachment therapy" (AT) is sometimes disparaged by attachment theoreticians and those who incorporate an attachment framework into their therapeutic work, and is not considered substantially relevant to the work of attachment theory. As described, one of the problems with AT is the view held by its practitioners that virtually all problems of childhood are the products of attachment deficits and can be resolved through the application of prescribed techniques, thus rendering the model incapable of differential diagnosis or treatment. Although some see the therapy as powerful and successful, reaching children and adolescents in ways that other therapies cannot, others shun this form of therapy and go so far as to warn us against its dangers (for instance, Mercer, 2002). In part, this is because AT uses some controversial or unproven techniques, such as holding therapy and corrective attachment therapy, which often involves intrusive, coercive, and boundary-less practices that include tickling, pinching, and pointed and sometimes relentless, sarcastic and demeaning questions and comments.

In fact, Speltz (2002) argues that there is little connection between AT and attachment theory, and links the theoretical roots of AT more to the early work of psychologist Robert Zaslow than to the ideas of John Bowlby. In 1972, Zaslow lost his license to practice psychology due to physical injuries suffered by a patient undergoing "Z-process therapy," the intrusive and physically coercive rage reduction therapy that gave rise to holding therapy. Coercive therapies, such as those associated with attachment therapy techniques, have led to significant physical injury and, in several cases, death. Accordingly, Speltz writes that coercive attachment therapy techniques, and particularly holding therapy, pose potential risks for psychological and physical harm, and have no potential benefits at all, despite dramatic, but short-term changes, in the patients (usually children). Mercer (2001) describes attachment therapy as both unvalidated and unconcerned with the ethics of physical contact during therapy, and recommends legislation that makes techniques of AT, such as holding therapy, unavailable.

However, Kelly (in press) writes that "the field of (AT) continues to grow and evolve," increasingly including interventions based on common principles and theories of attachment and healthy development. She asserts that it is not synonymous with holding therapy, and describes "attachment-focused" therapeutic techniques covering a wide range of clinical interventions with infant–parent dyads, children, and adults. She describes the goals of AT as accessing and modifying experiences that provide the basis for insecure internal working models, writing that "nurturing holding can often provide direct experiential access to these often unconscious, nonverbal memories and beliefs." Nevertheless, despite support for the model, holding therapy, as used today, continues to be a sometimes powerful, but nonetheless invasive and controversial, technique, and is often far from nurturing in application. Similarly, AT continues to apply broad and undifferentiated descriptions to attachment-related difficulties and related treatment, as described in Chapter 9. Consequently, as we describe treatment for attachment difficulties in the remainder of this book, we are not discussing "attachment therapy," but instead an attachment-informed therapy.

Rather than practicing a prescribed attachment therapy based on a specified model or set of techniques, most clinicians recognizing and addressing attachment difficulties use an attachment-informed framework by which psychodynamic and cognitive interventions can be applied with attachment as a target of treatment. A framework (but not a specified model or school) of attachment-informed therapy is most often integrated into broader psychodynamic therapies, and is perhaps simply therapy seen through an attachment lens and guided by an attachment framework. The implications of such an attachment-informed framework are clear, in that unless we are providing an attachment-focused therapy for the parent–child dyad during the earliest stages of the relationship (the first months or first few years), we are talking about a "catch up" model. Here, the role of the therapist is to first assess the nature and quality of attachment in the individual, and then to assess whether the level and quality of attachment is pathological or disordered, in which case the role of the therapist is to bring about change. The approach here is developmentally sensitive and contextual, and assessment and treatment will take a different course with an 8-year-old as opposed to a 30-year-old.

AN ATTACHMENT-INFORMED FRAMEWORK

For the therapist focusing on building attachment, coherence, and a more secure internal working model, interaction and behaviors are understood through an attachment lens. Behaviors are reframed and seen as attachment-seeking rather than attention-seeking, and healthy, non-pathological behaviors are recognized as possible only in light of a sense of security—exploration behaviors are activated only when attachment behaviors are deactivated. Behavioral episodes that otherwise appear irrational are recognized and understood as emotional, and even neurobiological, episodes sparked and fueled by poorly processed and unintegrated perceptions in the patient. The development of a "secure base" injected into the internal working model is paramount.

In an attachment-based model, the infant–mother relationship (or equivalent, involving an alternative primary caregiver) sets the pace for representations of self and others and the foundation for all relationships that follow. Emotional and cognitive schemata that foreshadow and trigger behavior are neurologically hard wired and embedded into a mental map, activated by biologically established drives. Through an attachment-informed framework, we seek causes and explanations for current behavior, at both a psychodynamic and cognitive level, an understanding of the transactions and interactions between the internal mentalized world and the external physical world, and recognize social relationships as the outcome of this interaction, driven by emotional and cognitive processes. In our work with clinical populations, the application of attachment theory thus becomes a psychology of social, emotional, and cognitive deficits. In the treatment setting, as described by Sroufe et al. (1999), attachment theory becomes a theory of psychopathology in which ideas about attachment inform us of the cause and development of functional deficits and help us to define appropriate treatment interventions.

In applying an attachment perspective, we must ask how children experience and internalize representations of their parents, not simply as their parents but as representatives of all adults and authority, and how they come to see themselves reflected through the eyes and behaviors of their parents. How do these children experience attunement and also learn to be attuned to others, learn to be regulated by others and to eventually regulate themselves, and identify with not just family goals and values but eventually with social values and norms as well? In aspiring to social values and norms, such as social belonging, social relatedness, social attractiveness, and sexuality, how do these children experience their ability to actually achieve such goals? Have their particular attachment experiences provided them with the capacity to be patient, tolerate frustration, and feel personally and socially successful, or does socially unacceptable (i.e., socially deviant) behavior represent their best course of action for adhering to social norms and acquiring socially desirable goals, as described by strain and social control theory?

The attachment-informed framework thus provides a lens through which to see, interpret, evaluate, and make sense of human behavior that may otherwise make little sense to us. This is of special importance as we work with sexually reactive children and juvenile sexual offenders whose sexual behaviors are often closely tied in with a range of other antisocial and socially deficient behaviors, and who are often emotionally very troubled, and not infrequently psychiatrically and functionally disturbed. Although we seek simple explanations for their sexually abusive behaviors, there often are no clear or obvious answers and we also recognize that these behaviors and relationships cannot be separated from their other behaviors and relationships, which are often just as, if not more, troubled.

The attachment lens provides a way of seeing things otherwise invisible, or another view of behavior and motivation that, when viewed from another perspective, may look quite different. For instance, understanding callous and unemotional behavior through an attachment lens may reveal an avoidant and dismissive attachment stance that is adaptive and defensive in origin, rather than having antisocial or psychopathic roots. It was described in Chapter 5 that, through the attachment-informed lens, things may look different. Anxiety may reflect a deeply rooted lack of personal competence whose origins lie in the failure to develop a sense of self-efficacy and a resulting need to be taken care of and protected by others; dependence on others and a need for reassurance may indicate failure to develop a sense of self-agency; and impulsive or frustration-driven behaviors may indicate an incapacity for self-regulation. Each of these may be seen as a failure in the early parent–child relationship and the product of attachment deficits. Similarly, callousness and lack of empathy may reflect the failure to experience and thus develop attunement with others and the parallel development of metacognition, and lack of moral development may be associated with a failure to form attachments to the larger society, secondary to lack of secure attachment with parents.

Early lack of accurate, nurturing, or responsive care, in which the child experiences adult caregivers as insensitive, unresponsive, or punishing and abusive, are neurally embedded into synaptic circuits, perhaps resulting in the uncertainty and anxiety that we see as characteristic of the insecurely attached child, serving only to ensure that the growing child continues to experience the world as unresponsive and unsettling. That's because the experiences and expectations of the child are expressed through his or her behavior and interactions with others, thus serving to shape the environment itself and reinforce and repeat the very experiences that led to insecure attachment in the first place. The child's behaviors in the environment stimulate responses from others that reinforce the child's behavior and experience. The rejecting child is rejected by others, the shy child becomes invisible, the needy child is avoided, and the angry child angers others. This is canalization at work, or the self fulfilling cycle in action.

Similarly, the oppositional and defiant behaviors that we experience in many troubled children may actually reflect an incapacity or unwillingness to trust or yield to authority, not because the child is intrinsically defiant, angry, or stubborn but because of uncertainty about adults, the possible outcome of inadequate, neglectful, or abusive parenting, or disruptions, inconsistencies, or instabilities in early attachment relationships. Erratic behaviors that are inexplicable and appear to be out of touch with the current situation, such as intermittent explosive disorder, for instance, or sudden and unexplained mood or behavioral changes, may be the expression of patterns of disorganized attachment or easily triggered neural circuits, primed for and triggered into quick action as a result of repeated early experiences or adaptation to early environmental conditions. We can understand such behaviors as global and rapid right brain emotional responses that lack the cognitive processing component which is the specialty of the left brain, perhaps representing both the morphological and structural development of the brain and a lack of integration between hemispheres. Troubling and troubled behaviors, therefore, including those that are sexually abusive of others, may appear and be understood differently when viewed through an attachment lens.

An attachment-informed framework can offer another view of behavior that may otherwise challenge explanation, and add insight and additional perspectives to what we already know. We are thus capable of recognizing emotional triggers and behavioral patterns that might otherwise remain unrecognized, and define treatment interventions that match an attachment-informed formulation of the case. This framework can provide a roadmap for treatment that recognizes the importance and critical quality of the treatment relationship and the treatment environment in bringing about change in the attachment-troubled patient, helping us to understand and define the relationship between clinician and patient, as well as the actual modes, techniques, and interventions of treatment.

ATTACHMENT-ACTIVATED BEHAVIORAL DISTURBANCE

Beverly James (1994) describes ways in which attachment deficits create problem, and sometimes inexplicable, behavior in the insecure child. In some cases, she describes children seeking out and engaging in antisocial and dangerous situations or responding to positive or neutral events with provocative, destructive behavior. She asserts that in the insecurely attached child, these behaviors provide relief from escalating anxiety because the child has no viable attachment relationship to which he or she can turn for assurance, protection, relief, or regulation. In particular, she describes an *alarm/numbing response* process which, she proposes, explains many of the puzzling behaviors seen in children with attachment disturbances. She suggests that this process is triggered by perceived stress, and helps children with few internal resources to cope with otherwise intolerable anxiety.

The *alarm* response is triggered by feelings of helplessness, easily stimulated by environmental cues identified with prior traumatizing events. These include external events, as well as associations that a child may have formed between current feelings and past experiences. James's description is reminiscent of the neural kindling and priming process described in Chapters 5 and 15, again tying attachment experiences and responses to their neural counterparts. James writes that the *numbing* response follows alarm as the child attempts to interrupt escalating alarm through a process of emotional numbing, "in the only way available to those who cannot modulate affect arousal" (p. 19). For those who are unable to numb themselves to their feelings, James argues that *provocative* behavior follows, in which children who are unable to experience relief through numbing, engage in escalating behavior in order to increase their internal alarm process, specifically to activate the numbing response to the point where they are able to "thus gain relief from their unbearable anxiety" (p. 20). From a neural perspective, the brain is flooded with stress response neurochemicals until a level of saturation is reached and the stress system is deactivated, resulting in a parasympathetic relaxed state.

In keeping with a model in which metacognition is limited, as well as poor internalization of security and other resources related to the attachment process, James describes the alexithymic child experiencing an internal alarm, but unable to recognize or understand why the alarm is sounding. She describes a subsequent physiological, and resulting behavioral, reaction that responds directly to the alarm. Here, James is describing a right-brained response without benefit of a left brain cognitive process. Neurally, the sympathetic nervous system has been activated, and the child must rely on physiological changes, rather than cognitively or consciously initiated processes, to activate the parasympathetic nervous system.

Although theoretical, James's model is nonetheless very useful in both visualizing the internal events that may lead to troubled behavior (and perhaps especially in children with disorganized forms of attachment) and in recognizing that the behaviors may actually serve a purpose for the child in ameliorating the anxiety that gives rise to the behavior. In addition, James provides us with a way to understand that the solution to behaviors like these lie in providing a treatment that is informed by attachment theory. It is thus focused on the development of security in attachment figures, security in self, and modes of self-expression and self-regulation that can provide the child with other sources for emotional and behavioral control, and a return to a state of emotional comfort.

However, in order to produce change through treatment, she writes that five conditions must be present: safety, protective environment, therapeutic parenting,[1] attachment-informed clinical skills, and a therapeutic relationship. In any circumstances, James notes that children who have learned not to trust adults and are insecurely attached, and especially those who are avoidant, may not show signs of a bonded therapeutic relationship for many months.

ATTACHMENT-INFORMED TREATMENT

In terms of treatment, attachment-informed therapy does not stand out as a "model." For the most part, it represents a set of ideas and practices, offering a lens through which client difficulties may be seen and a framework and perspective that individual clinicians may bring to bear in their practices. This fits in well with a model of eclectic or integrated therapy in which the clinician is able to easily and freely switch gears in terms of both technique and even perceptual frameworks, as required by a pantheoretical model of treatment. A main emphasis of attachment-informed therapy is to understand insecure attachment and obstructions to secure attachment, and assess whether any of these obstacles can be removed, perhaps through individual, family, or group therapy, or even through medication. A second emphasis is to revive and re-engage social behavior that may have become detached. A third is to help the individual to reorganize attachment systems, and a fourth is to eliminate ambiguity and incoherence from attachment narratives, or the expression of internal working models. Another is, of course, to improve self-esteem, as we discuss the development of the secure personality, through increased self-agency and self-efficacy.

---

[1] Therapeutic parenting can be provided by staff in residential treatment programs, and implies the provision of an emotionally safe and responsive environment, consistent and supportive relationships, and caring, structured, and tolerant guidance.

Not surprisingly, as attachment theory is essentially a psychodynamic and interactional model, the therapeutic relationship comes squarely back into the foreground in attachment-informed therapy. Although cognitive-behavioral work is important in sex-offender-specific issues, and will remain central to any sex-offender-specific treatment program, rather than teaching or discussing concepts of attachment in a cognitive-behavioral or psychoeducational mode, the therapist uses interactional techniques imparted through the therapeutic alliance. It is through this relationship, as well as other techniques and practices of treatment, that a treatment environment and a relationship are established that can help to rebuild attachment and develop the sort of coherence and right–left brain integration thought to be reflective of a secure internal working model. Ultimately, the emphasis in an attachment-informed therapy is on the development of an understanding, supportive, and caring relationship, marked by attunement between the therapist and the patient.

Although cognitive distortions play a significant role, not only in the onset of sexual abuse but perhaps even more so in the continuation and maintenance of sexually abusive behavior, they are not a central target in attachment-informed treatment. Hudson and Ward (2000) suggest, for instance, that sexual offending might occur impulsively, whereas cognitive distortions and the suppression of empathy may follow, sustaining the ability to re-offend rather than serving as a cause of sexual abuse. On one level in treatment, we *must* target cognitive distortions in order to prevent further abuse. But on another level, it is insecure attachment and attachment deficits that are central to treatment, the wellspring, one may argue, from which cognitive distortions develop in the first place.

Consequently, in an attachment-informed therapy, rather than technique or content (as in cognitive-behavioral therapy or dialectical behavior therapy, for instance), the relationship between the clinician and the patient is primary, as is the treatment environment in which the relationship develops and treatment unfolds. For the therapist focusing on building attachment, a more secure internal working model, and narrative coherence and a stable sense of self,[2] interactions and behaviors are viewed and understood through an attachment lens. Healthy and non-pathological behaviors are recognized as possible only when the client feels secure. Hence, the exploration behaviors we wish to stimulate in our clients are activated only when attachment behaviors and their neurological counterparts, sparked by insecurity, anxiety, and fear, are deactivated. Behavioral episodes that otherwise appear irrational are recognized and understood as emotional, and even neurobiological, episodes fueled by poorly processed and unintegrated perceptions in the patient. Seen through this attachment lens, the development of a "secure base" introjected into the internal working model of the juvenile sexual offender is paramount. Simply put, built on an attachment framework, in our clients the goals of treatment include developing:

- A sense of experienced security (secure base) from which to explore and grow.
- Confidence (security) in and connection to important figures who are accurately and consistently responsive, and thus trustworthy.
- A secure and coherent sense of self, including the experience of self-agency and self-efficacy.
- A balance in the use of affective and cognitive problem-solving strategies.

---

[2] In Tulving's terms, autonoetic awareness; see Chapter 4.

- The use of cooperative and non-coercive strategies to get needs met in social interactions with others.
- The capacity for perspective taking and the unlocking of empathy for others.
- The capacity to tolerate and regulate frustration and disappointment.
- A higher level of moral understanding, reasoning, and decision making.
- The experience of connection and relatedness to other people.

This brief list will not be new to anyone who provides a form of holistic, integrated treatment to troubled young people, built on treating the juvenile as a "whole" person rather than as a "sexual offender." The difference may simply be in the application of a framework that recognizes many of these features as attachment-dependent, based upon earlier experiences that have limited the capacity of the youth to engage in healthy and satisfying social relationships.

This framework, coupled with an understanding of the neurobiology of attachment, allows the practitioner to recognize and understand behavioral, social, and even sexual difficulties as the sequelae, at least in part, of earlier attachment experiences. The goal of this treatment, in the final analysis, cannot be the re-establishment of early childhood attachment experiences with a primary caregiver, as that opportunity has passed. Although through family therapy and other forms of family work, we can restore, reinvigorate, and restructure family relationships, we can never travel back through time to the days when attachment first developed and the internal working model first began to form. The goal, instead, is the rehabilitation (and, if you like, the recalibration) of the *current* internal working model, providing for the juvenile the capacity for self-regulation and a sense of self-efficacy and security that will serve as the basis for all current and future experiences of self and others, and hence current and future relationships and behaviors.

This requires an understanding, definition, and application of the concept of attachment that makes it relevant to adolescents, rather than simply applying ideas about attachment in infancy or early childhood, or even the attachment needs of adults. Through an attachment perspective, we recognize that in treatment:

- There is a need for empathic attunement to the client.
- The client must see his or her value in the minds of other people.
- The client must experience important others as capable and competent.
- Seemingly irrational behaviors can be understood as variants of insecure or disorganized attachment strategies, triggered under specific conditions.
- Change requires giving up prior adaptive strategies.
- Change comes slowly.
- Healthy, or secure, attachment requires a secure base.
- The development of a secure base results from life experience.
- The brain is plastic, and neural pathways can develop with new experience and practice.

SECURITY IN TREATMENT

In fact, discussing attachment-informed treatment without discussing secure personality is like asking what is the sound of one hand clapping, particularly as attachment is conceptualized and measured in terms of security (and insecurity). In this respect attachment and the experience of security are virtually synonymous, and as we work to renew and rebuild attachment, we recognize increased attachment through increased security in relationships and in self. If the individual is generally not secure in relationships then it's likely that he or she is insecure in general. Similarly, insecure individuals are likely to experience insecure relationships. In order to produce security in the individual, then, we have to be able to produce emotionally secure, attuned, and responsive environments. This is, after all, the very medium through which the child's sense of security is built in the first place.

Particularly because we are playing catch up in our attachment work with juvenile sexual offenders, we must recognize that security in attachment and self, although eventually residing within the individual, is the result of the interaction between the individual and the environment. If security of attachment does not already reside within our clients, and we cannot simply instill secure attachment within the individual, then we *must* ensure an emotionally secure treatment environment if we are to produce emotionally secure individuals.

The next chapter describes the treatment environment within which attachment-informed treatment takes places, and the attachment-informed treatment relationships that target and facilitate changes in attachment status and experience.

CHAPTER 17

The Attachment-informed Treatment Environment

Attachment-informed treatment does not occur in a vacuum, and one can describe key principles that underlie such treatment. Of special note, however, in discussing an attachment-informed model of treatment for juvenile sexual offenders, we are *not* discussing a new model of treatment. In fact, as described, there is no "model" of attachment-based therapy.

Instead, in reviewing and considering factors that underlie and are common to effective treatment we see an approach that fits exactly with attachment-oriented clinical work. The elements in an attachment-informed approach to treatment are those already found in integrated treatment programs that treat the adolescent as a "whole" child, rather than simply as a juvenile sexual offender (for instance, see Longo, 2002; Rich, 2003), and an attachment-informed model provides nothing new in this regard. It is an *ideational* shift that an attachment-informed perspective adds to our treatment, in how we understand the personal development and behavior of sexually reactive children and juvenile sexual offenders, and how we envision our treatment relationships, treatment interventions, and the treatment environment. It is an approach, perspective, and understanding that makes an attachment-informed therapy useful, and not a technique or particular model.

On this note, Slade (1999) writes that she is not making a case for a specific *type* of therapy, and specifically an "attachment therapy." Instead, she points out that an understanding of the nature and dynamics of attachment informs and offers therapists a broad view of human functioning that has the potential to change the way they think about and respond to their clients, as well as how they understand the dynamics of the therapeutic relationship. Brisch (1999) writes, also, that training clinicians in attachment theory will expose them to entirely new ways of thinking.

COMMON TREATMENT FACTORS IN THE THERAPEUTIC PROCESS

Norcross (2000) has written that the clinician–client relationship accounts as much for treatment outcome as particular treatment techniques, and Lambert (1992) and associates (Asay & Lambert, 1999; Lambert & Bergin, 1993) have written that *most* of what happens in successful treatment is unrelated to treatment model or technique, related instead to factors that are common to all therapy. According to Lambert (1992), of the four elements most commonly associated with treatment efficacy, model and technique account for only 15% of the variance in treatment outcome, with most treatment success resulting from client factors (40%), therapeutic alliance (30%), and the self-healing placebo effects of expectancy and hope (15%).

In describing therapies that cut across and integrate therapeutic forms, Holmes and Bateman (2002) have written that "common factors such as the therapeutic relationship, the creation of hope, explanations, a pathway to recovery, and opportunities for emotional release remain important explanatory variables for the similar outcomes of different therapies in the same conditions" (p. 8). The essential elements in these common factors, accounting for 85% of treatment outcome (Lambert, 1992), are the highly interpersonal factors introduced by the therapist and the client together, embodied in the therapeutic alliance that forms between them and in which the work of treatment is accomplished. The four factors identified by Lambert, which he believes are common to all forms of effective treatment, illustrate the power of the therapeutic environment, especially pertinent to any discussion of attachment-informed therapy.

1. *Extra-therapeutic client factors* are those factors not related to the therapy itself that the client brings to the therapeutic relationship. Lambert and colleagues (Asay & Lambert, 1999; Lambert, 1992; Lambert & Bergin, 1993) report that 40% of therapeutic success is related to extra-therapeutic factors. Writing that it is the client who makes treatment effective, rather than the therapist or technique, Tallman and Bohart (1999) describe the capacity of the client as the "engine that makes therapy work" (p. 91). Particularly relevant to the role of the clinician in attachment-informed treatment, Keijsers, Schaap, and Hoogduin (2000) write that this includes the client's perception of the therapist as self-confident, skillful, and active.

2. *The therapeutic alliance* accounts for 30% of the variance in treatment outcome (Lambert, 1992), regardless of treatment orientation. This idea is supported by many in the field, including cognitive-behavioral therapists, who believe that the client–clinician relationship is a critical factor in any form of therapy.[1] Again, of special importance in attachment-oriented therapy, this includes items such as caring, warmth, acceptance, affirmation, empathy, encouragement, positive regard, and authenticity. In addition, Lambert and Bergin (1993) describe reassurance, structure, advice, cognitive learning and cognitive mastery, changing expectations for personal effectiveness, modeling and success experience as important factors in the therapeutic alliance.

3. *Expectancy and hope.* Lambert (1992) asserts that the client's belief in therapy and expectation that he or she can and will change, accounts for 15% of treatment results.

4. *Therapeutic model and technique* is responsible for only 12% to 15% of the variance across therapies according to Norcross (2000), and Lambert (1992) estimates that only 15% of treatment outcome is the result of technique. Similarly, Kazdin and Bass (1989) have written that techniques either do not play a powerful role or, if they do, research methods are not powerful enough to detect them.

---

[1] For instance, Bachelor and Horvath, (1999), A. T. Beck (1979), J. S. Beck (1995), Dryden (1989), Hubble, Duncan, and Miller (1999), Maione and Chenail (1999), Meichenbaum (1985), and Thase and Beck (1993).

Thus, factors related to the client and therapist engaged in the treatment relationship are not only represented as the operating variables common to all effective treatment, but also more important than specific ideas and techniques of treatment associated with a particular therapeutic type (i.e., cognitive-behavioral or psychodynamic therapy). This idea is especially important as we consider the centrality and role played by the therapeutic relationship in attachment-oriented treatment. Further, the interrelationship of and interaction between factors 1, 2, and 3, independent of technique (factor 4), is further strengthened when we consider the role and impact of a successful therapeutic alliance on clients and what they subsequently bring into therapy over time, as well as their increasing sense of expectation, hope, and personal satisfaction and success.

Hence, although the roots of attachment theory lie in psychoanalysis, and particularly object relations theory, the elements that are critical to an attachment-informed therapy result from common factors that underlie good therapy, regardless of whether it is psychodynamic or cognitive-behavioral. In studies designed to identify the relationship of treatment elements to treatment outcome, effective therapists used both psychodynamic and cognitive-behavioral elements in their treatment (Ablon & Jones, 1998; Castonguay, Goldfried, Wiser, Raue, & Hayes, 1996; Kerr, Goldfried, Hayes, Castonguay, & Goldsamt, 1992). It is the elements common to *both* forms of treatment that are most probably responsible for efficacy in treatment, rather than technique or ideology.

THE ATTACHMENT-INFORMED THERAPIST

Slade (1999) writes that an attachment-informed approach informs, rather than defines, clinical thinking, providing a way for the clinician to think about early patterns of emotional regulation and behavior, helping them to better understand the developmental experience and behaviors of their clients. She writes that attending to the manner in which attachment themes and organization are consciously and unconsciously expressed, changes how therapists observe their clients and make sense of their cases, recognizing that the ability of the client to work with his or her therapist is profoundly shaped by the client's level of attachment security.

In a similar vein, Marrone (1998) writes that attachment-informed therapists engage in treatment in much the same way as other psychotherapists, but the incorporation of attachment theory into their framework is likely to influence their therapeutic technique and style. He describes the attachment-oriented therapist as being able to recognize the client as a whole person with both pathological and healthy attributes, and through the therapeutic relationship allowing the client to freely explore and develop a sense of autonomy and personal values. In order to accomplish these tasks, a central task for the therapist is to become a source of security for the client, or a secure base (Bowlby, 1988; Brisch, 1999), demanding "great sensitivity and empathy as the therapist adjusts to or feels his way into the patient's . . . attachment needs" (Brisch, 1999, p. 78). This aspect of therapeutic empathy is central to the therapeutic relationship, described by Rogers (1980) as essential to the facilitative treatment environment through which individuals are able to recognize and modify their attitudes, behaviors, and self-concepts. For this personal development to occur in the treatment environment, however, Rogers describes the requirement of three necessary elements.

The first attribute of the facilitative climate involves the authenticity of the clinician, or "congruence." The therapist is genuine, transparent, and honest in the therapeutic relationship, "putting up no professional front or personal façade . . . (in which) the client can see right through what the therapist *is* in the relationship" (Rogers, 1980, p. 115). In other words, the client experiences the therapist as real and present, engaged in the therapeutic relationship. Rogers' second condition for facilitative growth involves creating in the client a sense of feeling accepted, cared for, and prized—a condition termed "unconditional positive regard." In attachment terms, this means that the client feels seen and recognized, and by the therapist in particular, who in this scenario is the attachment figure, or caregiver. The effect of these first two conditions is the creation of attunement, central to the early attachment experience, and equally central to the role of therapy in attachment-informed treatment. The therapist is recognized and experienced by the client as present and honest, who in turn experiences a sense of being recognized, understood, and valued by the therapist. The third facilitative aspect of the therapeutic relationship, and central to the idea of attunement, is empathic understanding, in which "the therapist senses accurately the feelings and personal meanings that the client is experiencing and communicates this understanding to the client" (p. 116).

Rogers (1980) describes empathy in therapy as the ability of the therapist to enter the perceptual world of the client, understanding and demonstrating sensitivity to the phenomenological experiences and meanings of the client. He describes the ideal therapist as, "first of all, empathic" (p. 146), in which empathic understanding is provided freely, and not drawn from, the therapist. Rogers writes that empathy is correlated with self-exploration and personal development, in which empathy experienced early in the relationship predicts later success. Of great importance, Rogers warns that brilliance and diagnostic perspectives are unrelated to empathy, and that "clients are better judges of the degree of empathy than are therapists" (p. 149).

THE ROLE OF THE THERAPIST

Bowlby (1980) points out that unless a therapist can enable the client to feel secure, therapy cannot begin, a point echoed by Marrone (1998) who describes sensitivity and responsiveness in the clinician as an essential condition for viable therapy. Bowlby writes that the therapist's role is "analogous to that of a mother who provides her child with a secure base from which to explore the world. The therapist strives to be reliable, attentive, and sympathetically responsive to his patient's explorations and, so far as he can, to see and feel the world through his patient's eyes, namely to be empathic" (1980, p. 140). The therapist's job, according to Bowlby, is to provide the conditions under which self-healing can best take place, thus creating the facilitative treatment environment described by Rogers in his work. Holmes (2001) suggests that the overall goals of attachment-informed therapy are those of *intimacy* and *autonomy*, and that in psychotherapy the capacity for intimacy arises out of attunement between therapist and client. Autonomy, on the other hand, develops from the client's ability to express and overcome dissatisfaction and, where difficulty is inevitable, learn how to experience and tolerate sorrow and express grief.

Allan Schore (1994) adds a neurobiological perspective to the role and tasks of therapy, in which he proposes that models of psychological change must incorporate the idea that brain structure is shaped and reshaped by emotional experience, including the emotional experience of therapy. To this end, he describes the importance of, in effect, brain-to-brain communication between the clinician and client. This idea is of great pertinence to an attachment perspective given Stern and Siegel's assertion that it is through a similar process that infant–mother attachment occurs, and by which early developing brain structures are influenced by the attachment process. Schore describes the requirement that the therapist become attuned to the patient, in resonance with the "crescendos and decrescendos of the patient's affective state" (p. 449), providing a mirroring and reflective function for the client. Writing that for many clients the therapeutic relationship creates, for the first time, an optimal environment for the development of neural structures that can efficiently regulate affect, Schore describes the ability of the clinician to become psychobiologically attuned to the patient's unconscious state as important to the therapeutic process.

Diana Fosha (2003) describes this, perhaps more simply, with respect to the clinician's ability to access and engage in an unspoken emotional connection with the client, in which "therapeutic discourse (is) conducted in a language that the right hemisphere speaks" (p. 229).

THE THERAPEUTIC RELATIONSHIP

In fact, regardless of theoretical focus or technique, all forms of therapy take place within the context of the therapeutic relationship (Castonguay et al., 1996), described by Dryden (1989) in terms of the emotional *bonds* of the relationship itself, shared *goals* which define the reasons for the relationship, and *tasks* which clarify the boundaries of the relationship and define the roles of both client and therapist. First conceived by Edward Bordin (1976), the integration of these three constituent elements (relationship bond, working goals, and defining tasks) result in a working alliance between therapist and client, which together define the strength of the therapeutic relationship.

Parish and Eagle (2003) write that a therapeutic relationship clearly has many qualities of an attachment relationship. In their study of 105 adults engaged in treatment, Parish and Eagle found that therapy clients admired and sought proximity to their therapists, found their therapists to be emotionally available, evoked mental representations of their therapists in the therapist's absence, and experienced their therapists as a secure base that helped them to feel confident outside of therapy. Clients formed strong emotional connections towards their therapists and regarded them as unique and irreplaceable. An additional similarity between an attachment relationship and a therapeutic relationship is the asymmetrical nature of the relationship (see Chapter 5), in which the therapist is not likely to experience the same sort of bond as the client, nor have the same needs. Further, Amini et al. (1996) write that therapy works *because* it is an attachment relationship "capable of regulating neurophysiology and altering underlying neural structure" (p. 232).

Mallinckrodt, Gantt, and Coble (1995) consider attachment theory as a useful way to understand the process of psychotherapy. They write that the therapist gains access to the client's internal working model when the client demonstrates attachment patterns in the therapeutic relationship, thus illuminating and making visible working models which may then become conscious and subject to change. Amini et al. (1996) thus propose that the therapeutic relationship works as a "directed attachment relationship whose purpose is the revision of the implicit emotional memory of (earlier) attachment" (p. 213).

Drawn from the work of Brisch, Holmes, Bowlby, Marrone, Schore, and others we can identify 14 aspects of the therapeutic relationship, specifically from the perspective of the therapist's role in the relationship.

1. The therapist is experienced by the client as a dependable, consistent, and responsive emotional support who is reliably available.
2. The therapist facilitates a therapeutic relationship in which the client can develop security in the therapeutic relationship, form a bond with the therapist, and freely engage in self-expression.
3. The therapist encourages both self-dependency and help-seeking in the client.
4. The therapist provides a secure base through which the client can experience a sense of being recognized and connected, and from which the client may safely engage in psychological exploration, recognizing, expressing, and working through problems.
5. The therapist uses attachment-related interactions in the therapeutic relationship as a means to understand the client and the client's attachment patterns and strategies, using these to shape and guide treatment interventions most appropriate for each client.
6. The therapist becomes attuned to the client's emotional and attachment-related states, remaining aware of the need for emotional connection, described by Fosha (2003) as "bottom–up processing" from an experiential perspective rather than "the top–down approach of most cognitive and insight-oriented therapies" (p. 229).
7. The therapist helps the client to recognize and explore attachment relationships and strategies for maintaining connections.
8. The therapist helps the client to recognize that current relationships, experiences, values, ideas, and attitudes are related to, and in many cases the result of, prior experiences, including early and ongoing attachment relationships.
9. The therapist challenges and stretches the client, remaining in the proximal learning zone but creating opportunities for new learning.
10. The therapist creates and recognizes boundaries, and maintains an appropriate level of closeness that fits the needs and capacities, and the particular attachment style and needs, of each individual client.
11. The therapist remains aware of counter-transference issues, or those feelings that arise in the therapist as a result of the therapeutic relationship, using these to better understand the client and the therapeutic relationship, guide treatment interventions, and maintain appropriate treatment boundaries.
12. The therapist maintains freedom of movement in the relationship, maintaining permeable boundaries, but able to move in and out of engagement with the client as needed.
13. The therapist helps the client develop the capacity to experience and tolerate difficulty, uncertainty, and doubt.
14. The therapist sensitively dissolves the therapeutic bond when appropriate, so that it will serve as a model for handling separations in life.

Although writing about work with traumatized clients, Allen's (1995) description of the barriers to an effective therapeutic relationship is also pertinent to attachment work. He writes that the therapist must overcome three obstacles to the therapeutic relationship: (i) distrust of authority figures, (ii) dependency, which is especially difficult because, as he points out, psychotherapy requires a degree of dependency, and (iii) boundary difficulties, essential in any circumstances but especially so in working with those who have had traumatic or otherwise difficult relationships with parents and other caregivers.

It is in the therapeutic relationship that these obstacles are faced and must be overcome, and it is through the special relationship embodied in the therapeutic alliance and the safe boundaries within relationship that client growth is sparked and enhanced. Allen (1995, p. 242) writes that in psychotherapy,

> touch itself is problematic. Psychotherapy is a *verbal* process. The comfort comes from being heard and understood . . . Physical comforting is highly desirable, but it should come from *other* relationships. The therapy process can help build the needed trust to make that possible.

TREATMENT STRUCTURE

Day and Sparacio (1989) frame the therapeutic alliance within a therapeutic structure that provides safety and protection for both client and clinician. Structure provides order and consistency to the therapeutic relationship and process, defines roles, and communicates expectations for both clinician and juvenile.

Similarly, James (1994) describes the protective environment as one in which the client feels emotionally safe enough to explore difficult or frightening issues. She writes that, in this environment, a therapeutic alliance is achieved only when the purpose, structure, and methods of treatment are understandable, consistent, and predictable. Whether in the therapeutic relationship that exists between clinician and client, or within the larger treatment environment, the capacity of the client to rely on the therapeutic process is enhanced when treatment staff demonstrate a professional demeanor that embodies confidence in the client, an expectation of success, and empathic warmth, and in which roles are clarified, structure and rules are discussed and understood, and the treatment process is explained, including what the client can expect and what is expected from the client.

Modifying Day, Sparacio, James, and Dryden (who describe structural aspects of the therapeutic relationship), and always recognizing that structure cannot substitute for clinician competence, effective therapeutic structure is:

- Flexible and open to modification.
- Guided by a rationale that can be explained, without unnecessary or purposeless rules.
- Clear in rules and expectations for staff and clients.
- Neither overstructured, rigid, nor punitive.
- Shaped by client need for structure.
- Sensitive to client needs, readiness, tolerance level, and resistance.
- Empathic with and valuing of the client.
- Supportive of and confident in client capacity for change.
- Provided by treatment staff who maintain a professional demeanor.

THE TREATMENT MILIEU

In the alarm/numbing process described by James (1994), the child has not internalized the image of a safe attachment figure, and thus has few internal resources to deal with or accurately recognize and assess situations, or form appropriate and successful solutions to problems. In a neurobiological model, this is a right-brained response. The role of the therapist in this case is to build, or begin to build, a treatment environment which eventually will give rise to the development of both secure attachment and personal security in the client. Between the therapist and the client, this environment is embodied in the therapeutic relationship. For the child at home, the family is the backdrop to treatment and for this reason it is likely that family treatment will be required as well, ideally with an attachment-oriented approach. However, for the child in foster care or residential treatment, the living environment becomes an active part of treatment, and not just a backdrop. In residential care, in particular, this active living environment becomes the treatment milieu, not just the context in which treatment occurs but an active aspect and critical element of treatment in which, in addition to the relationship between therapist and client, attachment will develop and flourish or, in the wrong treatment circumstances, will fail to develop.

In fact, James (1994) describes individual therapy as inadequate in the treatment of attachment deficits, because such treatment cannot be limited to only one or several hours each week. Instead, attachment treatment "must pervade the child's total environment because the child's disturbed behavior, emotional distress, and fear that adults will not protect and care for (the child) may not emerge during weekly therapy sessions" (p. 59). James writes that it is within the treatment milieu (whether in the home, foster care, or residential treatment) that "therapeutic parenting" occurs in which the focus of attention is on the child, provided by caring, responsive, and attuned adults who are not only able to recognize and understand underlying attachment issues that drive behaviors, but are also able to respond appropriately. It is within the attachment-informed treatment environment as a whole, and not individual therapy, that opportunities for success and responsibility taking are provided, wrapped up in an environment that is structured and supportive, and in which attunement and understanding are central. This represents a treatment environment in which clients are recognized, opportunities for success and the development of self-efficacy are available, and the client has the capacity to accept and demonstrate responsibility and thus develop a sense of self-agency.

Applying Bronfenrenner's model of the human ecological environment (Chapter 15) to the treatment milieu, and the network of relationships, transactions, and interactions that occur between individuals and systems within that environment, allows a means to analyze the operations, communication, and efficacy of the treatment system. It also offers a way for us to understand how clients are affected by the entire treatment environment and how treatment as a *whole*, and not just treatment in the relationship between client and therapist, affects the quality of the client's experience in treatment and the effectiveness of that treatment. That is, in an attachment-based model, the quality of the treatment milieu as attachment-sensitive and supportive is critical, and an attachment perspective must, as James points out, be pervasive throughout the treatment environment.

Children and adolescents in residential treatment, in particular, are exposed to and live within this treatment milieu. It is imperative, then, if an attachment-based model of treatment is to be effective, that all staff, and at every level of treatment, understand, sub-scribe to, and enact an attachment-oriented approach. Although security in attachment resides, at some level, within the individual, embedded in the internal working model, attachment is nevertheless experienced, enacted and developed in the social environment or, in this case, the treatment milieu. Here, the capacity for attachment is dispositional, not in the juvenile, but in the interaction between the child and the people in the envi-ronment. In attachment problems at the level of the therapeutic milieu, rather than the ther-apeutic relationship, we must look for problems in the structure, communication, and teamwork of the treatment team that plans and carries out the treatment, and the ability of team members to enact an attachment-based model.

THE FIRST LINE OF TREATMENT: INTERACTIONS IN THE TREATMENT ENVIRONMENT

The treatment environment results from the interactions that occur between individuals involved in the treatment process, both clients and staff, and includes words, relationships, emotions, and, of course, behaviors. For treatment to be successful, such a climate must foster and support its goals and methods, and indeed in residential treatment the treatment environment is *part* of the treatment method, and may be referred to as a "facilitative climate." Before words and before conscious awareness, the environment, its structures, its relationships, and its interactions are first experienced through physical perception rather than cognitive/psychological language-based interpretation. The treatment environ-ment is the first line of treatment, and must be recognized as such.

In the treatment environment, although clients must be held responsible for their own behavioral choices, we must remember that behavioral difficulties are often the result of poorly regulated interactions with others. Sometimes, this involves their interactions with staff. In such cases, although behaviors are generated by the client, the behaviors origi-nate in an interaction with another person. Here, we recognize again that the capacity to develop and experience attachment lies not only within the individual, but also in the inter-actions between the child and the people in the environment. It is important, then, in pro-viding supervision, containment, and structure for juvenile sexual offenders, that staff realize that client behaviors are sometimes the result of an actual or perceived interaction with another person, *including staff*. If staff fail to recognize this, in their attempts to work with a client having a difficult time, they may themselves actually escalate a situation, resulting in some negative outcome for which the child may be held completely respon-sible. In reality, however, the often predictable behavioral outcome is actually the product of the client–staff relationship. It is important that staff recognize their own role in inter-actions that produce a negative behavior, or at least examine the possibility that client behavior may have been partly catalyzed by client–staff interaction. In the therapeutic milieu, we recognize treatment growth *and* setbacks as the product, at least in part, of the environment.

CONCLUSION: THE ATTACHMENT-INFORMED ENVIRONMENT

Attachment theory and understanding the attachment process in both its development and its effect on current emotions, thoughts, and behaviors offers a powerful means for making sense of emotional and behavioral development, social connection and relatedness, the power of the therapeutic relationship, and the development of treatment interventions aimed at rehabilitation and reconnection. "Optimally," Slade writes, listening for and tuning into attachment patterns "should add to therapists' ways of listening to and understanding clinical material" (p. 590). Nevertheless, we recognize that attachment is not the only way to see the client or provide treatment. As Slade (1999) reminds us, attachment does not define all aspects of human experience, just as an attachment-informed approach to therapy cannot replace other, equally important and equally meaningful, formulations of human behavior.

As noted, we're not proposing anything new in the sense of a "new" model of attachment-based sex offender treatment. Instead, it is the provision of juvenile sexual offender treatment *within* the shroud of an attachment-informed environment that is important, and perhaps new. Here, all aspects of behavior, and the treatment relationship itself, are seen through an attachment lens and therapists and other treatment staff are guided by attachment-oriented principles of treatment and relationship building. To juvenile sex offender treatment models that have already become increasingly well rounded and holistic, attachment-informed treatment adds an important dimension by adding the component of social relatedness.

CHAPTER 18

Implications for Treatment

It is clear, from a nationwide study of outpatient and residential programs treating adult and juvenile sexual offenders in the United States (McGrath, Cumming, & Burchard, 2003), that cognitive-behavioral, psychoeducational, and relapse prevention planning models continue to predominate treatment by far. Nevertheless, between 80 and 95% of adult programs provide treatment in intimacy and relationship skills, social skills training, and victim empathy, as do between 75 and 97% of adolescent treatment programs, with a lower emphasis than adult programs on empathy and a higher emphasis on family support. Of juvenile sexual offender residential treatment programs, 81% focus on the juvenile's own history of victimization, 80% provide relaxation or stress management, 40% art therapy, and 16% drama therapy. In the treatment of juvenile sexual offenders, then, we are seeing programs that treat far more than simply sexually abusive behaviors, and provide far more than cognitive-behavioral and psychoeducational treatment alone, thereby recognizing that their clients are in need of a range of treatment services.[1]

Leaders in the field, such as Robert Longo and Gail Ryan, urge the development of holistic juvenile sexual offender treatment programs that address multiple aspects in the treatment and development of the youth, and we are seeing the implementation of integrated models that attack treatment from many angles. Through the provision of cognitive-behavioral therapy we explore, challenge, and restructure thinking and related behaviors that contribute to sexually abusive and other antisocial behavior, as well as self-defeating behavior. Through psychoeducation, we provide a common language and teach concepts that can help to rehabilitate behavior and acquire coping and other social skills. Through psychodynamic and insight-oriented therapies we link current behaviors, relationships, social interactions, and emotional experiences with root causes and psychological needs, and through family therapies we explore and reconstruct family relationships and support systems. In our provision of relapse prevention planning, we establish a means for self-awareness, help-seeking, self-control, and harm avoidance post-treatment. In adding expressive, experiential, and recreational therapies to an integrated treatment model, we allow for non-verbal learning and expression, and through multimodal treat-

---

[1] In fact, given the broad range of treatment services offered, it may be that programs report cognitive-behavioral and relapse prevention approaches as the predominant model of treatment because the survey format elicits this response, due to its design and structure.

ment that includes individual, group, and family treatment, as well as psychopharmacology, we ensure multiple mechanisms for treatment delivery and treatment approaches and interventions capable of covering much ground.

By blending these different treatments and allowing a pantheoretical approach to guide treatment in which no single theory predominates, we create integrated models of treatment, illustrated in Figure 18.1, "Dappled," in the words of Holmes and Bateman (2002), "in the sense that they bring together elements from single tradition therapeutic modalities in an organized and systematic way, in order to enhance therapeutic efficiency" (p. 1). They describe integration as wedding together strands of different therapies into a new and coherent whole, as opposed to eclecticism which can be idiosyncratic and without theory.

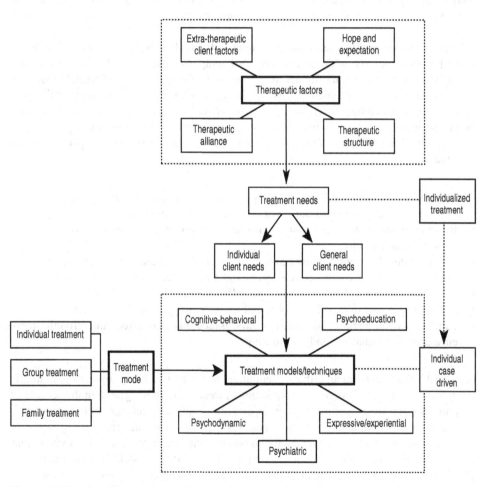

Figure 18.1 Blending common therapeutic approaches with treatment interventions in a multimodal, multitechnique, multitask, pantheoretical treatment model

COMPREHENSIVE AND HOLISTIC TREATMENT

Treatment of the whole child means viewing the problem of juvenile sexual offending from many angles, and attacking through treatment and rehabilitation as many of those problems as possible, or at least identifying them as significant factors to be addressed. To be effective, sexual-offender-specific treatment includes both specific interventions explicitly aimed at sexual offending behavior *and* interventions aimed at collateral or other conditions and factors that directly contribute to, influence, or maintain sexually abusive behavior. Ryan (1999b) describes *offense-specific interventions* as those that focus on elements and patterns directly related to sexual offending, and *holistic preventative interventions* focused on increased self-control and efficacy, and general issues. She writes that the struggle "is to combine the specific and the holistic into comprehensive models that can differentially diagnose and treat offenders while respecting the unique developmental and contextual realities of each individual" (p. 427), noting that not every sexually abusive juvenile requires the same treatment or will respond in the same way.

Explicit abuse-specific treatment, then, an essential and central component of the treatment process, directly addresses sexual offending thoughts, beliefs, and behaviors. Other components of sexual offender treatment can be thought of as collateral, but are also aimed at the presenting problem of sexual offending behaviors. In fact, whether aimed at *explicit* sexual offending behaviors or *comorbid* and *collateral* conditions, all sexual-offender-specific treatment is intended to extinguish and eliminate sexual aggression. In treating the whole person, or in holistic treatment, we treat not just abuse-specific behaviors, but also:

- The sexual offenses that brought the youth into treatment in the first place.
- Comorbid psychiatric conditions that may be affecting the youth.
- Behavioral and relationship issues that shape and influence self-perception and interpersonal relationships.
- Issues of developmental trauma and life-changing experiences that may have a profound effect on the youth's development and current behavior.
- Issues of self-identity, self-concept, and self-esteem.
- Social skills and the experience of social mastery and personal competency.
- Family, environmental, and other systemic issues that may affect and strongly influence thinking, behavior, and relationships.

In sexual offender treatment that is comprehensive and holistic, multimodal, multidisciplinary, and multitheoretical components of treatment are integrated in the sense that they are part of a larger treatment program, and not simply a loosely strung together bunch of treatments. This implies coordination among the parts, communication among members of the treatment team that deliver each component, and a coherent model and vision that ensures that each modality is a single component of a larger model. These elements are all embodied within the treatment milieu, described in Chapter 17 as the ecological environment in which treatment is implemented and experienced, and the medium through which treatment ideas are transmitted and received.

THE FIRST LINE OF TREATMENT: ATTACHMENT IN THE TREATMENT MILIEU

As described in Chapter 17, in the therapeutic milieu, we recognize treatment growth, as well as treatment setbacks, partly as the product of the environment itself and the interactions it embodies. Indeed, especially in foster and residential care, this treatment environment is the first line of attachment-oriented treatment.

In framing a blended and integrated model of treatment within a treatment environment that recognizes attachment needs and difficulties, and fosters social connection and the development of attached relationships, we create an *attachment-informed treatment environment*, shown in Figure 18.2. Here, treatment occurs in a caring and supportive manner, through an attachment-friendly environment in which relationships are genuine, respectful, and supportive while at the same time being structured and challenging, and in which the message that comes through is one of care, concern, understanding, and attunement. In this environment, individuals are experienced and treated as individuals, and not simply

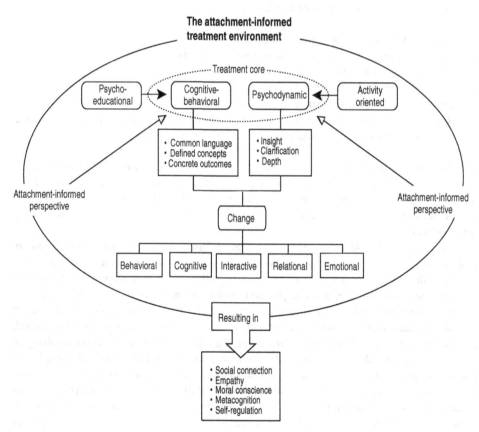

Figure 18.2   Integrated treatment occurring within and guided by the attachment framework, forming an ecological system that reinforces and provides attachment at all levels, resulting in elements of social relatedness

"sexual offenders" or troubled children who all share the same backgrounds and behaviors, and in which, despite commonalities, the needs of clients are based on an assessment and interpretation of their individual needs, through the process of clinical formulation.

In this treatment environment, we recognize that although we cannot undo the past, we can influence the future through our actions in the present.

FORMULATING AND INDIVIDUALIZING TREATMENT

To be effective in the assessment and treatment of juvenile sexual offenders and in the assignment of risk for sexual re-offense, a central aspect of sexual-offender-specific evaluation, clinicians must develop a comprehensive understanding of each youth they assess. Making sense of the gathered data and using those data to generate clinical hypotheses and treatment plans requires that clinicians have the skills of clinical formulation. That is, clinicians must be able to synthesize and reduce what they have discovered about the client into a description that:

1. Explains the development of the youth.
2. Identifies factors influential in shaping personality and behavior.
3. Describes behaviors that bring the youth into treatment.
4. Attributes causes for those behaviors.
5. Prognosticates on future behaviors.
6. Recommends treatment interventions that are most likely to alter pathological trajectory and promote positive change.

In effect, in formulating the case, therapists create a clinical theory about the juvenile sexual offender. Like all theories, this must be able to describe past conditions that led to the phenomenon, explain current occurrences of the phenomenon, predict future occurrences and conditions under which the phenomenon will recur, and define control interventions.

Drake and Ward (2003a) write that formulation-based approaches to treatment require that therapists understand psychological problems and vulnerabilities for individual clients, rather than "manualized" assessment that offers cookbook approaches for understanding behavior. In formulation, planned treatment interventions are individualized, resulting from different case formulations. Despite the prevailing perspective that adult sexual offenders share common dysfunctions and can thus be treated through prescribed, manualized treatment, Drake and Ward argue that this is a limited position resulting in treatment that is weak, poorly targeted, and fails to meet individual needs. Although it is reasonable to assume that most adult sexual offenders have dysfunctions involving intimacy, sexual behavior, emotional regulation, and cognitive distortions, they write that individualized case formulation is likely to improve understanding and lead to a more precise, finely tuned, and precise treatment. For a sexual offender, they write, case formulation illuminates the specific developmental factors that made *that* specific individual vulnerable to sexual offending, leading to the development of distinct therapeutic interventions for that individual.

BUILDING AN ATTACHMENT-INFORMED MODEL

Creeden (2005) writes that the focus on cognitive-behavioral/relapse prevention treatment model overlooks or fails to recognize neurological obstacles that create difficulty in attachment-disordered juvenile sexual offenders. In Creeden's opinion, such neurobiological challenges, in many cases, result from early trauma and attachment-related experiences (the possible mechanisms of which are described in Chapter 15). He supports and describes a residential treatment program for juvenile sexual offenders that engages clients in phases of treatment that address developmental trauma and attachment difficulties.

The *containment* phase focuses on relaxation, stress management, and attunement and the development of interoceptive skills (the ability to be in touch with and recognize internal states, physical and emotional), using biofeedback; the use of slow movement, such as yoga and tai chi; movement and music therapies that allow individuals to become attuned; and the development of organizational and problem-solving skills. The second phase described by Creeden involves *deconditioning traumatic responses and re-establishing social connection*, which focuses on the development of metacognitive capacity, in this case, based on social interactions between clients and staff who serve as primary caregivers. This reinforces the idea that the child is being attended to rather than monitored, and includes the use of physical touch, described by Creeden (in press) as a fundamental aspect of the process by which children become attached, and central to the idea of developing healthy, rather than sexualized, touch. Experiential treatment experiences also play an important role in this phase of treatment, including art, drama, music, and movement therapies.

The third and final phase in the model described by Creeden is *restructuring personal traumatic schemes*, in which the model employs techniques such as Eye Movement Desensitization and Reprocessing (EMDR) as a means to drain trauma of its power, and other cognitive-behavioral and restructuring treatments are also used. Although the model possesses a sequential quality, Creeden (in press) notes that the treatment is not necessarily linear, but is instead interactive and developmental in which clients move back and forth through different phases, revisiting particular issues with the development of different levels of personal coping, organizational, and other psychological skills.

Creeden is describing a program that, like most treatment for juvenile and adult sexual offenders, has no long-term or empirical evidence of its effect, and is hence based on theoretical assumptions only. Nevertheless, he connects treatment interventions with a model of neurobiological development, and demonstrates how one might construct a program or define program elements that recognize and are intended to directly address attachment-based issues. In adding new components, such as yoga, drama therapy, and EMDR, to what are by now standard methods and techniques of sex-offender-specific treatment; by reframing and recasting into an attachment-related light some of the typical practices of residential life, such as activities of daily living and recreational activities; and by emphasizing attachment and caregiving relationships in the treatment environment, Creeden succeeds in defining and describing an attachment-informed treatment milieu in which the treatment of juvenile sexual offending is cradled. In this regard, he demonstrates an intentionality and purpose in treatment, in which specific treatment tasks are identified and specifically directed towards trauma and attachment recovery.

In his model, Creeden does not describe the foundation upon which all stages, phases, or elements of attachment-related treatment must be built. According to attachment theory, this is, of course, the development of the secure base. Returning to a common factors model, although Creeden is describing activities and methods connected to each phase of his model, beneath each of these lies the element of trust that must exist in the therapeutic relationship and be experienced by the client in the treatment environment. As such, building trust and a treatment bond may be considered a "stage" in a treatment model, or a theme that runs throughout treatment. Treatment elements such as relaxation, trauma resolution, biofeedback, and attunement to rhythm, for instance, have value in an attachment-based model *only* when they are built upon or contribute to the establishment of the attachment bond and the secure base that paves the way for the exploration of self, others, and relationships that Creeden is ultimately describing in his model.

BUILDING BLOCKS: STEPS AND PHASES IN ATTACHMENT-RELATED TREATMENT

The model described by Creeden is actually an activity model aimed at resolving trauma and activating attachment experiences, focused on building skills of social connection and self-regulation. That is, the model describes activities that are applied within each phase, aimed at addressing, resolving, and/or developing specific internalized processes assumed to be associated with trauma and attachment issues and the development of social skills and social affiliation.

However, an attachment-informed treatment *model* must first focus on the steps by which attachment security is established and internalized. In this respect, such a treatment model defines sequential steps, or phases, that focus on particular aspects of attachment formation, and recognizes the goal of each step as the development of those particular aspects. An attachment-informed model thus recognizes the building blocks of attachment that signal the development, deepening, and internalization of attachment structures, patterns, and strategies, mirroring Bowlby's phases of attachment (Chapter 3).

Phase 1: Containment and Stabilization

Without intending to borrow Creeden's term, which appears to have a different meaning, the first step in an attachment-informed model involves the containment of emotional and behavioral episodes triggered by insecurity and reactivity to the environment, driven by the attachment behavioral system. Attachment behaviors reflect insecurity and are sparked by anxiety, are characterized by proximity seeking and behaviors designed to get the attention of an attachment figure, are antithetical to exploratory behaviors, and signal a lack of secure base. Active attachment elements that are a focus during this treatment phase include establishing a sense of safety in the child and ensuring his or her proximity to reliable and responsive attachment figures. A focus, then, is on the de-activation of attachment behavior once the child feels that he or she is safe, and increasing his or her capacity for self-regulation. Therefore, phase one focuses on the stabilization and containment of emotion, anxiety, and often destructive behavior, as well as the development of the secure base from which the child can explore emotions, thoughts, and behaviors, and engage in new relationships and activities. This phase reflects Bowlby's first attachment phase of early and initial pre-attachment, involving orientation and primitive attachment signals.

Like all attachment treatment work, the tasks of this step most effectively occur in an emotionally safe treatment environment, capable of tolerating and absorbing the child's behaviors, and recognizing the source and meaning of behaviors as attachment-derived and attachment-seeking. This environment is attuned to the child, well-regulated, not reactive to the child's behaviors, and able to "hold" the child's behavior, thus serving as the facilitative environment essential for effective treatment.

Phase 2: Engagement and Exploration

This step focuses on and leads to the building and expansion of the behaviors, social skills, and relationships developed during the first phase of treatment. Although connections and relationships form with treatment staff and peers during the first phase, the emphasis and main focus of that phase is on stabilizing behaviors and creating emotional containment and self-regulation. That first phase represents a primary building block in the formation of secure attachment and the experience of felt security that paves the way for further development. Thus, although engagement and exploration are present in phase one, acting on the secure base and engaging in healthy and secure exploration becomes possible only after the child has stabilized and anxiety-driven behaviors are contained. The child experiences security and a sense of safety, exhibiting less insecurity and fewer attachment behaviors, thus signaling a movement in attachment building to this second phase,

Remember, *attachment behaviors* are triggered by the attachment behavioral system and reflect anxiety and insecurity, as opposed to *behaviors that reflect attachment*, such as secure relationships with parents, peers, and others. Therefore, we are looking, not for attachment behaviors, but for behaviors that indicate attachment. That simple rewording has much significance. Attachment-seeking behaviors signal insecurity, whereas behaviors that reflect attachment signal security, and do not include the proximity and attention-seeking behaviors triggered by uncertainty and insecurity. Acting on the secure base and engaging in healthy and secure exploration becomes possible only after the child has stabilized and is thus more secure and safe, resulting in fewer attachment behaviors. In phase two, engagement, exploration, and relationships expand, embracing Bowlby's second phase of attachment-in-the-making, and by the end of this phase are beginning to incorporate Bowlby's third phase of clear cut attachment.

Phase 3: Connection and Partnership

During this phase, attached treatment relationships and social connections are more fully formed, in which the child feels an attachment bond and is more clearly involved in a partnership with treatment staff. In its earliest appearance, this step in attachment building reflects Bowlby's phase of clear cut attachment and during its further development, in which clients are secure in their treatment relationships and working with their therapists and other treatment staff; the phase embraces the elements of Bowlby's fourth and final phase of goal-corrected partnership. Building on a more established sense of security in self and others, this step expands on the work started in phase two, continuing to develop self-confidence (self-efficacy and self-agency), metacognition (awareness and under-standing of self and others), and self-regulation. However, in phase three, in older chil-dren and particularly in adolescents, attachment work focuses on the exploration of personal and social values and the development of perspective-taking, moral decision making, empathy, and social belonging.

Phase 4: Security and Social Relatedness

In terms of attachment-building, as the child comes close to and enters this phase, he or she is likely to be close to discharge from treatment, where the gains of the phase will be most relevant post-discharge and for the rest of his or her life. Here, the goals are to fully cement and ensure the internalization of self-confidence, recognition of others, and social connection. Phase 4 represents an ongoing embodiment of representations of self and others, reflected and demonstrated in a combination of self-agency, self-efficacy, proso-cial behaviors, and healthy and socially appropriate relationships.

Summary

These four phases, or steps, in attachment-related treatment, describe a developmental pro-gression in which attachment representations and patterns and beliefs about self and others are shaped, reshaped, and internalized in a rehabilitated internal working model. They do not capture the stages of attachment briefly described in Chapter 5, which reflect the content, purpose, and goals of attachment during different periods in human development. Whereas, attachment stages describe the changing needs of attachment, with respect to the functions of attachment, the nature of attached relationships, and the role of attachment figures at different developmental ages, the phases in attachment building describe the building blocks of attachment-related treatment. This involves, not the meaning of attach-ment during adolescence, for instance, or who becomes an attachment figure and why, but *how* attachment patterns and the experience of attachment is rehabilitated in attachment-disturbed youths and how insecure attachment is transformed into something that more resembles "earned" security. Nevertheless, as we work with these steps, or phases, of attachment building, we need to be sensitive to the developmental and chronological age of clients, recognizing that attachment needs and relationships for a 6-year-old are going to be quite different from those of a 16-year-old.

ASSESSING ATTACHMENT

Built into any attachment model must be an assessment of attachment. However, although it may be useful to use a tool that recognizes and classifies attachment patterns, we have seen already that such tools are weak (Chapter 8) when it comes to both operationalizing and measuring attachment in adults, and even more limited in assessing attachment in adolescents. However, in this case, I am thinking of assessment not so much as a tool for assessing an attachment style or assigning an attachment classification but, rather, as a means for assessing the quality and status (rather than category) of attachment. Even if we are able to develop stronger attachment classification tools, the psychosocial assessment that leads to clinical understanding and case formulation is a particularly useful means for such assessment. This is especially true when guided by a structured instrument, such as the *Inventory for Attachment-informed Analysis of Behaviors (IAAB)* or *Attached Relationship Inventory (ARI)* described in Chapter 10, or the *Dimensions of Attachment Assessment Scale (DAAS)* described in Chapter 8, that identifies areas to be assessed and, in effect, questions to be asked.

To the attachment-informed evaluator, the psychosocial assessment brings patterns of attachment and attachment history to life, not through inventories, self-reports, or psychometric tools, but through the observation of patterns of attachment which will become evident to us as we observe and interpret behavior through an attachment lens, as shown in the case study presented in Chapter 10. In assessment, we have to apply a particular way of looking *for* and *at* behaviors that inform us, as Holmes (2001) and Slade (1999) note, of what attachment looks like in real life. In treatment, if we have a basis for observing and recording our observations about assessment, we can see and reflect upon how dimensions of attachment change over time, and we can certainly evaluate and re-evaluate aspects and classifications of attachment using tools such as the Inventory of Parent and Peer Attachment or other similar tools (described in Chapter 8), or tools we may develop for the purpose. However, tools developed for the purpose of assessment should enhance, inform, and add to psychosocial assessment, rather than being used *as* the assessment. This is true, for instance, in the case of the Adult Attachment Interview which requires clinical interpretation, albeit guided by a structured coding system. This clinical focus is precisely why it's such a strong tool.

In fact, other than perhaps assigning a client to an attachment category or some other measure correlated to attachment status, it is most likely that formal instruments will simply validate or confirm our clinical assessments of attachment. For example, it would be unusual and unexpected if someone we clearly experienced as securely attached was assessed by an attachment measure as insecure, or, conversely, if we found through evaluation that someone we considered to be insecure was actually secure. In other words, we are likely to find that formal evaluation of attachment simply corroborates what we already know. If it doesn't, something may be wrong with the tools we are using, the way we are using them, or our clinical ability to understand and recognize attachment.

In terms of assessment, attachment is a "soft" target. That is, it is not easily observed and is not something we can easily measure, and we have already described many of the instruments used to measure assessment. However, in the case of clients who we know and can observe directly (as opposed to individuals in a research population who may be unknown to us), formal assessment instruments simply provide a means of placing individuals into a particular assessment category. Although they do this in a more consistent and efficient manner than can most clinicians, such instruments do not inform us about aspects of client attachment status, related attachment history, or relevant treatment interventions. Frankly, with respect to the assessment of attachment style, it's not clear that we will ever be able to define clear cut categories or types of attachment that are capable of fully capturing the nuances and textures of attachment, other than recognizing that there is a continuum that runs between secure attachment at one end, and insecure attachment at the other. Along this continuum, people are more or less secure in their attachment, and even this changes in different circumstances, in different relationships and situations, and at different points in life. Our goal in treatment, of course, is to move people as close to secure attachment as possible, for as much of the time as possible, and in as many relationships and situations as possible.

Aside from assigning an attachment classification, however, we can recognize changes in attachment status and patterns by selecting attachment instrument(s), or measures that infer attachment, to be used pre- and post-treatment. Similarly, we can use tools such as the DAAS, IAAB, and ARI to gather information and reflect upon and help to define treatment. Through these means, we can use assessment tools to help to apply an approach to assessment and treatment that reflects attachment theory. Additionally, developing and using assessment measures that both recognize what needs to be changed and whether or not it has changed, also helps us to shape and define what it is we are trying to change.

PHASE-RELATED TREATMENT ACTIVITIES

In the phase model of attachment building described here, treatment interventions related to specific phases reinforce the formation and internalization of attachment rather than serve as activities or interventions used to directly address trauma or attachment issues. Although most treatment activities are common to all phases, simply developing and expanding over time in treatment, some activities are clearly more related to certain phases than others. Phase one (containment and stabilization) interventions, for instance, will focus on and involve reassuring and calming activities that include staff responsiveness, availability, and proximity in a manner appropriate to the age of the client, that establish a sense of safety and structure, aiming for the development of self-regulation. Activities and interventions most relevant to the second phase (engagement and exploration) will increasingly include those intended to foster responsibility taking, aimed at building a sense of self-agency and self-efficacy, and establishing the groundwork for metacognition, at least with respect to self-reflectivity. During the third phase (connection and partnership), interventions will be aimed at building treatment relationships in which clients are actively working *with* the therapists and other treatment staff, enhancing and capitalizing upon the strengths that the client brings to treatment (extra-therapeutic treatment factors), as well as a sense of hope and expectancy, and the therapeutic relationship itself. Finally, as shown in Figure 18.3, phase 4 (security and social relatedness) activities will most focus on fully internalizing gains in attachment and social connection, understanding self and others, and preparing the client for attached relationships in the post-treatment world.

More specifically, informed by attachment and child development in general, no matter how provided, a number of specific treatment components will be incorporated into an attachment-based model. They may be provided through psychodynamic, cognitive-behavioral, psychoeducational, or experience-based treatment, and one way or another must also be present, modeled, and experienced both in the therapeutic relationship and, in residential treatment, the therapeutic milieu.

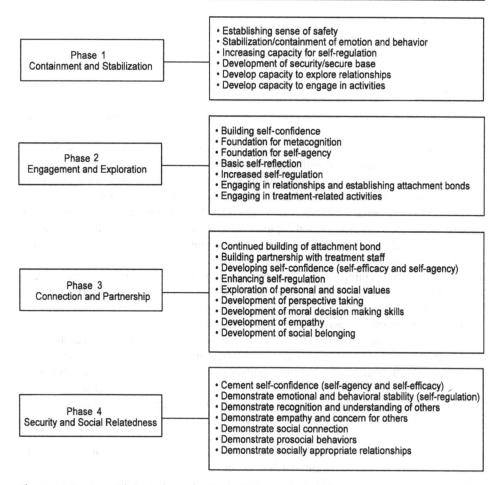

Figure 18.3 Steps/phases of attachment building and related tasks

COMPONENTS IN ATTACHMENT-BASED TREATMENT

All treatment components are wrapped and delivered within a treatment environment that is attuned to and responsive to clients, and in which they are recognized and understood. In this environment, opportunities are available for taking responsibility, realizing potential, and experiencing success, and thus building self-agency and self-efficacy. Although there are many elements to be transmitted to and nurtured in the client engaged in attachment-based treatment, several stand out as essential components, including the development of empathy, metacognition, morality, and self-regulation. Beyond these treatment components, however, which are related specifically to the attachment goal, treatment for juvenile sexual offenders is, of course, sex offender specific. This includes cognitive-behavioral, psychoeducational, and psychodynamic treatment specifically directed towards sexually abusive behavior, as well as treatment that recognizes and addresses important collateral issues such as trauma resolution, anger management, self-expression, and psychiatric comorbidity.

1. *Empathy training and development* includes a focus on the cognitive components of empathy such as the capacity to recognize and identify emotions in others and perspective taking, and affective components that include exploring and identifying with the distress of the other person (through role plays, for instance, and victim clarification exercises).
2. *Metacognitive skill development* is related to empathy development in its emphasis on recognizing the emotional and cognitive states of self and others, but also involves the ability to *think* about thoughts and feelings and recognize how one's own mind and the minds of others work, thus enhancing theory of mind in the client.
3. *Moral decision making and behavior* is also related to empathy and perspective taking, involving value clarification and exploration of personal and social values, the attachment of values to behavioral decisions, the consequences of behavior and its impact on others, and acceptance of personal responsibility.
4. *Self-regulation* training provides clients with a means to manage and release stress, including "mindless" methods which include techniques of guided imagery, yoga, and recreation, and expressive therapies that are wordless in their effects. Stress management and regulation can also employ cognitive approaches that allow clients to recognize and learn how to manage and maintain control over affect, such as the stress inoculation techniques developed by Meichenbaum (1977, 1985). These include cognitive-behavioral strategies for problem recognition and solution, cognitive restructuring, environmental monitoring, and relaxation. Similarly, Linehan's (1993) distress tolerance model teaches clients cognitive strategies for recognizing, tolerating, and managing difficulty and emotional discomfort.

In describing these elements of an attachment-based treatment, there is no intention to describe *how* they should be taught or delivered, or the actual nature of the treatment intervention. They may be delivered through individual or group therapy, activity-oriented and expressive therapies, cognitive-behavioral treatment, psychodynamic therapy, or workbook-driven curricula, and many excellent resources already exist from which to draw ideas, materials, and techniques. In each case, however, treatment interventions and activities must be age appropriate and, perhaps more to the point, age relevant from a developmental perspective. In addition, no matter how constructed and delivered, given the preconscious aspect of the attachment experience, consideration should be given to the need for wordless, brain-based learning.

BRAIN-BASED LEARNING

Jensen (2000) describes brain-based learning as a teaching approach that is designed to directly tap into the natural learning capacity of the brain, recognizing that learning is complex and operates along multiple and simultaneous paths. In this model, the richer and the more varied the types of learning stimuli, the more likely that learning will occur on some level. He describes stages by which learning occurs at the neural level, from the acquisition and consolidation of new information; the interconnection of new information with already learned information, adding context and meaning; integration into memory, and thus retention; to finally functional integration resulting from the transfer and application of new information to actual behavior, or activity and practice related directly to newly acquired information.

We also recognize that brain-based learning is emotional, and that people learn better under the right emotional conditions. This does not mean that low stress creates the best learning environment. It may at times, but at other times, such as on a high ropes course or when things are happening all at once and require immediate solutions, a different type of learning may occur that is only available under those learning conditions. This is a form of state-based learning that may occur best, or only occur, under certain conditions that promote neurochemical changes in the brain and body which in turn, allow specific learning to occur. Brain-based learning, then, additionally means matching the learning task with the physical and emotional learning environment. However, we also know that although the brain processes many stimuli at once, stress triggers right brain activities before left brain processing and, in the poorly integrated brain, stress may overwhelm learning. Accordingly, we want to ensure graduated learning experiences that can help our clients to develop self-regulatory skills before we can expect them to learn under high-stress conditions.

The challenge of brain-based learning is to imagine and create treatment interventions that promote the tasks of attachment building, including self-regulation, mentalization, and attachment itself, through activities that reach directly to the brain.

EMPATHY IN THE ATTACHMENT-BASED TREATMENT ENVIRONMENT

We have described the centrality of empathy in social relatedness, its relationship to attachment, and its importance in the ability to feel connected and attached to others. We have noted also that although the capacity for empathy appears to be present in a rudimentary form during infancy and early childhood, it is only during adolescence that the capacity for empathy begins to unfold, particularly with the development of abstraction and perspective-taking skills.

Carl Rogers (1980) writes that empathy dissolves alienation, allowing those who feel empathy for others to feel like "part of the human race" (p. 151) and those who experience empathic understanding to feel valued, cared for, and accepted. These are the very qualities that we wish to instill, develop, or unlock in the treatment of juvenile sexual offenders. They are also the same qualities that juvenile sexual offenders must experience from others in their environment, whether in their own homes, in the therapeutic relationship, or in the larger treatment milieu of the residential program.

Rogers (1980) tells us that an empathic way of being, central to the treatment relationship and the treatment milieu, can be learned from empathic persons, and that "perhaps the most important statement of all is that the ability to be accurately empathic is something that can be developed by training" (p. 150). However, Fernandez and Serran (2002) write that although there are numerous empathy training programs for clients, "the first step to teaching clients empathy is to recognize, understand, and model empathy" (p. 131).

Accordingly, we recognize that being the *subject* of empathy is the first step in the development of the capacity to *be* empathic. Indeed, Eagle and Wolitzky (1997) consider empathy to be closely related to the experiences of attunement and sensitive responsiveness that we also consider critical to the development of attachment in our clients. Warner (1997) describes empathic understanding as crucial in therapy with clients whose ability to contain and process their own experiences has been weakened due to empathic failures in their early development. Hence, she describes the therapist's empathy to be curative, developing and strengthening the client's own capacity to relate to others.

Feshbach (1997) notes that not only is the client's experience of the therapist's empathy likely to enhance the effectiveness of treatment, but therapeutic empathy also provides the clinician with clues about the experiences and emotions of the client. Fernandez and Serran (2002) note that therapeutic empathy not only informs the clinician about the client, but also provides the clinician with the motivation to help the client. In fact, it is generally believed that the capacity of treatment staff to recognize and empathically respond to distress in the client influences the development of empathy (Anderson & Dodgson, 2002), clarifying once again that the attachment experiences and elements we wish to develop in juvenile sexual offenders are dispositional in his interactions with others *before* they become dispositional in him. In teaching empathy, then, it is the therapist and treatment staff who must demonstrate empathy, described by Fernandez and Serran as integral to the therapeutic relationship.

Through the warmth, concern, support, caring, safety and structure provided by the empathic therapist and treatment staff, children and adolescents in treatment are seen and *feel* seen. In turn, they are enabled to see, not only themselves, but other people as well, beginning first with the other person in the attachment relationship—in this case, the therapist. Despite the label of juvenile sexual offender, our clients are first children and adolescents, as they are the entire time they are with us in treatment. Thus, kids who have often felt uncared for, unloved, unsupported, misunderstood, and disconnected may, through treatment and the treatment environment, reclaim their humanity and begin to feel a sense of connection to others.

RELATIONSHIPS IN THE TREATMENT ENVIRONMENT

The effectiveness of sex-offender-specific treatment is influenced not just by the things we teach our clients, but by the things they bring into treatment with them, and the way in which they participate in treatment. It is also very much affected by our interactions with our clients. This idea clearly has ramifications for the therapeutic relationship and the larger relationship environment, particularly in residential treatment. Of course, relationships and interactions for juvenile sexual offenders living at home with their natural families during treatment are of tremendous significance, but in residential care, the ecology of the treatment environment takes on a different flavor. In this setting, the job of treatment staff is to rebuild and teach attachment, not to become substitute parents. Nevertheless, through the transference inherent in the therapeutic relationship, clinicians and other treatment staff may play a parental role in their capacity to emotionally hold the client and form attachment, and be experienced by clients as parent substitutes, filling some of the same purposes and operating through some of the same mechanisms as a primary attachment relationship (Amini et al., 1996; Parish & Eagle, 2003).

In the attachment work of the therapeutic relationship, the job of the clinician is to help the client to learn *how* to become attached. This, by necessity, means *becoming* attached. Nevertheless, we should not expect youth in treatment, and perhaps residential treatment most of all where relationships can be long term, to develop the same sort of attachments that they may develop in the ideal circumstances as a child. This is partly because the treatment environment is contrived, and relationships within it are defined by the structure and purpose of treatment. No matter how strong the relationship between client and therapist or other treatment staff, it is never going to be the same as, or replace, relationships with parents, friends, or partners. In fact, recognizing that attachment styles are adaptive, we should expect clients to always demonstrate a somewhat cautious and distant attachment because of the nature of the relationship itself.

Nevertheless, we should watch out for client relationships with therapists that are distant and avoidant because they signal client mistrust and uncertainty in the therapeutic alliance, but we must be equally aware of relationships in which clients are becoming too close or too enmeshed with their clinicians or other staff, suggesting an unrealistic understanding or expectation of the relationship. It is not unusual for clients to want to be adopted by treatment staff, for instance, not to mention having sexual and romantic fantasies. The role of the clinician is to be aware of these dynamics, recognizing also that therapeutic relationships can take months (and in some cases, well over a year) to develop, as well as the inevitability of setbacks in the therapeutic relationship and the need to repair these ruptures in the therapeutic relationship as they develop (Siegel, 1999, 2003).

FAMILY TREATMENT

We cannot discuss attachment treatment without recognizing the family as the *source* of attachment, and usually the cause of attachment difficulties. However, most of the time, treatment with juvenile sexual offenders does not directly involve the family, especially if treatment occurs in residential care, even in the treatment of attachment deficits. This may seem like an odd thing to say, particularly as the family is so central to attachment and also because the victim of the juvenile sexual offender is frequently a member of the family. In fact, in residential care, the family is relatively removed from the treatment of juvenile sexual offenders, other than when it is directly engaged in a treatment activity, such as family therapy. In the course of treatment in the residential setting, however, family therapy and other forms of family treatment involvement usually represent a very small slice of the entire treatment program.

Nevertheless, at an implicit or explicit level, the treatment of attachment will and must always include the family. Of course, this is most obviously the case in the provision of family therapy. Attachment theory is certainly relevant to understanding family dynamics, and, as we have seen, family patterns of attachment are believed to be transmitted intergenerationally. Minimally, understanding the attachment patterns and behaviors of the parents can be of enormous value in understanding the development and history of attachment in children. However, although the attachment-informed family therapist can easily apply an attachment perspective to family work, attachment work is more clearly and closely geared to working with individuals,[2] as it is individuals within whom attachment resides. Again, this is especially true in the residential setting. Kozlowska and Hanney (2002) write of the difficulty in conceptualizing the relationship between attachment theory and theories of family therapy, as well as whether attachment theory and family systems theory can be merged in a single model of therapy or must remain distinct. In a similar vein, James (1994) writes that attachment-based family therapy is not traditional family therapy, instead treating the attachment work of the child *within* a framework of family therapy, combining the two modes of treatment. Regardless, we can apply an attachment approach to working with families, both to better understand family systems and the functioning of individuals within the family, and as a means to help the family change interactional patterns. In effect, consistent with a model of family systems, in which the family *unit*, and not the individual, is the patient, it is the pattern of attachment within the family as a whole that must be the target for treatment in an attachment-informed family therapy.[3]

In many respects, family therapy resembles attachment treatment. Not least of all, this is because family systems can be conceived of in terms remarkably similar to attachment classifications of secure and insecure attachment. Defined by Minuchin (1974) in terms of boundaries, *adaptive* families are well balanced with clear boundaries, are mutually sensitive, have open communication, are supportive, and allow independence among family members; in attachment terms, this is a secure family whose members experience secure attachment. The *disengaged* family is described as avoidant, under-involved, and insensitive, sounding like the avoidantly attached individual, and the *enmeshed* family is the counterpart of the ambivalent or anxiously attached individual, described as over-involved, intrusive, ambivalent, and resistant to independence and boundaries. As in attachment-based treatments, effective family therapy also operates through a therapeutic alliance, in this case formed between the clinician and the family. This requires "joining" with the family (Minuchin, 1974; Minuchin & Fishman, 1981), in which the clinician must understand and accept the organization and style of the family, "following their path of communication, discovering which ones are open, which are partly closed, and which are entirely blocked" (Minuchin, 1974, p. 123). Through this process, the clinician is thus able to develop a secure base, described by Byng-Hall (1999) as critical for family therapy, and by which the family may engage in difficult emotional interactions.

Byng-Hall (1999) writes that the capacity of family members to feel understood in family therapy is central to the development of a secure attachment to the therapist, who may then, in an unthreatening manner, help family members to learn about themselves as individuals within the family and as a whole family, making "sense out of what may be otherwise perplexing" (p. 636). The secure base created through the therapeutic alliance allows family members to safely engage in and explore conflicts, and understand their own narrative history. Byng-Hall (1991) describes the "family script" as the family's shared expectations of how family roles are to be performed in various contexts, described by Marvin and Stewart (1990) as family "working models" that consist of shared expectations and plans, and a primary means by which family structure is maintained. These

---

[2] Except in the case of young children, for whom attachment work is always going to involve the primary caregiver(s), and especially very young children.

[3] For a review and discussion of family therapy in the treatment of juvenile sexual offenders, see Rich (2003).

scripts, or models, are developed through the repetition of family behavior that becomes familiar to all family members, including those not directly involved in the behavior, and used to predict and determine the next step in the usual sequence of interactions. Byng-Hall writes that it is through understanding the family script, which also contains representations of family attachment bonds, that the clinician can come to understand the family and work with it to understand and bring about structural change. Through direct and indirect work with the family, the clinician is able to understand family communication and attachments. During family sessions the therapist is presented with the opportunity to see such patterns at work, revealing these to family members, creating what Byng-Hall (1991) refers to as family "interactional awareness."

Marvin and Stewart (1990) write that attachment-based family therapy addresses attachment and interactional patterns among *all* members of the family system, and not just dyadic interactions between pairs within the family. As the templates for all attachment relationships are derived from the initial parent–child relationship and the family interactions that follow, they propose that attachment *cannot* be understood fully except as an outcome of a family network of organized relationships. Therefore, attachment-informed family therapists focus on patterns that organize relationships, physical proximity, and contact among all family members in a way that should increase the protection of family members from danger but clearly does not in all cases. This is, of course, especially true in work with the families of juvenile sexual offenders, where the victim is often another family member, and the juvenile sexual offender may himself have been victimized at an earlier time by a family member or close friend of the family. Relevant to a family therapy orientation, a major focus must be on *current* and recurrent patterns of family attachment and interactions, distinguishing between the actual behavior of family members and the effects and function of that of behavior in family interactions.

Marvin and Stewart also recommend that attachment-informed family therapists recognize behavioral regulatory patterns within the family, and the methods that the family (remember, in family therapy, we, in effect, treat the *family* as the patient, as a unit rather than as individuals within the unit) uses to reinforce existing communication systems that regulate and maintain behavior, presumably also including attachment patterns. In particular, they consider that these behavioral, communication, and attachment patterns are contained within and regulated by family scripts, or family-shared internal working models. Avoidant families, for instance, may use distance, coercion, and intentional emotional manipulation to maintain family boundaries and control relationships and roles; anxious, or enmeshed, families may engage in boundary-less, anxiety-provoking, or affective strategies to establish and maintain family connection and limit the ability of family members to develop independently of the family. Regulatory family patterns are described by June Sroufe (1991) who connected the level of family control and affect to resiliency and self-control in adolescent children, concluding that both under- and over-control in children are outcomes of emotionally unsafe families. Chambers et al. (2000) similarly implicated high levels of parental control with affective difficulties in adolescent children, linking the quality of parental care, control, and protection with adolescent psychosocial functioning.

Noting that attachment-based family therapy treats attachment within a family therapy framework, James (1994) writes that children with attachment problems need help connecting to families, and that families can benefit from exploring and understanding who they are as a group. She describes attachment-based family therapy providing a support-ive, structured, and guiding treatment environment in order to: (i) develop individual identity and help to build family relationships, (ii) address family experiences that have contributed to dysfunctional behavior and insecure attachment in the child, as well as limitations in the child's ability to trust others, (iii) mourn damaged and lost family relationships, and (iv) revise, create, and maintain new family relationships. Similarly, Diamond and Stern (2003) describe attachment-based family therapy as focused on repairing ruptured relationships between children and their parents by facilitating discus-sion and interactions about family experiences that have damaged trust, and ongoing con-flicts that have resulted. This is, of course, of particular importance, in families of juvenile sexual offenders, where both the perpetrator and the victim are often members of the same family.

Here, therapy serves a reparative function in families with damaged attachment bonds which, after initial disclosures and descriptions of feelings, eventually involves a parent–child dialogue and the development of more mutual, mature, and reciprocal family relationships. James writes that structured family therapy, which may include shared expe-riential and expressive activities as well as verbal interventions, helps to build family iden-tity, sorting through how things are done in the family, why, and how, and helps to increase family cohesion through a process by which family members reclaim one another and, in particular, the family "claims" the child, increasing security, cohesion, and identity.

Family involvement in the treatment of juvenile sexual offenders must always be con-sidered a central element in any circumstances. In attachment-based treatment in particu-lar, family involvement and treatment is not only inevitable, but important in recognizing and addressing changes in attachment status. If we can improve and enhance the sense of attachment among family members, it will no doubt increase the chances of healthier attachment and connection in the children of those families with whom we work. In turn, in keeping with the principle of equifinality, changes in the attachment status of in-dividual family members will influence changes in the attachment status of other family members, and the family as whole. On a final note, regardless of attachment goals, the recognition and resolution of attachment issues, the clinician should bear in mind these essential principles of family therapy:

1. *The family is the patient.* The clinician must not become distracted or pulled into a view of family problems centered on one individual.
2. *The orientation is in the present.* Family therapy is centered on current functioning, and not the past.
3. *The family is a system equally affected by all members.* The family is a system of interacting people and events, and the development of attitudes, ideas, relationships, and behaviors is the product of the interactional system in which no family member stands alone or unaffected.
4. *Family systems interact with external systems.* Families do not exist in a vacuum and are in constant interaction with the larger neighborhood, community, and cultural systems of which they are a part.
5. *Family culture and multigenerational transmission.* Ideas, attitudes, beliefs, values, and behaviors are shared and transmitted through the family structure, or family culture.

6. *Families are dynamic.* Families, and their internal and external relationships, are constantly changing over time.
7. *Individuation of family members.* In healthy families, members constantly move towards a state of differentiation and individuality without loss of family connection and closeness.

CONCLUSION: RECONSTRUCTING ATTACHMENT

We have come to understand by now that attachment interventions are more than just those interventions and techniques used solely by the individual therapist to build an attached relationship with, and instill a sense of attachment in, the client. Instead, attachment is built through interventions and experiences that permeate the child's ecological environment, that operate on an underlying biological model that resides in the neural substrata, and that attachment building occurs in the environment and through the interactions between the caregiver and the client. Attachment, in this respect is a felt experience, imparted not through words or even behaviors, but through mutual interaction and the hidden dynamics and regulators present in such interactions.

The rebuilding, reshaping, and creation of neural connections and psychological experiences that promote prosocial and affiliative behaviors, and ultimately the attachment experience, is brain based. Attachment building is not based upon people's words or best intentions, no matter how well crafted or well intended. Attachment, then, is more than simply forming attachments with other people. It represents the process by which we are introduced to others and to ourselves, form a sense of identity, and experience and build enduring affinities and connections with others which involve social relatedness and lead to social connection. Through attachment we become social beings.

Of special relevance, attachment is not learned through the spoken word but through perception and experience, developed and embedded through hidden regulators present in our environment. To build attachment, we must recognize that these regulatory and developmental mechanisms are also found within the therapeutic environment and in the treatment milieu, or must be if we are to establish new attachment pathways. As attachment experiences are realized on a preconscious basis and through implicit memory before they enter consciousness or become explicit, we have come to understand that, at its most fundamental level, attachment is a preconscious and implicit process. Our verbal therapy, whether cognitive-behavioral or psychodynamic, can bring attachment more clearly into awareness. But before this can occur we have to treat the development or restoration of attachment at the emotionally experienced, and not the cognitive, level. In this regard, verbal and expressive therapies through the use of their words or experiences do not produce the change we are looking for; they merely serve as the vehicle through which we are trying to influence and bring about change in the internal working model. Using an attachment model, we are really attempting to provide brain-to-brain contact. The therapeutic relationship is thus enormously important, as the crucible within which re-engagement occurs.

When we fold treatment interventions aimed at building and strengthening attachment into a treatment milieu that embodies and transmits ideas of attachment and social connection, we arrive at a seamless program in which the attachment orientation is pervasive and felt throughout the treatment environment, as James (1994) suggests it must be. In this treatment environment, security in relationships is prime, the source from which the development of attunement, empathy, metacognition, self-regulation, and self-responsibility flows. This treatment environment, while minimizing risk factors that contribute to sexual recidivism through programs such as cognitive-behavioral treatment, psychoeducation, and relapse prevention planning, also enhances protective factors by instilling a sense of security in self and trust in others and in relationships, and a subsequent change in the self-view of the juvenile sexual offender. Attachment-based treatment is not going to replace cognitive-behavioral or psychodynamic therapy, nor can it. The attachment-informed model is something that must be integrated *into* existing multimodal and multitheoretical models of treatment, informing and further enhancing integrating and holistic treatment.

With respect to how long it takes to bring about changes in attachment representations and social relatedness, there is no simple answer. Just as sexual offender work takes place in multiple treatment settings, with later treatment building on earlier treatment, and it is not clear how much sex-offender-specific treatment is *enough*, so too is it difficult to say how long attachment-based treatment takes and when it is over. MacDonald (1985) describes the greatest plasticity in human development occurring prior to age 2, writing that after this time and increasingly so, considerable time and energy "must be expended to reverse the effects of early experience," describing the child as "increasingly refractory to change from environmental sources" (p. 104). This certainly suggests that the younger the child, the less difficult to change experiences already integrated in neural templates, arguing, of course, for early intervention. However, MacDonald certainly does not rule out ongoing plasticity, although notes that the longer we wait the more difficult it is to produce change in already established neurobiological systems. As adolescent brains are continuing to develop, as attachment relationships are continuing to change and form during adolescence, and as new cognitive processes are coming on line during adolescence, we can hope for renewed opportunities to introduce change and incorporate new experiences into the developing adolescent brain and personality.

Any work on reconstructing attachment is a worthwhile enterprise. But, no matter how well designed or how intensive, treatment cannot simply fill in blanks in attachment, correct attachment deficits, or transform insecure into secure attachment in short-term treatment, and certainly not through the use of workbook assignments, attachment exercises and roleplays, or discussion alone. It is likely, then, that significant attachment work takes place only over extended periods of time, as attachment experiences develop and the internal working model gradually accommodates and adapts to these new experiences. If we are to work with attachment deficits in the treatment of sexually reactive children and juvenile sexual offenders, we should expect this work to start to take hold in months, not weeks, and be worked through over the course of many more months, passing into the one- and two-year mark. Nevertheless, without studies designed to measure baseline attachment (pre-treatment) and track change through treatment over time, there is no empirical basis for making such a statement. However, it is not likely that we will be able to produce significant changes in attachment patterns in six months, whereas we might make a dent at the nine-month mark. In the end, we must judge the length of time it takes to produce healthier attachments and more secure identities by the behaviors, social interactions, and relationships we see demonstrated by our clients, which we can hope to see enacted during the course of juvenile sex-offender-specific treatment.

If we are witness to the internalization of self-agency, self-efficacy, and prosocial values, reflected over time in the behavior of our clients, then we can see success in treatment, at least insofar as attachment is concerned. And, if we have succeeded in increasing secure attachment and social relatedness to others, then we can reasonably presume that we have diminished the possibility that the client will engage in further sexually abusive behavior. In such circumstances, we will have succeeded in helping the juvenile sexual offender to become more secure in his internal working model and more secure in his relationships with others. However, we cannot fool ourselves into thinking that the development or the establishment of "earned" security is a simple task, no matter how caring, supportive, careful, and attuned we are in our treatment. Our best work offers no guarantee that we can undo perhaps significant damage caused, as Schore and others suggest, to the neurological system that contains representations of attachment.

CHAPTER 19

Conclusions: Getting Connected

Marshall recognized, more than 15 years ago, the value of attachment theory as an explanatory factor in the causation or development of sexually abusive behavior. Nevertheless, despite a recent and markedly increasing interest in (and even "discovery" of) attachment as a causative or contributing factor in the development of sexually abusive behavior, a well-informed understanding of attachment theory seems to be missing in our exploration of possible links. I hope that this book has helped to remedy this problem, and provided the reader with a thorough overview of attachment theory and its possible links to sexually abusive behavior.

However, we have also discussed the weaknesses of attachment theory, both as a theory of human development across the life span and in its limitations as an adequate explanation for sexually abusive behavior in adults or juveniles. I hope we have thus come to recognize that attachment theory does not adequately provide an explanation for the development of sexually abusive behavior, although attachment may certainly be a contributing factor in the development of all sorts of life problems, antisocial and sexually abusive behavior included. Concluding that attachment deficits or insecure attachments lead to sexual aggression is questionable at best, and the idea that insecure attachment is any more relevant to adult sexual offenders than any other criminal population is not only specious, but quite possibly, it seems, inaccurate. Thus far, we are able to draw the same sort of conclusions about the relationship between attachment classifications and juvenile sexual offending.

That is, attachment deficits and insecure attachment may be a necessary condition for the development of juvenile sexual abuse in many children and adolescents, but it is certainly not a sufficient condition. Insecure and impaired attachment seems no more relevant or specific to juvenile sexual offenders than non-sexual juvenile delinquents or non-criminal, but troubled adolescents. Although attachment difficulties appear common to troubled, clinical, and criminal populations, they do not seem to be specific to any particular subpopulation within that larger group, and certainly not to juvenile sexual offenders. Further, substantial problems with the coherence and consistency of attachment theory itself demonstrates that we lack a full or clear understanding about the nature of attachment, certainly past early childhood, limiting its value as a tool to be applied to causative explanations for sexually abusive behavior.

In discussing an attachment-informed approach to the treatment of juvenile sexual offenders, I am proposing that attachment deficits are not *the* thing that leads to sexually abusive or other antisocial behaviors, just as attachment-related treatment is not *the* thing that will prevent sexual offense recidivism. Instead, I conclude, not that attachment deficits are irrelevant to our understanding of sexual abuse, but that insecure attachment and related attachment difficulty is just one element in a complex pathway that, for some, leads to sexual aggression. Nevertheless, although attachment is not *the* thing that leads to sexually abusive behavior, if understood and applied carefully attachment theory offers a powerful and useful way to understand current functioning and behavior in light of social connectedness and internalized representations of self and others. That is, although attachment difficulties are not the direct cause of sexually abusive behavior, attachment theory is nonetheless capable of providing an important explanatory link in understanding the etiology of sexual aggression.

Similarly, attachment-based treatment is not likely to solve or cure the problem. However, it does offer a powerful means for understanding prior behaviors and development, as well as helping to instill a sense of self, others, and values that may go a long way towards preventing future sexually abusive behavior, as well as other antisocial and self-destructive behaviors. Such treatment may also enhance the possibility and likelihood that our kids will lead healthier "good lives,"[1] of particular relevance when we realize that juvenile sexual offenders are more likely to engage in ongoing *non*-sexual behavioral problems than sexually abusive behavior. Hence, the treatment of attachment deficits and related difficulties in juvenile sexual offenders is relevant to and addresses the *whole* person, rather than just his sexually offensive behaviors.

As the reader cannot fail to have noticed, much of this book has been about attachment theory, rather than juvenile sexual offending. This is because attachment theory is a model of psychological development whose ideas we must apply to sexually abusive youth. Once learned, I hope that the reader will be able to apply the ideas and nuances of attachment-driven identity formation. Perhaps more importantly, I hope the reader will be able to apply an attachment-informed framework to understanding the subtleties that drive behavior, including, but not exclusively, sexually abusive behavior, that can then help us to understand our clients and how to plan treatment interventions. It is unlikely, however, that an attachment-informed treatment alone is going to reclaim those youth who have been attachment deprived, or who have troubled attachments. But just as attachment difficulties set the path for later difficulties in life, an attachment-informed therapy and the rehabilitation of attachment, social connection, and social relatedness can only set the path for positive outcomes, although without other forces acting upon that pathway there is no guarantee that life will continue to unfold in a prosocial manner.

We've come to understand attachment, then, as a less straightforward and far more complex and amorphous construct than we perhaps imagined. In many ways, it is the ultimate reflection of the relationship between the individual and society, because attachment seems to reside both within the individual and in the interaction between the individual and his or her environment. From an ecological perspective, we see that individuals do not exist alone and that everything about the individual as a social being, attachment included, is a reflection of the interactions and transactions between individuals and their environment, as well as transactions and interactions *within* the environment.

---

[1] The term is borrowed from the "good lives" model for the treatment and rehabilitation of adult sexual offenders, described by Ward and Stewart (2003).

We see also how attachment, to some degree, sets the pace for and shapes the pathway along which we develop. This is a self-reinforcing pathway, to a great degree dependent upon how the foundations for the pathway were first laid. However, although we can see certain trajectories developing, even early in life, we recognize that forces other than attachment act upon the pathway to reshape, redirect, or solidify it, in a positive or negative direction. Although we understand that insecure attachment itself is not pathological, as we move along our self-reinforcing developmental pathways, the combination of insecure attachment and other risk factors generates, in some cases, pathological thinking, behavior, and relationships. Attachment theory also allows us to see that people are able to victimize others either because they fail to experience other people *as* people (and, therefore, can objectify and turn them into objects, sometimes at will, as when we switch off our empathy), or because people's own needs are so great that they are blinded to the needs of others.

Attachment theory is not a technique. Instead, it is a tool that can help us to recognize *how* connections are made, how they are damaged, and how they took shape in each individual with whom we work. An attachment-informed framework can help us to better see and understand our clients, and help us to recognize how to re-form or re-activate that sense of being understood and thus become more attached to others. Attachment theory can teach us how to build our treatment programs, so that behind technique lies connection. It is actually far more useful to think of attachment work as being aimed at the internal working model, rather than attachment per se. If you accept the idea that a mental map exists, such as the IWM—itself neurologically hard wired into the brain—then we are dealing with a far more concrete construct than "attachment." In this case, attachment is embedded within the IWM, and does not stand alone. By working on our understanding of the IWM and by seeking to reform the experiences, representations, and mental scripts contained within the IWM, we can more clearly grasp how we may actually change patterns of social connection and relatedness, and hence the experience of attachment. We cannot change or re-create prior attachment experiences and the formation of the early mental working model, but we *can* work with the current working model to promote change and rehabilitate attitudes, expectation, relationships, and behavior.

In the end, attachment theory is found not to be the white horse that appears on the treatment horizon to bring us the answers we seek, nor, as Greenberg (1999) warned, the "Holy Grail of psychopathology." Nevertheless, it does offer tremendous power and amplifies the capacity of the clinician and treatment team to understand human behavior and relationships, and over time implement treatment interventions that we hope will lead to change. I end this book as I began it in the introduction. It is not through our therapeutic technique that we are likely to produce changes in antisocial behavior or close the gap between people that allows one person to take advantage of and victimize another. Treatment technique allows us to reach and deliver messages to those parts of the human psyche that underlie behavior, but it is attachment to others and social relatedness that dissolves the emotional distance and detachment that must exist between perpetrator and victim for crime to occur. It is through the driving force of relationships and *feeling* connected to others that we are most likely to bring about change and stand the best chance of eliminating sexually abusive behavior.

Bibliography

Abel, G. G., Osborn, C. A., & Twigg, D. A. (1993). Sexual assault through the life span: Adult offenders with juvenile histories. In H. E. Barbaree, W. L. Marshall, & S. M. Hudson (Eds), *The juvenile sex offender* (pp. 104–117). New York: Guilford.

Ablon, J. S. & Jones, E. E. (1998). How expert clinicians' prototypes of an ideal treatment correlate with outcome in psychodynamic and cognitive-behavioral therapy. *Psychotherapy Research, 8*, 71–83.

Adam, K. S., Sheldon-Keller, A. E., & West, M. (2000). Attachment organization and vulnerability to loss, separation, and abuse in disturbed adolescents. In S. Goldberg, R. Muir, & J. Kerr (Eds), *Attachment theory: Social, developmental, and clinical perspectives* (pp. 309–341). Hillsdale, NJ: The Analytic Press.

Adam, K. S., Sheldon-Keller, A. E., & West, M. (1996). Attachment organization and history of suicidal behavior in clinical adolescents. *Journal of Consulting and Clinical Psychology, 64*, 264–272.

Adolphs, R. & Damasio, A. R. (2000). Neurobiology at a systems level. In J. C. Borod (Ed.), *The neuropsychology of emotions* (pp. 194–213). New York: Oxford University Press.

Agnew, R. (1997). The nature and determinants of strain: Another look at Durkheim and Merton. In N. Passas & R. Agnew (Eds), *The future of anomie theory* (pp. 27–51). Boston, MA: Northeastern University Press.

Agnew, R. & Passas, N. (1997). *The future of anomie theory.* Boston, MA: Northeastern University Press.

Ainsworth, M. D. S. (1969). Object relations, dependency, and attachment: A theoretical review of the infant-mother relationship. *Child Development, 40*, 969–1025.

Ainsworth, M. D. S. (1988, January). *On Security.* Unpublished position paper from the Stony Brook Winter Attachment Conference, Stony Brook, NY. Retrieved August 2004 from SUNY Stony Brook Attachment Lab Website: http://www.psychology.sunysb.edu/attachment/pdf/mda_security.pdf.

Ainsworth, M. D. S. (1989). Attachments beyond infancy. *American Psychologist, 44* (4), 709–716.

Ainsworth, M. D. S., Blehar, M. C., Everett, W., & Wall, S. (1978). *Patterns of Attachment: A psychological study of the strange situation.* Hillsdale, NJ: Lawrence Erlbaum Associates.

Alexander, P. C. (1992). Application of attachment theory to the study of sexual abuse. *Journal of Consulting and Clinical Psychology, 60* (2), 185–195.

Allen, J. A. & Land, D. (1999). Attachment in adolescence. In J. Cassidy & P. R. Shaver (Eds), *Handbook of attachment: Theory, research, and clinical application* (pp. 319–335). New York: Guilford.

Allen, J. G. (1995). *Coping with trauma: A guide to self understanding.* Washington, DC: American Psychiatric Press.

Allen, J. P., Hauser, S. T., & Borman-Spurrell, E. (1996). Attachment theory as a framework for understanding sequelae of severe adolescent psychopathology: An 11-year follow-up study. *Journal of Consulting and Clinical Psychology, 64*, 254–263.

Allen, J. P., Marsh, P., McFarland, C., McElhaney, K. B., Land, D. J., Jodl, K. M., & Peck, S. (2002). Attachment and autonomy as predictors of the development of social skills and delinquency during midadolescence. *Journal of Consulting & Clinical Psychology, 70* (1), 56–66.

Allen, J. P., Moore, C., Kuperminc, G., & Bell, K. (1998) Attachment and adolescent psychosocial functioning. *Child Development, 69*, 1406–1419.

Allen, J. S., Bruss, J., & Damasio, H. (2004, May–June). The structure of the human brain. *American Scientist, 92*, 246–253.

Amen, D. G. (1998). *Change your brain, change your life.* New York: Three Rivers Press.

American Psychiatric Association (2000). *Diagnostic and statistical manual of mental disorders* (4th edn text revision). Washington, DC: Author.

Amini, F., Lewis, T., Lannon, R., Louie, A., Baumbacher, G., McGuiness, T., & Schiff, E. Z. (1996). Affect, attachment, memory: contribution toward psychobiologic integration. *Psychiatry, 59*, 213–239.

Anderson, D. & Dodgson, P. G. (2002). Empathy deficits, self-esteem, & cognitive distortions in sexual offenders. In Y. Fernandez (Ed.), *In their shoes* (pp. 73–90). Oklahoma City, OK: Wood "N" Barnes Publishing.

Anthony, E. J. (1987). Risk, vulnerability, and resilience: An overview. In E. J. Anthony & B. J. Cohler (Eds), *The invulnerable child* (pp. 3–48). New York: Guilford.

Armsden, G. C. & Greenberg, M. T. (1987). The inventory of parent and peer attachment: Relationships to well-being in adolescence. *Journal of Youth and Adolescence, 16*, 427–454.

Armsden, G. C., McCauley, E., Greenberg, M. T., Burke, P. M., & Mitchell, J. R. (1990). Parent and peer attachment in early adolescent depression. *Journal of Abnormal Child Psychology, 18*, 683–697.

Asay, T. P. & Lambert, M. L. (1999). The empirical case for the common factors in therapy: Quantitative finding. In M. A. Hubble, B. L. Duncan, & S. D. Miller (Eds), *The heart and soul of change: What works in therapy* (pp. 23–55). Washington, DC: American Psychological Association.

Association for Treatment & Training in the Attachment of Children (2004). *Attachment and reactive attachment disorder.* Retrieved October 2004 from http://www.attach.org.

Atkinson, L. & Goldberg, S. (2004). Applications of attachment: The integration of developmental and clinical traditions. In L. Atkinson & S. Goldberg (Eds), *Attachment issues in psychopathology and intervention* (pp. 3–25). Mahwah, NJ: Erlbaum.

Bachelor, A. & Horvath, A. (1999). The therapeutic relationship. In M. A. Hubble, B. L. Duncan, & S. D. Miller (Eds), *The heart and soul of change: What works in therapy* (pp. 133–178). Washington, DC: American Psychological Association.

Bailey, S. (2000). Sadistic, sexual and violent acts in the young. In C. Itzen (Ed.), *Home truths about child sexual abuse: Influencing policy and practice* (pp. 200–221). London: Routledge.

Baker, E. & Beech, A. R. (2004). Dissociation and variability of adult attachment dimensions and early maladaptive schemas in sexual and violent offenders. *Journal of Interpersonal Violence, 19*, 1119–1136.

Balbernie, R. (2001). Circuits and circumstances: The neurobiological consequences of early relationship experiences and how they shape behaviour. *Journal of Child Psychotherapy, 27*, 237–255.

Balbernie, R. (2002). *The importance of the early years and evidence-based practice.* London: The Child Psychotherapy Trust.

Baldwin, M. W. & Fehr, B. (1995) On the instability of attachment style ratings. *Personal Relationships, 2*, 247–261.

Bartholomew, K. (2004). *Self-report measures of adult attachment.* Retrieved October 2004 from Simon Fraser University, Department of Psychology, Bartholomew Research Lab, Website: http://www2.sfu.ca/psychology/groups/faculty/bartholomew/research/attachment/selfreports.htm.

Bartholomew, K. & Horowitz, L. M. (1991). Attachment styles among young adults: A test of a four-category model. *Journal of Personality and Social Psychology, 61* (2), 226–244.

Bartholomew, K. & Shaver, P. R. (1998). Methods of assessing adult attachment: Do they converge? In J. A. Simpson & W. S. Rholes (Eds), *Attachment theory and close relationships* (pp. 25–45). New York: Guilford.

Bates, J. E. & Bayles, K. (1988). Attachment and the development of behavior problems. In J. Belsky & T. Nezworski (Eds), *Clinical implications of attachment* (pp. 253–299). Hillsdale, NJ: Erlbaum.

Bear, M. F., Connors, B., & Paradiso, M. (1996). *Neuroscience: Exploring the brain.* Philadelphia, PA: Lippincott, Williams & Wilkins.

Beauregard, E., Lussier, P., & Proulx, J. (2004). An exploration of developmental factors related to deviant sexual preferences among adult rapists. *Sexual Abuse: A Journal of Research and Treatment, 16,* 151–161.

Beck, A. T. (1979). *Cognitive treatment and the emotional disorders.* New York: Meridian.

Beck, J. S. (1995). *Cognitive therapy: Basics and beyond.* New York: Guilford Press.

Beech, A. R. & Mitchell, I. J. (2005). A neurobiological perspective on attachment problems in sexual offenders and the role of selective serotonin re-uptake inhibitors in treatment of such problems. *Clinical Psychology Review, 25,* 153–182.

Belsky, J. (1999a). Interactional and contextual determinants of attachment security. In J. Cassidy & P. R. Shaver (Eds), *Handbook of attachment: Theory, research, and clinical application* (pp. 249–264). New York: Guilford.

Belsky, J. (1999b). Modern evolutionary theory and patterns of attachment. In J. Cassidy & P. R. Shaver (Eds), *Handbook of attachment: Theory, research, and clinical application* (pp. 141–161). New York: Guilford.

Belsky, J. & Nezworski, T. (1988). *Clinical implications of attachment.* Hillsdale, NJ: Erlbaum.

Belsky, J., Campbell, S. B., Cohn, J. F., & Moore, G. (1996). Instability of infant–parent attachment security. *Developmental Psychology, 32,* 921–924.

Belsky, J., Steinberg, L., & Draper, P. (1991). Childhood experience, interpersonal development, and reproductive strategy: An evolutionary theory of socialization. *Child Development, 62,* 647–670.

Benoit, D. & Parker, K. (1994). Stability and transmission of attachment across three generations. *Child Development, 65,* 1444–1456.

Blatz, W. E. (1966). *Human security: Some reflections.* Toronto, Canada: University of Toronto Press.

Bogaerts, S., Vervaeke, G., & Goethals, J. (2004). A comparison of relational attitude and personality disorder in the explanation of child abuse. *Sexual Abuse: A Journal of Research and Treatment, 16,* 37–47.

Bolen, R. M. (2000). Validity of attachment theory. *Trauma, Violence, and Abuse, 1,* 128–153.

Bordin, E. S. (1976). The generalizability of the psychoanalytical concept of the working alliance. *Psychotherapy: Theory, Research, and Practice, 16,* 252–260.

Borod, J. C. & Madigan, N. K. (2000). Neuropsychology of emotion and emotional disorders: An overview and research directions. In J. C. Borod (Ed.), *The neuropsychology of emotions* (pp. 3–28). New York: Oxford University Press.

Bowlby, J. (1969). *Attachment and loss, Vol. 1: Attachment* (2nd edn). New York: Basic Books.

Bowlby, J. (1973). *Attachment and loss, Vol. 2: Separation: Anxiety and anger.* New York: Basic Books.

Bowlby, J. (1979). *The making and breaking of affectional bonds.* London: Routledge.

Bowlby, J. (1980). *Attachment and loss, Vol. 3. Loss: Sadness and depression.* New York: Basic Books.

Bowlby, J. (1986). The nature of the child's tie to his mother. In P. Buckley (Ed.), *Essential papers on object relations* (pp. 153–199). New York: New York University Press.

Bowlby, J. (1988). *A secure base: Clinical applications of attachment theory.* London: Routledge.

Bremner, J. D., Innis, R. B., & Charney, D. S. (1995). MRI-based measurement of hippocampal volume in patients with combat-related posttraumatic stress disorder. *American Journal of Psychiatry, 152,* 973–981.

Bremner, J. D., Innis, R. B., & Charney, D. S. (1996). Dr. Bremner and colleagues reply: MRI-based measurement of hippocampal volume in patients with combat-related posttraumatic stress disorder. *American Journal of Psychiatry, 153,* 1658–1659.

Brennan, K. A., Clark, C. L., & Shaver, P. R. (1998). Self-report measurement of adult attachment: An integrative overview. In J. A. Simpson & W. S. Rholes (Eds), *Attachment theory and close relationships* (pp. 46–76). New York: Guilford.

Bretherton, I. & Munholland, K. A. (1999). Internal working models in attachment relationships: A construct revisited. In J. Cassidy & P. R. Shaver (Eds), *Handbook of attachment: Theory, research, and clinical application* (pp. 89–111). New York: Guilford.

Brisch, K. H. (1999). *Treating attachment disorders: From theory to therapy.* New York: Guilford.

Bronfenbrenner, U. (1979). *The ecology of human development: Experiments in human behavior.* Cambridge, MA: Harvard University Press.

Brown, J. D. & Keller, S. N. (2000, September/October). Can the mass media be healthy sex educators? *Family Planning Perspectives, 32,* 255–256.

Bruner, J. (1966). *Toward a theory of instruction.* Cambridge, MA: Belknap Press.

Buckley, P. (1986). *Essential papers on object relations.* New York: New York University Press.

Burk, L. R. & Burkhart, B. R. (2003). Disorganized attachment as a diathesis for sexual deviance: Developmental experience and the motivation for sexual offending. *Aggression and Violent Behavior, 8,* 487–511.

Burton, D. L. & Meezan, W. (2004). Revisiting recent research on social learning theory as an etiological proposition for sexually abusive male adolescents. *Journal of Evidence-based Social Work, 1,* 41–80.

Byng-Hall, J. (1991). The application of attachment theory to understanding and treatment in family therapy. In C. M. Parkes, J. Stevenson-Hinde, & P. Marris (Eds), *Attachment across the life cycle* (pp. 197–213). London: Routledge.

Byng-Hall, J. (1999). Family and couple therapy: Toward greater security. In J. Cassidy & P. R. Shaver (Eds), *Handbook of attachment: Theory, research, and clinical application* (pp. 625–645). New York: Guilford.

Cahill, L. (2003). Sex- and hemisphere-related influences on the neurobiology of emotionally influenced memory. *Progress in Neuro-psychopharmacology & Biological Psychiatry, 27,* 1235–1241.

Calder, M. C. (2000). *The complete guide to sexual abuse assessments.* Dorset, England: Russell House Publishing.

Carr, L., Iacoboni, M., Dubeau, M., & Mazziotta, J. C. (2003, April 29). *Proceedings of the National Academy of Sciences (PNAS), 100,* 5497–5502.

Carter, C. S., Lederhendler, I. I., & Kirkpatrick, B. (1997). Introduction. In C. S. Carter., I. I. Lederhendler, & B. Kirkpatrick (Eds), *The integrative neurobiology of affiliation* (pp. xiii–xviii). New York: The New York Academy of Sciences.

Castonguay, L. G., Goldfried, M. R., Wiser, S., Raue, P. J., & Hayes, A. M. (1996). Predicting the effect of cognitive therapy for depression: A study of unique and common factors. *Journal of Consulting and Clinical Psychology, 64,* 497–504.

Catalano, R. F., Haggerty, K. P., Oesterle, S., Fleming, C. B., & Hawkins, J. D. (2004). The importance of bonding to school for healthy development: Findings from the Social Development Research Group. *Journal of School Health, 74,* 252–261.

Chaffin, M. & Bonner, B. (1998, November). Don't shoot, we're your children. Have we gone too far in our response to adolescent sexual abusers and children with sexual behavior problems? *Child Maltreatment, 3,* 314–316.

Chambers, A., Power, K. G., Loucks, N., & Swanson, V. (2000). Psychometric properties of the Parental Bonding Instrument and its association with psychological distress in a group of incarcerated young offenders in Scotland. *Social Psychiatry and Psychiatric Epidemiology, 35,* 318–325.

Chisholm, J. S. (1996), The evolutionary ecology of attachment organization. *Human Nature, 7,* 1–38.

Chisholm, K. A. (2000). Attachment in children adopted from Romanian orphanages: Two case studies. In P. M. Crittenden & A. H. Claussen (Eds), *The organization of attachment relationships: Maturation, culture, and context* (pp. 171–189). Cambridge, England: Cambridge University Press.

Clarke, L., Ungerer, J. A., Chahoud, K., Johnson, S., & Stiefel, I. (2002). Attention deficit hyperactivity disorder is associated with attachment insecurity. *Clinical Child Psychology and Psychiatry, 7,* 179–198.

Clyman, R. B., Emde, R. N., Kempe, J. E., & Harmon, R. J. (1986). Social reinforcing and social looking among twelve-month-old infants. In T. B. Brazelton & M. W. Yogman (Eds), *Affective development in infancy* (pp. 75–94). Norwood, NJ: Ablex Publishing.

Cohen, L. B., DeLoache, J. S., & Strauss, M. S. (1979). Infant visual perception. In J. D. Osofsky (Ed.), *Handbook of infant development* (pp. 393–438). New York: John Wiley & Sons.

Colin, V. L. (1996). *Human attachment.* New York: McGraw-Hill.

Commission on Children at Risk (2003). *Hardwired to connect.* New York: Institute for American Values.

Connolly, M. (2004). Developmental trajectories and sexual offending. *Qualitative Social Work, 3,* 39–59.

Craik, K. J. W. (1952). *The nature of explanation.* Cambridge, England: Cambridge University Press.

Craissati, J., McGlurg, G., & Browne, K. (2002). Characteristics of perpetrators of child sexual abuse who have been sexually victimized as children. *Sexual Abuse: A Journal of Research and Treatment, 14,* 225–239.

Creeden, K. (2005). Integrating trauma and attachment research into the treatment of sexually abusive youth. In M. C. Calder (Ed.), *Children and young people who sexually abuse: New theory, research and practice developments* (pp. 196–210). Dorset, England: Russell House Publishing.

Creeden, K. (in press). The neurological impact of trauma and attachment experiences: Implications for understanding and treating sexual behavior problems. In Schwartz, B. K. (Ed.), *The sex offender: Volume 5.* Kingston, NY: Civic Research Institute.

Crittenden, P. M. (1997). Patterns of attachment and sexual behavior: Risk of dysfunction versus opportunity for creative integration. In L. Atkinson & K. J. Zucker (Eds), *Attachment and psychopathology* (pp. 47–93). New York: Guilford.

Crittenden, P. M. (2000a). A dynamic-maturational approach to continuity and change in patterns of attachment. In P. M. Crittenden & A. H. Claussen (Eds), *The organization of attachment relationships: Maturation, culture, and context* (pp. 343–383). Cambridge, England: Cambridge University Press.

Crittenden, P. M. (2000b). Attachment and psychopathology. In S. Goldberg, R. Muir, & J. Kerr (Eds), *Attachment theory: Social, developmental, and clinical perspectives* (pp. 367–406). Hillsdale, NJ: The Analytic Press.

Crittenden, P. M. (2000c). Introduction. In P. M. Crittenden & A. H. Claussen (Eds), *The organization of attachment relationships: Maturation, culture, and context* (pp. 1–10). Cambridge, England: Cambridge University Press.

Crittenden, P. M. (2001). Transformations in attachment relationships in adolescence: Adaptation versus need for psychotherapy (Transformaciones en las relaciones de apego en la adolescencia: Adaptación frente a necesidad de psicoterapia). *Revista de Psicoterapia, 12,* 33–62.

Crittenden, P. M. (in press). Why do inadequate parents do what they do? In O. Mayseless (Ed.), *Parenting representations: Theory, research, and clinical implications.* Cambridge, England: Cambridge University Press.

Crittenden, P. M. & Claussen, A. H. (2000). Adaptation to varied environments. In P. M. Crittenden & A. H. Claussen (Eds), *The organization of attachment relationships: Maturation, culture, and context* (pp. 234–248). Cambridge, England: Cambridge University Press.

Crowell, J. A. & Treboux, D. (1995). A review of adult attachment measures: Implications for theory and research. *Social Development, 4,* 294–327.

Crowell, J. A., Treboux, D., & Waters, E. (2002). Stability of attachment representations: The transition to marriage. *Developmental Psychology, 38,* 467–479.

Damasio, A. R. (1994). *Descartes' error: Emotion, reason, and the human brain.* NY: HarperCollins Quill.

Damasio, A. (1999). *The feeling of what happens: Body and emotion in the making of consciousness.* San Diego, CA: Harcourt.

Damasio, A. (2003). *Looking for Spinoza: Joy, sorrow, and the feeling brain.* San Diego, CA: Harcourt.

Davila, J., Burge, D., & Hammen, C. (1997). Why does attachment style change? *Journal of Personality and Social Psychology, 73* (4), 826–838.

Davis, M. H. (1996). *Empathy: A social psychological approach.* Boulder, CO: Westview Press.

Davis, D., Shaver, P. R., & Vernon, M. L. (2004). Attachment style and subjective motivations for sex. *Personality and Social Psychology Bulletin, 30,* 1076–1090.

Day, R. W. & Sparacio, R. T. (1989) Structuring the counseling process. In W. Dryden (Ed.), *Key issues for counselling in action* (pp. 16–25). London: Sage.

DeBellis, M. D., Baum, A. S., Birmaher, B., Keshavan, M. S., Eccard, C. H., Boring, A. M., Jenkins, F. J., & Ryan, N. D. (1999a). Developmental traumatology, Part I: Biological stress systems. *Biological Psychiatry, 45,* 1259–1270.

DeBellis, M. D., Keshavan, M. S., Clark, D. B., Casey, B. J., Giedd, J. N., Boring, A. M., Frustaci, K., & Ryan, N. D. (1999b). Developmental traumatology, Part II: Brain development. *Biological Psychiatry, 45,* 1271–1284.

Delson, N. (2003). *Using conscience as a guide: Enhancing sexual offender treatment in the moral domain.* Holyoke, MA: NEARI Press.

Diamond, G. S. & Stern, R. S. (2003). Attachment-based family therapy for depressed adolescents: Repairing attachment failures. In S. M. Johnson & V. E. Whiffen (Eds), *Attachment processes in couples and family therapy* (pp. 191–212). New York: Guilford.

Doren, D. M. (2002). *Evaluating sex offenders: A manual for civil commitments and beyond.* Thousand Oaks, CA: Sage.

D'Orazio, D. (2002). *A comparative analysis of empathy in sexually offending and non-offending juvenile and adult males.* Unpublished doctoral dissertation. California School of Professional Psychology at Alliant University, Fresno.

Drake, C. R. & Ward, T. (2003a). Practical and theoretical roles for the formulation based treatment of sexual offenders. *International Journal of Forensic Psychology, 1,* 71–84.

Drake, C. R. & Ward, T. (2003b). Treatment models for sexual offenders. In T. Ward, D. R. Laws., & S. M. Hudson (Eds), *Sexual deviance: Issues and controversies* (pp. 226–243). Thousand Oaks, CA: Sage.

Dryden, W. (1989). The therapeutic alliance as an integrating framework. In W. Dryden (Ed.), *Key issues for counselling in action* (1–15). London: Sage.

Dunn, J. (1987). The beginnings of moral understanding: Development in the second year. In J. Kagan & S. Lamb (Eds), *The emergence of morality in young children* (pp. 91–112). Chicago, IL: University of Chicago Press.

Dunn, J. (1993). *Young children's relationships: Beyond attachment.* Newbury Park, CA: Sage.

Durkheim, E. (1893/1997). *The division of labor in society.* New York: The Free Press.

Durkheim, E. (1897/1951). *Suicide: A study in sociology.* New York: The Free Press.

Eagle, M. & Wolitzky, O. (1997). Empathy: A psychoanalytic perspective. In A. C. Bohart & L. S. Greenberg (Eds), *Empathy reconsidered: New directions in psychotherapy* (pp. 217–244). Washington, DC: American Psychological Association.

Egeland, B. & Carlson, E. A. (2004). Attachment and psychopathology. In L. Atkinson & S. Goldberg (Eds), *Attachment issues in psychopathology and intervention* (pp. 27–48). Mahwah, NJ: Erlbaum.

Elbert, T., Heim, S., & Rockstroh, B. (2001). Neural plasticity and development. In C. A. Nelson & M. Luciana (Eds), *Handbook of developmental cognitive neuroscience* (pp. 191–202.). Cambridge, MA: Massachusetts Institute of Technology Press.

Eldridge, H. (2000). Patterns of sexual offending and strategies for effective assessment and intervention. In C. Itzen (Ed.), *Home truths about child sexual abuse: Influencing policy and practice* (pp. 313–334). London: Routledge.

Elliott, D. (1994). *National Youth Survey* [United States]: Wave III, 1978. [Computer file.] ICPSR version. Boulder, CO: University of Colorado, Behavioral Research Institute [producer], 1986. Ann Arbor, MI: Inter-university Consortium for Political and Social Research.

Elliot, D. S., Williams, K. R., & Hamburg, B. (1998). An integrated approach to violence prevention. In D. S. Elliot, B. A. Hamburg, & K. R. Williams (Eds), *Violence in American schools: A new perspective* (pp. 379–386). Cambridge, England: Cambridge University Press.

Emde, R. N., Johnson, W. F., & Easterbrooks, M. A. (1987). In J. Kagan & S. Lamb (Eds), *The emergence of morality in young children* (pp. 245–176). Chicago, IL: University of Chicago Press.

Erikson, E. H. (1959/1980). *Identity and the life cycle*. New York: Norton.

Evergreen Center (2004). *What is attachment disorder?* Retrieved October, 2004, from http://www.attachmentexperts.com/whatisattachment.html.

Fagan, J. & Wilkinson, D. L. (1998). Social contexts and functions of adolescent violence. In D. S. Elliot, B. A. Hamburg, & K. R. Williams (Eds), *Violence in American schools: A new perspective* (pp. 55–93). Cambridge, England: Cambridge University Press.

Fago, D. P. (2003). Evaluation and treatment of neurodevelopmental deficits in sexually aggressive children and adolescents. *Professional Psychology: Research and Practice, 34,* 248–257.

Fairbairn, W. R. D. (1952). *Psychoanalytic studies of the personality*. London: Tavistock/Routledge.

Fernandez, Y. (2002). *In their shoes*. Oklahoma City, OK: Wood "N" Barnes Publishing.

Fernandez, Y. M. & Marshall, W. L. (2003). Victim empathy, social self-esteem, and psychopathy in rapists. *Sexual Abuse: A Journal of Research and Treatment, 15,* 11–26.

Fernandez, Y. M., Marshall, W. L., Lightbody, S., & O'Sullivan, C. (1999). The child molester empathy measure: Description and examination of its reliability and validity. *Sexual Abuse: A Journal of Research and Treatment, 11,* 17–31.

Fernandez, Y. M. & Serran, G. (2002). Empathy training for therapists and clients. In Y. Fernandez (Ed.), *In their shoes* (pp. 110–131). Oklahoma City, OK: Wood "N" Barnes Publishing.

Feshbach, N. D. (1997). Empathy: The formative years—implications for clinical practice. In A. C. Bohart & L. S. Greenberg (Eds), *Empathy reconsidered: New directions in psychotherapy* (pp. 33–59). Washington, DC: American Psychological Association.

Fields, R. D. (2004, April). The other half of the brain. *Scientific American, 290,* 54–61.

Fischer, D. & Beech, A. R. (1999). Comparison of sex offenders to nonoffenders on selected psychological measures. *International Journal of Offender Therapy and Comparative Criminology, 43,* 473–491.

Fonagy, P. (1999a). Male perpetrators of violence against women: An attachment theory perspective. *Journal of Applied Psychoanalytic Studies, 1,* 7–27.

Fonagy, P. (1999b). Psychoanalytic theory from the viewpoint of attachment theory and research. In J. Cassidy & P. R. Shaver (Eds), *Handbook of attachment: Theory, research, and clinical application* (pp. 595–624). New York: Guilford.

Fonagy, P. (2001a). *Attachment theory and psychoanalysis*. New York: Other Press.

Fonagy, P. (2001b, March). *Male perpetrators of violence against women: An attachment theory perspective*. Paper presented to the meeting of the Dallas Society of Psychoanalytic Psychology, Dallas, TX.

Fonagy, P. (2004). The developmental roots of violence in the failure of mentalization. In F. Pfafflin & G. Adshead (Eds), *A matter of security: The application of attachment theory to forensic psychiatry and psychotherapy* (pp. 13–56). London: Jessica Kingsley Publishers.

Fonagy, P., Leigh, T., Steele, M., Steele, H., Kennedy, G., Mattoon, M., Target, M., & Gerber, A. (1996). The relation of attachment status, psychiatric classification, and response to psychotherapy. *Journal of Consulting and Clinical Psychology, 64,* 22–31.

Fonagy, P., Steele, M., Steele, H., Leigh, T., Kennedy, R., Mattoon, G., & Target, M. (2000). Attachment, the reflective self, and borderline states: The predictive specificity of the Adult Attachment Interview and pathological emotional development. In S. Goldberg, R. Muir, & J. Kerr (Eds), *Attachment theory: Social, developmental, and clinical perspectives* (pp. 233–278). Hillsdale, NJ: The Analytic Press.

Fonagy, P., Target, M., Steele, M., Steele, H., Leigh, H., Levinson, A., & Kennedy, R. (1997a). Morality, disruptive behavior, borderline personality disorder, crime, and their relationships to security of attachment. In L. Atkinson & K. J. Zucker (Eds), *Attachment and psychopathology* (pp. 223–274). New York: Guilford.

Fonagy, P., Target, M., Steele, M., & Steele, H. (1997b). The development of violence and crime as it relates to security of attachment. In J. D. Osofsky (Ed.), *Children in a violent society* (pp. 150–177b). New York: Guilford.

Forth, A. E., Kosson, D. S., & Hare, R. D. (2003). *Hare PCL: Youth version. Technical manual*. North Tonawanda, NY: Multi-Health Systems (MHS).

Fosha, D. (2003). Dyadic regulation and experiential work with emotion and relatedness in trauma and disorganized attachment. In M. F. Solomon & D. J. Siegel (Eds), *Healing trauma: Attachment, mind, body, and brain* (pp. 221–281). New York: Norton.

Fraley, R. C. & Shaver, P. R. (2000). Adult romantic attachment: Theoretical developments, emerging controversies, and unanswered questions. *Review of General Psychology, 4*, 132–154.

Fraley, R. C. & Spieker, S. J. (2003). What are the differences between dimensional and categorical models of individual differences in attachment? Reply to Cassidy (2003), Cummings (2003), Sroufe (2003), and Waters and Beauchaine (2003). *Developmental Psychology, 39*, 423–429.

Fraley, R. C. & Waller, N. G. (1998). Adult attachment patterns: A test of the typological model. In J. A. Simpson & W. S. Rholes (Eds), *Attachment theory and close relationships* (pp. 77–114). New York: Guilford.

France, K. G. & Hudson, S. M. (1993). The conduct disorders and the juvenile sexual offender. In H. E. Barbaree, W. L. Marshall, & S. M. Hudson (Eds), *The juvenile sex offender* (pp. 225–234). New York: Guilford.

Frick, P. J., Cornell, A. H., Barry, C. T., Bodin, S. D., & Dane, H. A. (2003a). Callous-unemotional traits and conduct problems in the prediction of conduct severity, aggression, and self-report of delinquency. *Journal of Abnormal Child Development, 31*, 457–470.

Frick, P. J., Cornell, A. H., Bodin, S. D., Dane, H. A., Barry, C. T., & Loney, B. R. (2003b). Callous-unemotional traits and developmental pathways to severe aggressive and antisocial behavior. *Developmental Psychology, 39*, 246–260.

Gainotti, G. (2000). Neuropsychological theories of emotion. In J. C. Borod (Ed.), *The neuropsychology of emotions* (pp. 214–236). New York: Oxford University Press.

Giedd, J. N. (2002). *Inside the teenage brain.* Retrieved December 2004 from http://www.pbs.org/wgbh/pages/frontline/shows/teenbrain/interviews/.

Giddens, A. (1984). *The constitution of society: Outline of the theory of structuration.* Berkeley, University of California Press.

Gilligan, C. & Wiggins, G. (1987). In J. Kagan & S. Lamb (Eds), *The emergence of morality in young children* (pp. 277–305). Chicago, IL: University of Chicago Press.

Giovenardi, M., Padoin, M. J., Cadore, L. P., & Lucion, A. B. (1997). Hypothalamic paraventricular nucleus, oxytocin, and maternal aggression in rats. In C. S. Carter, I. I. Lederhendler, & B. Kirkpatrick (Eds), *The integrative neurobiology of affiliation* (pp. 606–609). New York: The New York Academy of Sciences.

Gläscher, J. & Adolphs, R. (2003). Processing of the arousal of subliminal and supraliminal emotional stimuli by the human amygdala. *The Journal of Neuroscience, 23*, 10274–10282.

Goldberg, E. (2001). *The executive brain: Frontal lobes and the civilized mind.* New York: Oxford University Press.

Goldberg, S. (1997). Attachment and childhood behavior problems in normal, at-risk, and clinical samples. In L. Atkinson & K. J. Zucker (Eds), *Attachment and psychopathology* (pp. 171–195). New York: Guilford.

Goldberg, S. (2000a). *Attachment and development.* London: Arnold Publishers.

Goldberg, S. (2000b). Introduction. In S. Goldberg, R. Muir, & J. Kerr (Eds), *Attachment theory: Social, developmental, and clinical perspectives* (pp. 1–15). Hillsdale, NJ: The Analytic Press.

Greenberg, M. T. (1999). Attachment and psychopathology in childhood. In J. Cassidy & P. R. Shaver (Eds), *Handbook of attachment: Theory, research, and clinical application* (pp. 469–496). New York: Guilford.

Greenberg, M. T. & Speltz, M. L. (1988). Attachment and the ontogeny of conduct problems. In J. Belsky & T. Nezworski (Eds), *Clinical implications of attachment* (pp. 177–218). Hillsdale, NJ: Erlbaum.

Greenberg, M. T., DeKlyen., Speltz, M. L., & Endriga, M. C. (1997). The role of attachment processes in externalizing psychopathology in young children. In L. Atkinson & K. J. Zucker (Eds), *Attachment and psychopathology* (pp. 196–222). New York: Guilford.

Greenberg, M. T., Siegel, J., & Leitch, C. (1983). The nature and importance of attachment relationship to parents and peers during adolescence. *Journal of Youth and Adolescence, 12*, 373–386.

Griffin, D. & Bartholomew, K. (1994). Models of the self and other: Fundamental dimensions underlying measures of adult attachment. *Journal of Personality and Social Psychology, 67*, 430–445.

Grossmann, K. E. (2000). The evolution and history of attachment research and theory. In S. Goldberg, R. Muir, & J. Kerr (Eds), *Attachment theory: Social, developmental, and clinical perspectives* (pp. 85–121). Hillsdale, NJ: The Analytic Press.

Grossmann, K. E. & Grossmann, K. (1981). Parent–infant attachment relationship in Bielefeld: A research note. In K. Immelmann, G. W. Barlow, L. Petrinovich, & M. Main (Eds), *Behavioral development: The Bielefeld interdisciplinary project* (pp. 694–699). Cambridge, England: Cambridge University Press.

Grossmann, K. & Grossmann, K. E. (2000). Parents and toddlers at play: Evidence for separate qualitative functioning of the play and the attachment system. In P. M. Crittenden & A. H. Claussen (Eds), *The organization of attachment relationships: Maturation, culture, and context* (pp. 13–37). Cambridge, England: Cambridge University Press.

Hanson, R. K. & Morton-Bourgon, K. (2004). *Predictors of sexual recidivism: An updated meta-analysis.* (Catalog No. PS3-1/2004-2E-PDF), Public Works and Services, Canada.

Hanson, R. F. & Spratt, E. G. (2000). Reactive attachment disorder: What we know about the disorder and implications for treatment. *Child Maltreatment, 5,* 137–145.

Hare, R. D. (1993). *Without conscience: The disturbing world of the psychopaths among us.* New York: Guilford.

Hart, S. D., Watt, K. A., & Vincent, G. M. (2002). Commentary on Seagrave and Grisso: Impressions of the state of the art. *Law and Human Behavior, 26,* 241–246.

Hawkins, J. D., Herrenkohl, T. I., Farrington, D. P., Brewer, D., Catalano, R. F., Harachi, T. W., & Cothern, L. (2000, August). Predictors of youth violence. *OJJDP Bulletin,* Washington, DC: US Department of Justice, Office of Juvenile Justice and Delinquency Prevention.

Hayslett-McCall, K. L. & Bernard, T. J. (2002). Attachment, masculinity, and self-control: A theory of male crime rates. *Theoretical Criminology, 6,* 5–33.

Hesse, E. (1999). The adult attachment interview: Historical and current perspectives. In J. Cassidy & P. R. Shaver (Eds), *Handbook of attachment: Theory, research, and clinical application* (pp. 395–433). New York: Guilford.

Hilburn-Cobb, C. (2004). Adolescent psychopathology in terms of multiple behavioral systems: The role of attachment and controlling strategies and frankly disorganized behavior. In L. Atkinson & S. Goldberg (Eds.), *Attachment issues in psychopathology and intervention* (pp. 95–135). Mahwah, NJ: Erlbaum.

Hinde, R. A. (1982). Attachment: Some conceptual and biological issues. In C. M. Parkes & J. Stevenson-Hinde (Eds), *The place of attachment in human behavior* (pp. 60–76). New York: Basic Books.

Hofer, M. A. (2000). Hidden regulators: Implications for a new understanding of attachment, separation, and loss. In S. Goldberg, R. Muir, & J. Kerr (Eds), *Attachment theory: Social, developmental, and clinical perspectives* (pp. 203–230). Hillsdale, NJ: The Analytic Press.

Hofer, M. A. & Sullivan, R. M. (2001). Toward a neurobiology of attachment. In C. A. Nelson & M. Luciana (Eds), *Handbook of developmental cognitive neuroscience* (pp. 599–616). Cambridge, MA: Massachusetts Institute of Technology Press.

Hoffman, M. L. (1976). Empathy, role-taking, guilt, and development of altruistic motives. In T. Lickona (Ed.), *Moral development and behavior* (pp. 124–143). New York: Holt, Rinehart, & Winston.

Hoffman, M. L. (1987). The contribution of empathy to justice and moral judgment. In M. Eisenberg & J. Strayer (Eds), *Empathy and its development* (pp. 47–80). Cambridge, England: Cambridge University Press.

Hoffman, M. L. (2000). *Empathy and moral development: Implications for caring and justice.* Cambridge, England: Cambridge University Press.

Holmes, J. (2001). *The search for the secure base: Attachment theory and psychotherapy.* Hive, England: Brunner-Routledge.

Holmes, J. (2004). Disorganized attachment and Borderline Personality Disorder: A clinical perspective. *Attachment & Human Development, 6,* 181–190.

Holmes, J. & Bateman, A. (2002). *Integration in psychotherapy: Models and methods.* Oxford, England: Oxford University Press.

Hubble, M. A., Duncan, B. L., & Miller, S. D. (1999). *The heart and soul of change: What works in therapy.* Washington, DC: American Psychological Association.

Hudson, S. M. & Ward, T. (1997). Intimacy, loneliness, and attachment style in sexual offenders. *Journal of Interpersonal Violence, 12*, 323–339.

Hudson, S. M. & Ward, T. (2000). Interpersonal competency in sex offenders. *Behavior Modification, 24*, 494–527.

Hunter, J. A., Figueredo, A. J., Malamuth, N. M., & Becker, J. V. (2004). Developmental pathways in youth sexual aggression and delinquency: Risk factors and mediators. *Journal of Family Violence, 19*, 233–242.

Insel, T. R. (2000). Toward a neurobiology of attachment. *Review of General Psychiatry, 4*, 176–185.

Institute for Attachment and Child Development (2004). *What is attachment disorder?* Retrieved October 2004 from http://www.instituteforattachment.org./whatisit.htm.

Jahromi, L. B., Putnam, S. B., & Stifter, C. A. (2004), Maternal regulation of infant reactivity from 2 to 6 months. *Developmental Psychology, 40,* pp. 477–487.

James, B. (1994). *Handbook for treatment of attachment-trauma problems in children.* New York: The Free Press.

Jensen, E. (2000). *Brain-based learning.* San Diego, CA: The Brain Store.

Johnson, S. M. (2003). Introduction to attachment: A therapist's guide to primary relationships and their renewal. In S. M. Johnson & V. E. Whiffen (Eds), *Attachment processes in couples and family therapy* (pp. 3–17). New York: Guilford.

Johnson-Laird, P. N. (1983). *Mental models: Towards a cognitive science of language, inference, and consciousness.* Harvard, MA: Harvard University Press.

Kagan, J. (1979). Overview: Perspectives on human infancy. In J. D. Osofsky (Ed.), *Handbook of infant development* (pp. 1–25). New York: John Wiley & Sons.

Kagan, J. (1984). *The nature of the child.* New York: Basic Books.

Kagan, J. (1996). Three pleasing ideas. *American Psychologist, 51* (9), 901–908.

Karen, R. (1994). *Becoming attached: First relationships and how they shape our capacity to love.* New York: Oxford University Press.

Kazdin, A. E. & Bass, D. (1989). Power to detect differences between alternative treatments in comparative psychotherapy outcome research. *Journal of Consulting and Clinical Psychology, 57*, 138–147.

Kear-Colwell, J. & Boer, D. P. (2000). The treatment of pedophiles: Clinical experience and implications of recent research. *International Journal of Offender Therapy and Comparative Criminology, 44*, 593–605.

Kear-Colwell, J. & Sawle, G. A. (2001). Coping strategies and attachment in pedophiles: Implications for treatment. *International Journal of Offender Therapy and Comparative Criminology, 45*, 171–182.

Keenan, T. & Ward, T. (2000). A theory of mind perspective on cognitive, affective, and intimacy deficits in child sexual offenders. *Sexual Abuse: A Journal of Research and Treatment, 12*, 49–60.

Keijsers, G. P. J., Schaap, C. P. D. R., & Hoogduin, C. A. L. (2000). The impact of interpersonal patient and therapist behavior on outcome in cognitive-behavior therapy: A review of empirical studies. *Behavior Modification, 24*, 264–297.

Kelly, V. (in press). Introduction to attachment therapy with children. In K. Seifert (Ed.), *Troubled children in a troubled world.* Champaign, IL: Research Press.

Kenny, M. E. (1987). The extent and function of parental attachment among first-year college students. *Journal of Youth and Adolescence, 16*, 17–29.

Kenny, M. E. (1994). Quality and correlates of parental attachment among late adolescents. *Journal of Counseling and Development, 72*, 399–403.

Kernberg, O. (1976). *Object-relations theory and clinical psychoanalysis.* New York: Jason Aronson.

Kerns, K. A., Tomich, P. L., Aspelmeier, J. E., & Contreras, J. M. (2000). Attachment-based assessments of parent–child relationships in middle childhood. *Developmental Psychology, 36*, 614–626.

Kerr, S., Goldfried, M. R., Hayes, A. M., Castonguay, L. G., & Goldsamt, L. A. (1992). Interpersonal and intrapersonal focus in cognitive-behavioral and psychodynamic-interpersonal therapies: A preliminary analysis of the Sheffield Project. *Psychotherapy Research, 4*, 266–276.

Kirby, D. (2001, November/December) Understanding what works and what doesn't in reducing adolescent sexual risk-taking. *Family Planning Perspectives, 33*, 276–281.

Knight, R. A. & Prentky, R. A. (1993). Exploring characteristics for classifying juvenile sexual offenders. In H. E. Barbaree, W. L. Marshall, & S. M. Hudson (Eds), *The juvenile sex offender* (pp. 45–83). New York: Guilford.

Knight, R. A. & Sims-Knight, J. E. (2003). The developmental antecedents of sexual coercion against women: Testing alternative hypotheses with structural equation modeling. In R. A. Prentky, E. S. Janus., & M. C. Seto (Eds), *Sexually coercive behavior: Understanding and management: Vol. 989. Annals of the New York Academy of Sciences* (pp. 72–85). New York: The New York Academy of Sciences.

Knight, R. A. & Sims-Knight, J. E. (2004). Testing an etiological model for juvenile sexual offending against women. In R. Geffner, K. C. Franey, T. G. Arnold, & R. Falconer (Eds), *Identifying and treating youths who sexually offend: Current approaches, techniques, and research*. New York: Haworth Press.

Kohlberg, L. (1976). Moral stages and moralization: The cognitive-developmental approach. In T. Lickona (Ed.), *Moral development and behavior: Theory, research and social issues* (pp. 31–53). New York: Holt, Rinehart, & Winston.

Kohut, H. (1977). *The restoration of the self*. New York: International University Press.

Kozlowska, K. & Hanney, L. (2002). The network perspective: an integration of attachment and family systems theories. *Family Process, 41*, 285–312.

Kunkel, D., Cope-Farrar, K., Biely, E., Farinola, W. J. M., & Donnerstein, E. (2001, February). *Sex on TV (2): A biennial report to the Kaiser Family Foundation*. Menlo Park, CA: The Henry J. Kaiser Family Foundation.

Lamb, M. E. (1987) Predictive implications of individual differences in attachment. *Journal of Consulting and Clinical Psychology, 55*, 817–824.

Lambert, M. J. (1992). Implications of outcome research for psychotherapy integration. In J. C. Norcross & M. R. Goldstein (Eds), *Handbook of psychotherapy integration* (pp. 94–129). New York: Basic Books.

Lambert, M. J. & Bergin, A. E. (1993). The effectiveness of psychotherapy. In A. E. Bergin & S. L. Garfield (Eds), *Handbook of psychotherapy and behavior change* (4th edn). (pp. 143–189). New York: John Wiley & Sons.

Laws, R. D., Hudson, S. M., & Ward, T. (2000). The original model of relapse prevention with sexual offenders: Promises unfulfilled. In D. R. Laws, S. M. Hudson, & T. Ward (Eds), *Remaking relapse prevention with sexual offenders: A sourcebook* (pp. 3–24). Thousand Oaks, CA: Sage.

LeDoux, J. (1996). *The emotional brain: The mysterious underpinnings of emotional life*. New York: Touchstone.

LeDoux, J. (2002). *Synaptic self: How our brains become who we are*. New York: Penguin.

Lee, J. K. P., Jackson, H. J., Pattison, P., & Ward, T. (2002). Developmental risk factors for sexual offending. *Child Abuse & Neglect, 26*, 73–92.

Levin, B. L., Hanson, A., Coe, R. D., & Taylor, A. (1998). *Mental health parity: 1998 National and state perspectives*. Tampa, FL: Louis de la Parte Florida Mental Health Institute.

LeVine, R. A. (2002, August). Attachment research as an ideological movement. In F. Rothbaum (Chair), *Attachment and culture: A debate*. Symposium conducted at the 17th biennial meeting of the International Society for the Study of Behavioural Development, Ottawa, Canada.

LeVine, R. A. & Miller, P. M. (1990). Commentary. *Human Development, 33*, 73–80.

Levy, T. M. (2000). *Handbook of attachment interventions*. San Diego: CA: Academic Press.

Levy, T. M. & Orlans, M. (2000). Attachment disorder as an antecedent to violence and antisocial patterns in children. In T. M. Levy (Ed.), *Handbook of attachment interventions* (pp. 1–26). San Diego, CA: Academic Press.

Lewis, D. O., Shanok, S. S., & Pincus, J. H. (1981). Juvenile male assaulters: Psychiatric, neurological, psychoeducational, and abuse factors. In D. O. Lewis (Ed.), *Vulnerabilities to delinquency* (pp. 89–105). Jamaica, NY: Spectrum.

Lewis, M. (1997). *Altering fate: Why the past does not predict the future*. New York: Guilford.

Libbey, H. P. (2004). Measuring student relationships to school: Attachment, binding, connectedness, and engagement. *Journal of School Health, 74*, 274–283.

Lieberman, A. F. & Pawl, J. H. (1988). Clinical applications of attachment theory. In J. Belsky & T. Nezworski (Eds), *Clinical implications of attachment* (pp. 327–351). Hillsdale, NJ: Erlbaum.

Lieberman, A. & Pawl, J. H. (1990). Disorders of attachment and secure base behavior in the second year of life: Conceptual issues and clinical intervention. In M. T. Greenberg, D. Cicchetti, & E. M. Cummings (Eds), *Attachment in the preschool years* (pp. 375–397). Chicago: University of Chicago Press.

Lifton, R. J. (1986). *The Nazi doctors: Medical killing and the psychology of genocide.* New York: Basic Books.

Lifton, R. J. (1993). *The protean self: Human resilience in an age of fragmentation.* Chicago, IL: The University of Chicago Press.

Lindsay, L. (2004) Sex offenders: Conceptualisation of the issues, services, treatment and management. In W. R. Lindsay, J. L. Taylor, & P. Sturmey (Eds), *Offenders with developmental disabilities* (pp. 163–185). Chichester: John Wiley & Sons.

Linehan, M. M. (1993). *Cognitive-behavioral treatment of borderline personality disorder.* New York: Guilford.

Longo, R. E. (2002). A holistic approach to treating young people who sexually abuse. In M. C. Calder (Ed.), *Young people who sexually abuse: Building the evidence base for your practice* (pp. 218–230). Dorset, England: Russell House Publishing.

Looman, J., Abracen, J., DiFazio, R., & Maillet, G. (2004). Alcohol and drug abuse among sexual and nonsexual offenders: Relationship to intimacy deficits and coping strategy. *Sexual Abuse: A Journal of Research and Treatment, 16,* 177–189.

Lopez, F. G. & Glover, M. R. (1993). Self-report measures of parent–adolescent attachment and separation-individuation: A selective review. *Journal of Counseling and Development, 71,* 560–569.

Lyddon, W. J., Bradford, E., & Nelson, J. P. (1993). Assessing adolescent and adult attachment: A review of current self-report measures. *Journal of Counseling and Development, 71,* 390–395.

Lyle, P. N. (2003). *Adult male survivors of childhood sexual abuse: Attachment and sexualized coping in a non-offender sample.* Unpublished master's thesis, Auburn University, AL.

Lyn, T. S. & Burton, D. L. (2004). Adult attachment and sexual offender status. *American Journal of Orthopsychiatry, 74,* 150–159.

Lyn, T. & Burton, D. (in press). Attachment, anger, and anxiety of male sexual offenders. *The Journal of Sexual Aggression.*

Lyons-Ruth, K. (1996). Attachment relationships among children with aggressive behavior problems: The role of disorganized early attachment patterns. *Journal of Consulting and Clinical Psychology, 64,* 64–73.

Lyons-Ruth, K., Alpern, L., & Repacholi, B. (1993). Disorganized infant attachment classification and maternal psychosocial problems as predictors of hostile-aggressive behavior in the preschool classroom. *Child Development, 64,* 572–585.

Lyons-Ruth, K., Easterbrooks, M. A., & Cibelli, C. D. (1997). Infant attachment strategies, infant mental lag, and maternal depressive symptoms predictors of internalizing and externalizing problems of age 7. *Developmental Psychology, 33,* 681–692.

Lyons-Ruth, K., Melnick, S., Bronfen, E., Sherry, S., & Llanas, L. (2004). Hostile–helpless relational models and disorganized attachment patterns between parents and their young children: Review of research and implications for clinical work. In L. Atkinson & S. Goldberg (Eds), *Attachment issues in psychopathology and intervention* (pp. 65–94). Mahwah, NJ: Erlbaum.

MacDonald, K. (1985). Early experience, relative plasticity and social development. In S. Chess & A. Thomas (Eds), *Annual progress in child psychiatry and child development* (pp. 86–110). New York: Brunner/Mazel.

MacLean, P. D. (1978). A mind of three minds: Educating the triune brain. In J. S. Chall & A. F. Mirsky (Eds), *Education and the brain: The seventy-seventh yearbook of the National Society for the Study of Education* (pp. 308–342). Chicago, IL: University of Chicago Press.

Maguire, E. A., Gadian, D. G., Johnsrude, I. S., Good, C. D., Ashburner, J., Frackowiak, R. S. J., et al. (2000, April 11). Navigation-related structural change in the hippocampi of taxi drivers. *Proceedings of the National Academy of Sciences USA, 97,* 4398–4403.

Mahler, M. S., Pine, F., & Bergman, A. (1975). *The psychological birth of the human infant: Symbiosis and individuation.* New York: Basic Books.

Main, M. & Cassidy, J. (1988). Categories of response to reunion with the parent at age 6 predictable from infant attachment classifications and stable over a 1-month period. *Developmental Psychology, 24,* 415–426.

Main, M. & Solomon, J. (1986). Discovery of a new, insecure-disorganized/disoriented attachment pattern. In T. B. Brazelton & M. W. Yogman (Eds), *Affective development in infancy* (pp. 95–124). Norwood, NJ: Ablex Publishing.

Maio, G. R., Fincham, F. D., & Lycett, E. J. (2000). Attitudinal ambivalence toward parents and attachment style. *Personality and Social Psychology Bulletin, 26,* 1451–1464.

Maione, P. V. & Chenail, R. J. (1999). Qualitative inquiry: Research on the common factors. In M. A. Hubble, B. L. Duncan, & S. D. Miller (Eds), *The heart and soul of change: What works in therapy* (pp. 57–88). Washington, DC: American Psychological Association.

Malamuth, N. M. (2003). Criminal and noncriminal sexual aggressors: Integrating psychopathy into a hierarchical-mediational confluence model. In R. A. Prentky, E. S. Janus, & M. C. Seto (Eds), *Sexually coercive behavior: Understanding and management: Vol. 989. Annals of the New York Academy of Sciences* (pp. 33–58). New York: The New York Academy of Sciences.

Mallinckrodt, B., Gantt, D. L., & Coble, H. M. (1995). Attachment patterns in the psychotherapy relationship: Development of the Client Attachment to Therapist Scale. *Journal of Counseling Psychology, 42,* 307–317.

Marrone, M. (1998). *Attachment and interaction.* London: Jessica Kingsley Publishers.

Marsa, F., O'Reilly, G., Carr, A., Murphy, P., O'Sullivan, M., Cotter, A., & Hevey, D. (2004). Attachment styles and psychological profiles of child sex offenders in Ireland. *Journal of Interpersonal Violence, 19,* 228–251.

Marshall, L. (2002). The development of empathy. In Y. Fernandez (Ed.), *In their shoes* (pp. 36–52). Oklahoma City, OK: Wood "N" Barnes Publishing.

Marshall, W. L. (1989). Intimacy, loneliness, and sexual offenders. *Behaviour Research and Therapy, 27,* 491–503.

Marshall, W. L. (2002). Historical foundations and current conceptualizations of empathy. In Y. Fernandez (Ed.), *In their shoes* (pp. 1–15). Oklahoma City, OK: Wood "N" Barnes Publishing.

Marshall, W. L. & Marshall, L. E. (2000). The origins of sexual offending. *Trauma, Violence, and Abuse, 1,* 250–263.

Marshall, W. L. & Mazzucco, A. (1995). Self-esteem and parental attachments in child molesters. *Sexual Abuse: A Journal of Research and Treatment, 7,* 279–285.

Marshall, W. L., Barbaree, H. E., & Fernandez, Y. M. (1995). Some aspects of social competence in sexual offenders. *Sexual Abuse: A Journal of Research and Treatment, 7,* 113–127.

Marshall, W. L., Cripps, E., Anderson, D., & Cortoni, F. A. (1999). Self-esteem and coping strategies in child molesters. *Journal of Interpersonal Violence, 14,* 955–962.

Marshall, W. L. & Eccles, A. (1993). Pavlovian conditioning processes in adolescent sex offenders. In H. E. Barbaree, W. L. Marshall, & S. M. Hudson (Eds), *The juvenile sex offender* (pp. 118–142). New York: Guilford.

Marshall, W. L., Hamilton, K., & Fernandez, Y. (2001). Empathy deficits and cognitive distortions in child molesters. *Sexual Abuse: A Journal of Research and Treatment, 13,* 123–130.

Marshall, W. L., Hudson, S. M., & Hodkinson, S. (1993). The importance of attachment bonds in the development of juvenile sexual offending. In H. E. Barbaree, W. L. Marshall, & S. M. Hudson (Eds), *The juvenile sexual offender* (pp. 164–181). New York: Guilford.

Marshall, W. L., Hudson, S. M., Jones, R., & Fernandez, Y. M. (1995). Empathy in sex offenders. *Clinical Psychology Review. 15,* 99–113.

Marshall, W. L., Serran, G. A., & Cortoni, F. A. (2000). Childhood attachments, sexual abuse, and their relationship to adult coping in child molesters. *Sexual Abuse: A Journal of Research and Treatment, 12,* 17–26

Marvin, R. S. & Stewart, R. B. (1990). A family systems framework for the study of attachment. In M. T. Greenberg, D. Cicchetti, & E. M. Cummings (Eds), *Attachment in the preschool years: Theory, research, and intervention* (pp. 51–86). Chicago: The University of Chicago Press.

Maslow, A. H. (1968). *Toward a psychology of being* (2nd edn). New York: Van Nostrand Rheinhold.

Maslow, A. H. (1970). *Motivation and Personality* (2nd edn). Harper & Row.

Maté, G. (2000). *Scattered: How attention disorder originates and what you can do about it.* New York: Plume.

McCormack, J., Hudson, S. M., & Ward, T. (2002). Sexual offenders' perceptions of their early interpersonal relationships: An attachment perspective. *Journal of Sex Research, 39*, 85–93.

McGrath, R. J., Cumming, G. F., & Burchard, B. L. (2003). *Current practices and trends in sexual abuser management: The Safer Society 2002 nationwide survey.* Brandon, VT: Safer Society Press.

McLean Hospital (2003, November 8). *Adolescent stress can change brain during adulthood.* [Press release]. Belmont, MA: Author.

Mediascope Press (2001). *Issue briefs: Teens, sex and the media.* Studio City, CA: Author.

Mehler, J. & Dupoux, E. (1994). *What infants know: The new cognitive science of early development.* Cambridge, MA: Blackwell Publishers.

Meichenbaum, D. (1977). *Cognitive-behavioral modification: An integrative approach.* New York: Plenum Press.

Meichenbaum, D. (1985). *Stress inoculation training.* New York: Pergamon Press.

Meloy, J. R. (1992). *Violent attachments.* Northvale, NJ: Jason Aronson.

Mercer, J. (2001). Attachment theory using deliberate restraint: An object lesson on the identification of unvalidated treatments. *Journal of Child and Adolescent Psychiatric Nursing, 14*, 105–114.

Mercer, J. (2002). Attachment therapy: A treatment without empirical support. *The Scientific Review of Mental Health Practice, 1*, 9–6.

Miner, M. H. (2004). *Risk for sexual abuse: A study of adolescent offenders.* Grant R49 CE000265 (project period, 8/1/04–7/31/07). National Center for Injury Prevention and Control, Centers for Disease Control and Prevention, Atlanta, GA.

Miner, M. H. & Crimmins, C. L. S. (1997). Adolescent sex offenders: Issues of etiology and risk factors. In B. K. Schwartz & H. R. Cellini (Eds), *The sex offender: Corrections, treatment and legal practice* (pp. 9.1–9.15). Kingston, NJ: Civic Research Institute.

Miner, M. H. & Munns, R. (in press). Isolation and normlessness: Attitudinal comparisons of adolescent sex offenders, juvenile offenders, and nondelinquents. *International Journal of Offender Therapy and Comparative Criminology.*

Miner, M. H. & Swinburne-Romine, J. (2004, October). *Understanding child molesting in adolescence: Testing attachment-based hypotheses.* Presentation at the 8th International Conference of the International Association for the Treatment of Sexual Offenders, Athens, Greece.

Minuchin, S. (1974). *Families and family therapy.* Cambridge, MA: Harvard University Press.

Minuchin, S. & Fishman, C. H. (1981). *Family therapy techniques.* Cambridge, MA: Harvard University Press.

Mischel, W. & Mischel, H. N. (1976). A cognitive social-learning approach to morality and self-regulation. In T. Lickona (Ed.), *Moral development and behavior* (pp. 70–107). New York: Holt, Rinehart, & Winston.

Moretti, M. M. & Holland, R. (2003). The journey of adolescence: Transitions in self within the context of attachment relationships. In S. M. Johnson & V. E. Whiffen (Eds), *Attachment processes in couples and family therapy* (pp. 234–257). New York: Guilford.

Morris, J. S., Öhman, A., & Dolan, R. J. (1998). Conscious and unconscious emotional learning in the human amygdala. *Nature, 393*, 467–470.

Moulden, H. & Marshall, W. L. (2002). Empathy, social intelligence, and aggressive behavior. In Y. Fernandez (Ed.), *In their shoes* (pp. 53–72). Oklahoma City, OK: Wood "N" Barnes Publishing.

Mulloy, R. & Marshall, W. L. (1999). Social functioning. In W. L. Marshall, D. Anderson, & Y. Fernandez (Eds), *Cognitive-behavioral treatment of sexual offenders* (pp. 93–109). Chichester, England: John Wiley & Sons.

National Center for Infants, Toddlers, and Families (1994). *Diagnostic classification of mental health and developmental disorders of infancy and early childhood.* Washington, DC: Author.

National Task Force on Juvenile Sexual Offending (1993). The Revised Report on Juvenile Sexual Offending, 1993, of the National Adolescent Perpetration Network. *Juvenile and Family Court Journal, 44*, 1–120.

Norcross, J. C. (2000). Toward the delineation of empirically based principles in psychotherapy: Commentary on Beutler (2000). *Prevention and Treatment, 3*, Article 28. Retrieved July 2002 from http://www.journals.apa.org/prevention/volume3/pre0030028c.html.

Ochsner, K. N. & Schacter, D. L. (2000). A social cognitive neuroscience approach to emotion and memory. In J. C. Borod (Ed.), *The neuropsychology of emotions* (pp. 163–193). New York: Oxford University Press.

Office of Juvenile Justice and Delinquency Prevention (2000, May). *Children as victims*. (1999 National Report Series Bulletin NCJ 180753). Washington, DC: Office of Juvenile Justice and Delinquency Prevention, US Department of Justice.

Overall, N. C., Fletcher, G. J. O., & Friesen, M. D. (2003). Mapping the intimate relationship mind: Comparisons between three models of attachment representations. *Personality and Social Psychology Bulletin, 12*, 1479–1493.

Panksepp, J., Nelson, E., & Bekkedal, M. (1997). Brain systems for the mediation of social separation-distress and social-reward. In C. S. Carter., I. I. Lederhendler, & B. Kirkpatrick (Eds), *The integrative neurobiology of affiliation* (pp. 78–100s). New York: The New York Academy of Sciences.

Parish, M. & Eagle, M. N. (2003). Attachment to the therapist. *Psychoanalytic Psychology, 20*, 271–286.

Parker, G., Tupling, H., & Brown, L. B. (1979) A parental bonding instrument. *British Journal of Medical Psychology, 52*, 1–10.

Passas, N. (1997). Anomie, reference groups, and relative deprivation. In N. Passas & R. Agnew (Eds), *The future of anomie theory* (pp. 62–94). Boston, MA: Northeastern University Press.

Perry, B. D. & Marcellus, J. E. (1997). The impact of abuse and neglect on the developing brain. *Colleagues for Children, 7*, 1–14, Missouri Chapter of the National Committee to Prevent Child Abuse.

Perry, D. G., Perry, L. C., & Kennedy, E. (1992). Conflict and the development of antisocial behavior. In C. U. Shantz & W. W. Hartup (Eds), *Conflict in child and adolescent development* (pp. 301–329). Cambridge, England: Cambridge University Press.

Piaget, J. (1932/1997). *The moral judgment of the child*. New York: Simon & Schuster.

Piaget, J. (1937/1954). *The construction of reality in the child*. New York: Basic Books.

Piaget, J. & Inhelder, B. (1969). *The psychology of the child*. New York: Basic Books.

Pithers, W. D., Gray, A., Busconi, A., & Houchens, P. (1998). Children with sexual behavior problems: Identification of five distinct child types and related treatment considerations. *Child Maltreatment, 3*, 384–406.

Polan, H. J. & Hofer, M. A. (1999). Psychobiological origins of infant attachment and separation responses. In J. Cassidy & P. R. Shaver (Eds), *Handbook of attachment: Theory, research, and clinical application* (pp. 162–180). New York: Guilford.

Prendergast, W. E. (1993). *The merry-go-round of sexual abuse: Identifying and treating survivors*. New York: Haworth Press.

Prentky, R., Harris, B., Frizzell, K., & Righthand, K. (2000). An actuarial procedure for assessing risk with juvenile sexual offenders. *Sexual Abuse: A Journal of Research and Treatment, 12*, 71–93.

Print, B. & Morrison, T. (2000). Treating adolescents who sexually abuse others. In C. Itzen (Ed.), *Home truths about child sexual abuse: Influencing policy and practice* (pp. 290–312). London: Routledge.

Proeve, M. J. (2003). Responsivity factors in sexual offender treatment. In T. Ward., D. R. Laws., & S. M. Hudson (Eds), *Sexual deviance: Issues and controversies* (pp. 244–261). Thousand Oaks, CA: Sage.

Randolph, E. M. (2000). *Manual for the Randolph Attachment Disorder Questionnaire* (3rd edn). Evergreen, CO: The Attachment Center Press.

Rasmussen, L. A., Burton, J. E., & Christopherson, B. J. (1992). Precursors to offending and the trauma outcome process in sexually reactive children. *Journal of Child Sexual Abuse, 1*, 33–48.

Regier, D. A., Hirschfeld, R. M., Goodwin, F. K., Burke, J. D. Jr., Lazar, J. B., & Judd, L. L. (1988). The NIMH Depression Awareness, Recognition, and Treatment Program: Structure, aims, and scientific basis. *American Journal of Psychiatry, 145,* 1351–1357.

Restak, R. (2000). *Mysteries of the mind.* Washington, DC: National Geographic Society.

Restak, R. (2001). *The secret life of the brain.* New York: Dana Press.

Rich, P. (2003). *Understanding juvenile sexual offenders: Assessment, treatment, and rehabilitation.* New York, John Wiley & Sons.

Richters, M. M. & Volkmar, F. R. (1994). Case study: Reactive attachment disorder of infancy or early childhood. *Journal of the American Academy of Child and Adolescent Psychiatry, 33,* 328–32.

Righthand, S. & Welch, C. (2001, March). *Juveniles who have sexually offended: A review of the professional literature.* Washington, DC: Office of Juvenile Justice and Delinquency Prevention, US Department of Justice.

Rogers, C. R. (1980). *A way of being.* Boston, MA: Houghton Mifflin.

Rolls, E. T. (1999). The functions of the orbitofrontal cortex. *Neurocase, 5,* 301–312.

Ross, T. (2004). Attachment representation, attachment style, or attachment pattern? Usage of terminology in attachment theory. In F. Pfafflin & G. Adshead (Eds), *A matter of security: The application of attachment theory to forensic psychiatry and psychotherapy* (pp. 57–84). London: Jessica Kingsley Publishers.

Rothbaum, F., Weisz, J., Pott, M., Miyake, K., & Morelli, G. (2000). Attachment and culture: Security in the United States and Japan. *American Psychologist, 55,* 1093–1104.

Rutter, M. (1987). Psychosocial resilience and protective mechanisms. *American Journal of Orthopsychiatry, 57,* 316–331.

Rutter, M. (1997). Clinical implications of attachment concepts: Retrospect and prospect. In L. Atkinson & K. J. Zucker (Eds), *Attachment and psychopathology* (pp. 17–46). New York: Guilford.

Rutter, M. & O'Connor, T. G. (1999). Implications of attachment theory for child care policies. In J. Cassidy & P. R. Shaver (Eds), *Handbook of attachment: Theory, research, and clinical application* (pp. 823–844). New York: Guilford.

Ryan, G. (1999a). Recent develops and conclusions. In G. Ryan and Associates (Eds), *Web of meaning: A developmental-contextual approach in sexual abuse treatment* (pp. 133–151). Brandon, VT: Safer Society Press.

Ryan, G. (1999b). Treatment of sexually abusive youth: The evolving consensus. *Journal of Interpersonal Violence, 14,* 422–436.

Ryan, G. & Lane, S. (1997). *Juvenile sexual offending: Causes, consequences, and correction* (new and rev. edn). San Francisco, CA: Jossey-Bass.

Salkind, N. J. (1994). *Child development* (7th edn). Fort Worth, TX: Harcourt.

Saltaris, C. (2002). Psychopathy in juvenile offenders: Can temperament and attachment be considered as robust developmental precursors? *Clinical Psychology Review, 22,* 729–752.

Schachner, D. A. & Shaver, P. R. (2004). Attachment dimensions and sexual motives. *Personal Relationships, 11,* 179–195.

Schank, R. & Abelson, R. (1977). *Scripts, plans, goals, and understanding: An inquiry into human knowledge structures.* Hillsdale, NJ: Erlbaum.

Schank, R. C. (1999). *Dynamic memory revisited.* Cambridge, England: Cambridge University Press.

Scharfe, E. (2003). Stability and change of attachment representations from cradle to grave. In S. M. Johnson & V. E. Whiffen (Eds), *Attachment processes in couples and family therapy* (pp. 64–84). New York: Guilford.

Schore, A. N. (1994). *Affect regulation and the origin of the self: The neurobiology of emotional development.* Hillsdale, NJ: Erlbaum.

Schore, A. N. (1999). Foreword. In J. Bowlby, *Attachment and loss, Vol. 1: Attachment* (2nd edn.) (pp. xi–xxv). New York: Basic Books.

Schore, A. N. (2001a). Effects of a secure attachment relationship on right brain development, affect regulation, and infant mental health. *Infant Mental Health Journal, 22,* 7–66.

Schore, A. N. (2001b). The effects of early relational trauma on right brain development, affect regulation, and infant mental health. *Infant Mental Health Journal, 22,* 201–269.

Schore, A. (2002). Dysregulation of the right brain: A fundamental mechanism of traumatic attachment and the psychopathogenesis of posttraumatic stress disorder. *Australian and New Zealand Journal of Psychiatry, 36,* 9–30.

Schore, A. N. (2003). Early relational trauma, disorganized attachment, and the development of a predisposition to violence. In M. F. Solomon & D. J. Siegel (Eds), *Healing trauma: Attachment, mind, body, and brain* (pp. 107–167). New York: Norton.

Schuengal, C., Bakermans-Kranenburg, M. J., van Ijzendoorn, M. H., & Blom, M. (1999). Unresolved loss and infant disorganization: Links to frightening maternal behavior. In J. Solomon & C. George (Eds), *Attachment disorganization* (pp. 71–94). New York: Guilford.

Schuengel, G., Bakermans-Kranenburg, M. J., & van Ijzendoorn, M. H. (1999). Frightening maternal behavior linking unresolved loss and disorganized infant attachment. *Journal of Consulting and Clinical Psychology, 67,* 54–63.

Seagrave, D. & Grisso, T. (2002). Adolescent development and the measurement of juvenile psychopathy. *Law and Human Behavior, 26,* 219–239.

Seidman, B., Marshall, W., Hudson, S., & Robertson, P. (1994). An examination of intimacy and loneliness in sex offenders. *Journal of Interpersonal Violence, 9,* 518–534.

Seifert, K. (2003a, Summer). Attachment, family violence, and disorders of childhood and adolescence. *Paradigm, 8* (3), 14–15, 18.

Seifert, K. (2003b, September/October). Childhood trauma: Its relationship to behavioral and psychiatric disorders. *The Forensic Examiner, 12* (9/10), 27–33.

Seto, M. C. & Lalumière (in press). Conduct problems and juvenile sexual offending. In H. E. Barbaree & W.L. Marshall (Eds), *The juvenile sex offender* (2nd edn) New York: Guilford.

Shaver, P. R., Hazan, C., & Bradshaw, D. (1988). Love as attachment: The integration of three behavioral systems. In R. J. Sternberg & M. Barnes (Eds), *The psychology of love* (pp. 68–99). New Haven, CT: Yale University Press.

Shonkoff, J. P. & Phillips, D. A. (Eds) (2000). *From neurons to neighborhoods: The science of early childhood development.* Report of the Committee on Integrating the Science of Early Childhood Development. Washington, DC: National Academy Press.

Shweder, R. A., Mahapatra, M., & Miller, J. G. (1987). Culture and moral development. In J. Kagan & S. Lamb (Eds), *The emergence of morality in young children* (pp. 1–83). Chicago, IL: University of Chicago Press.

Siegel, D. J. (1999). *The developing mind: How relationships and the brain interact to shape who we are.* New York: Guilford.

Siegel, D. J. (2001). Toward an interpersonal neurobiology of the developing mind: Attachment relationships, "mindsight," and neural integration. *Infant Mental Health Journal, 22,* 67–94.

Siegel, D. J. (2003). An interpersonal neurobiology of psychotherapy: The developing mind and the resolution of trauma. In M. F. Solomon & D. J. Siegel (Eds), *Healing trauma: Attachment, mind, body, and brain* (pp. 1–56). New York: Norton.

Siegert, R. & Ward, T. (2003). Back to the future? Evolutionary explanations of rape. In T. Ward, D. R. Laws., & S. M. Hudson (Eds), *Sexual deviance: Issues and controversies* (pp. 45–64). Thousand Oaks, CA: Sage.

Slade, A. (1999). Attachment theory and research. Implications for the theory and practice of individual psychotherapy with adults. In J. Cassidy & P. R. Shaver (Eds), *Handbook of attachment: Theory, research, and clinical application* (pp. 575–594). New York: Guilford.

Slade, A. (2004). Two therapies: Attachment organization and the clinical process. In L. Atkinson & S. Goldberg (Eds), *Attachment issues in psychopathology and intervention* (pp. 181–206). Mahwah, NJ: Erlbaum.

Smallbone, S. W. (2005). Attachment insecurity as a predisposing and precipitating factor for young people who sexually abuse. In M. C. Calder (Ed.), *Children and young people who sexually abuse: New theory, research and practice developments* (pp. 4–16). Dorset, England: Russell House Publishing.

Smallbone, S.W. (in press-a). An attachment-theoretical revision of Marshall and Barbaree's Integrated Theory of the Etiology of Sexual Offending. In W.L. Marshall, Y.M. Fernandez, & L.E. Marshall (Eds), *Sexual offender treatment: controversial issues.* New York: John Wiley & Sons.

Smallbone, S.W. (in press-b). Social and psychological factors in the development of delinquency and sexual deviance. In H. E. Barbaree, & W.L. Marshall (Eds). *The juvenile sex offender* (2nd edn) New York: Guilford.

Smallbone, S. W. & Dadds, M. (1998). Childhood attachment and adult attachment in incarcerated adult male sex offenders. *Journal of Interpersonal Violence, 13,* 555–573.

Smallbone, S. W. & Dadds, M. (2000). Attachment and coercive sexual behavior. *Sexual Abuse: A Journal of Research and Treatment, 12,* 3–15.

Smallbone, S.W. & Dadds, M.R. (2001). Further evidence for a relationship between attachment insecurity and coercive sexual behavior. *Journal of Interpersonal Violence, 16,* 22–35.

Smallbone, S. W. & McCabe, B. (2003). Child attachment, childhood sexual abuse, and onset of masturbation among adult sexual offenders. *Sexual Abuse: A Journal of Research and Treatment, 15,* 1–9.

Smallbone, S.W. & Wortley, R.K. (2004). Onset, persistence and versatility of offending among adult males convicted of sexual offenses against children. *Sexual Abuse: A Journal of Research and Treatment, 16,* 285–298.

Smallbone, S.W., Wheaton, J., & Hourigan, D. (2003). Trait empathy and criminal versatility in sexual offenders. *Sexual Abuse: A Journal of Research and Treatment, 15,* 49–60.

Smith, P. K., Cowie, H., & Blades, M. (1998). *Understanding Children's Development* (3rd edn). Malden, Oxford, England: Blackwell.

Snyder, H. N. (2000, July). *Sexual assault of young children as reported to law enforcement: Victim, incident, and offender characteristics.* (NCJ 182990). Washington, DC: Bureau of Justice Statistics.

Solomon, J. & George, C. (1999a). The measurement of attachment security in infancy and childhood. In J. Cassidy & P. R. Shaver (Eds), *Handbook of attachment: Theory, research, and clinical application* (pp. 287–316). New York: Guilford.

Solomon, J. & George, C. (1999b). The place of disorganization in attachment theory: linking classic observations with contemporary findings. In J. Solomon & C. George (Eds), *Attachment disorganization* (pp. 3–32). New York: Guilford.

Spear, L. P. (2000). The adolescent brain and age-related behavioral manifestations. *Neuroscience and Biobehavioral Reviews, 24,* 417–463.

Spear, L. P. (2003). *The psychobiology of adolescence* (Working Paper 76–11). New York: Institute for American Values.

Speltz, M. L. (2002). Description, history, and critique of coercive attachment therapy. *The APSAC Advisor, 14,* 4–8.

Sroufe, J. W. (1991). Assessment of parent–adolescent relationships: Implications for adolescent development. *Journal of Family Psychology, 5* (1), 21–45.

Sroufe, L. A. (1988). The role of infant–caregiver attachment in development. In J. Belsky & T. Nezworski (Eds), *Clinical implications of attachment* (pp. 19–38). Hillsdale, NJ: Erlbaum.

Sroufe, L. A. (1995). *Emotional development: The organization of emotional life in the early years.* Cambridge, England: Cambridge University Press.

Sroufe, L. A., Carlson, E. A., Levy, A. K., & Egeland, B. (1999). Implications of attachment theory for developmental psychopathology. *Development and Psychopathology, 11,* 1–13.

Starzyk, K. B. & Marshall, W. L. (2003). Childhood family and personological risk factors for sexual offending. *Aggression and Violent Behavior, 8,* 93–105.

Stein, M. B., Koverola, C., Hanna, C., Torchia, M. G., & McClarty, B. (1997). Hippocampal volume in women victimized by childhood sexual abuse. *Psychological Medicine, 27,* 951–959.

Stern, D. N. (1985/2000). *The interpersonal world of the infant: A view from psychoanalysis and developmental psychology.* New York: Basic Books.

Stilwell, B. M. & Galvin, M. R. (1985). Conceptualization of conscience in 11–12 year olds. *Journal of the American Academy of Child and Adolescent Psychiatry, 24,* 630–636.

Stilwell, B. M, Galvin, M. R., Kopta, S. M., & Norton, J. A. (1994). Moral-emotional responsiveness: A two-factor domain of conscience functioning. *Journal of the American Academy of Child and Adolescent Psychiatry, 33,* 130–139.

Stilwell, B. M., Galvin, M. R., Kopta, S. M., Padgett, J. R., & Holt, J. W. (1997). Moralization of attachment: A fourth domain of conscience functioning. *Journal of the American Academy of Child and Adolescent Psychiatry, 36,* 1140–1147.

Stilwell, B. M., Galvin, M. R., Kopta, S. M., & Padgett, R. J. (1998). Moral volition: The fifth and final domain leading to an integrated theory of conscience understanding. *Journal of the American Academy of Child and Adolescent Psychiatry, 37,* 202–210.

Takahashi, T., Nowakowski, R. S., & Caviness, V. S. Jr. (2001). Neocorticol neurogenesis: Regulation, control points, and a strategy of structural variation. In C. A. Nelson & M. Luciana (Eds), *Handbook of developmental cognitive neuroscience* (pp. 3–22). Cambridge, MA: Massachusetts Institute of Technology Press.

Tallman, K. & Bohart, A. C. (1999). The client as a common factor: Clients as self-healers. In M. A. Hubble, B. L. Duncan, & S. D. Miller (Eds), *The heart and soul of change: What works in therapy* (pp. 91–131). Washington, DC: American Psychological Association.

Teicher, M. H. (2000, Fall). Wounds that won't heal: The neurobiology of child abuse. *Cerebrum, 2* (4), 50–67.

Teicher, M. H. (2002, March). Scars that won't heal: The neurobiology of child abuse. *Scientific American,* 68–75.

Thase, M. E. & Beck, A. T. (1993). An overview of cognitive therapy. In J. E. Wright, M. E. Thase, A. T. Beck, & J. W. Ludgate (Eds), *Cognitive therapy with inpatients* (pp. 3–34). New York: Guilford Press.

Thompson, R. A. (1999). Early attachment and later development. In J. Cassidy & P. R. Shaver (Eds), *Handbook of attachment: Theory, research, and clinical application* (pp. 265–286). New York: Guilford.

Thompson, R. A., Lamb, M. E., & Estes, D. (1982). Stability of infant–mother attachment and its relationship to changing life circumstances in an unselected middle-class sample. *Child Development, 53,* 144–148.

Thornton, D., Beech, A., Marshall, W. L. (2004). Pretreatment self-esteem and posttreatment sexual recidivism. *International Journal of Offender Therapy and Comparative Criminology, 48,* 587–599.

Tracy, J. L., Shaver, P. R., Albino, A. W., & Cooper, M. L. (2003). Attachment styles and adolescent sexuality. In P. Florsheim (Ed.), *Adolescent romance and sexual behavior: Theory, research, and practical implications* (pp. 137–159). Mahwah, NJ: Erlbaum.

Tronick, E. Z., Cohn, J., & Shea, E. (1986). The transfer of affect between mothers and infants. In T. B. Brazelton & M. W. Yogman (Eds), *Affective development in infancy* (pp. 11–25). Norwood, NJ: Ablex Publishing.

Tucker, D. M., Derryberry, D., & Luu, P. (2000). Anatomy and physiology of human emotion: Vertical integration of brain stem, limbic, and cortical systems. In J. C. Borod (Ed.), *The neuropsychology of emotions* (pp. 56–79). New York: Oxford University Press.

Tulving, E. (1985). How many memory systems are there? *American Psychologist, 40,* 385–398.

Turiel, E., Killen, M., & Helwig, C. C. (1987). In J. Kagan & S. Lamb (Eds), *The emergence of morality in young children* (pp. 155–243). Chicago, IL: University of Chicago Press.

Turner, R.A., Altemus, M., Enos, T., Cooper, B., & McGuinness, T. (1999). Preliminary research on plasma oxytocin in normal cycling women: Investigating emotion and interpersonal distress. *Psychiatry 62,* 97–113.

US Department of Health and Human Services (1999). *Mental health: A report of the Surgeon General.* Rockville, MD: US Department of Health and Human Services.

US Department of Health and Human Services (2001). *Youth violence: A report of the Surgeon General.* Rockville, MD: US Department of Health and Human Services.

Uvnäs-Moberg, K. (1997). Physiological and endocrine effects of social contact. In C. S. Carter., I. I. Lederhendler, & B. Kirkpatrick (Eds), *The integrative neurobiology of affiliation* (pp. 146–163). New York, The New York: Academy of Sciences.

Van der Kolk, B. A. (1987). *Psychological trauma.* Washington, DC: American Psychiatric Press.

Van Ijzendoorn, M. H. & Sagi, A. (1999). Cross-cultural patterns of attachment: Universal and contextual dimensions. In J. Cassidy & P. R. Shaver (Eds), *Handbook of attachment: Theory, research, and clinical application* (pp. 713–734). New York: Guilford.

Van Ijzendoorn, M. H. & Sagi, A. (2001). Cultural blindness or selective inattention? *American Psychologist, 56,* 824–825.

Vance, J. E. (1997). Aggressive youth: Healing biology with relationship. In C. S. Carter., I. I. Lederhendler, & B. Kirkpatrick (Eds), *The integrative neurobiology of affiliation* (pp. 587–589). New
York: The New York Academy of Sciences.

Vetlesen, A. J. (1994). *Perception, empathy, and judgment: An inquiry into the preconditions of
moral performance.* University Park, PA: Pennsylvania University Press.

Vygotsky, L. S. (1978). *Mind in society: The development of higher psychological processes.*
Cambridge, MA: Harvard University Press.

Ward, T. (2003). The explanation, assessment and treatment of child sexual abuse. *International
Journal of Forensic Psychology, 1*, 10–25.

Ward, T. & Sorbello, L. (2003). Explaining child sexual abuse: Integration and elaboration. In T.
Ward, D. R. Laws., & S. M. Hudson (Eds), *Sexual deviance: Issues and controversies* (pp. 3–20).
Thousand Oaks, CA: Sage.

Ward, T. & Stewart, C. A. (2003). Good lives and the rehabilitation of sexual offenders. In T. Ward,
D. R. Laws., & S. M. Hudson (Eds), *Sexual deviance: Issues and controversies* (pp. 21–44).
Thousand Oaks, CA: Sage.

Ward, T., Hudson, S. M., & Marshall, W. L. (1996). Attachment style in sex offenders: A preliminary study. *Journal of Sex Research 33*, 17–26.

Ward, T., Hudson, S. M., Marshall, W. L., & Siegert, R. (1995). Attachment style and intimacy
deficits in sexual offenders: A theoretical framework. *Sexual Abuse: A Journal of Research and
Treatment, 7*, 317–335.

Ward, T., McCormack, J., & Hudson, S. M. (1997). Sexual offenders' perceptions of their intimate
relationships. *Sexual Abuse: A Journal of Research and Treatment, 9*, 57–74.

Warner, M. S. (1997). Does empathy cure? A theoretical consideration of empathy, processing, and
personal narrative. In A. C. Bohart & L. S. Greenberg (Eds), *Empathy reconsidered: New directions in psychotherapy* (pp. 125–140). Washington, DC: American Psychological Association.

Waters, E. (1978). The reliability and stability of individual differences in infant–mother attachment.
Child Development, 49, 483–494.

Waters, E. & Beauchaine, T. P. (2003). Are there really patterns of attachment? Comment on Fraley
and Spieker (2003). *Developmental Psychology, 39*, 417–422.

Waters, E., Merrick, S., Treboux, D., Crowell, J., & Albersheim, L. (2000). Attachment security in
infancy and early adulthood: A twenty-year longitudinal study. *Child Development, 71*, 684–
689.

Webster, S. D. (2002). Assessing victim empathy in sexual offenders using the victim letter task.
Sexual Abuse: A Journal of Research and Treatment, 14, 281–300.

Weinfeld, N. S., Sroufe, L. A., Egeland, B., & Carlson, E. A. (1999). The nature of individual differences in infant–caregiver attachment. In J. Cassidy & P. R. Shaver (Eds), *Handbook of attachment: Theory, research, and clinical application* (pp. 68–88). New York: Guilford.

Weinrott, M. R. (1996, June). *Juvenile sexual aggression: A critical review* (Center Paper 005).
Boulder, CO: University of Colorado, Center for the Study and Prevention of Violence.

Weiss, R. S. (1982). Attachment in adult life. In C. M. Parkes & J. Stevenson-Hinde (Eds), *The place
of attachment in human behavior* (pp. 171–184). New York: Basic Books.

Werner, E. E. & Smith, R. S. (1992). *Overcoming the odds: High risk children from birth to adulthood.* Ithaca, NY: Cornell University Press.

Werner, E. E. & Smith, R. S. (2001). *Journeys from childhood to midlife: Risk, resilience, and recovery.* Ithaca, NY: Cornell University Press.

West, M., Rose, S., Spreng, S., & Adam, K. (2000). The Adolescent Unresolved Attachment Questionnaire: The assessment of perceptions of parental abdication of caregiving behavior. *The
Journal of Genetic Psychology, 16*, 493–503.

West, M., Rose, M. S., Spreng, S., Sheldon-Keller, A., & Adam, K. (1998). Adolescent Attachment
Questionnaire: A brief assessment of attachment in adolescence. *Journal of Youth and Adolescence, 27*, 661–673.

Wheeler, M. A., Stuss, D. T., & Tulving, E. (1997). Toward a theory of episodic memory: The frontal
lobes and autonoetic consciousness. *Psychological Bulletin, 121*, 331–354.

Winnicott, D. W. (1964). *The child, the family, and the outside world.* Harmondsworth, England:
Penguin Books.

Winnicott, D. W. (1986). The theory of the parent–child relationship. In P. Buckley (Ed.), *Essential papers on object relations* (pp. 233–253). New York: New York University Press.

Winnicott, D. W. (2002). *Winnicott on the child.* Cambridge, MA: Perseus.

World Health Organization (1992). ICD-10: *International statistical classification of diseases and related health problems* (10th revision, Vol. 1). Geneva, Switzerland: Author.

Yale, M. E., Messinger, D. S., Cobo-Lewis, A. B., & Delgado, C. F. (2003). The temporal coordination of early infant communication. *Developmental Psychology, 39*, 815–824.

Yurgelun-Todd, D. (2002). *Inside the teenage brain.* Retrieved December 2004 from http://www.pbs.org/wgbh/pages/frontline/shows/teenbrain/interviews/.

Zeanah, C. H. (1996). Beyond insecurity: A reconceptualization of attachment disorders in infancy. *Journal of Consulting and Clinical Psychology, 64*, 42–52.

Zeanah, C. H. Jr, Mammen, O. K., & Lieberman, A. F. (1993). Disorders of attachment. In C. H. Zeanah Jr (Ed.), *Handbook of infant mental health* (pp. 332–349). New York: Guilford.

Index